HOME CARE
for the
CHRONICALLY ILL
or DISABLED CHILD

HOME CARE
for the
CHRONICALLY ILL
or DISABLED CHILD

A Manual and Sourcebook
for Parents and Professionals

MONICA LOOSE JONES

Illustrations by Linda Trujillo

1817

HARPER & ROW, PUBLISHERS, New York

Cambridge, Philadelphia, San Francisco, London

Mexico City, São Paulo, Singapore, Sydney

HOME CARE FOR THE CHRONICALLY ILL OR DISABLED CHILD. Copyright © 1985 by Monica Loose Jones. Illustrations copyright © 1985 by Linda Trujillo. All rights reserved. Printed in the United States of America. No part of this book may be used or reproduced in any manner whatsoever without written permission except in the case of brief quotations embodied in critical articles and reviews. For information address Harper & Row, Publishers, Inc., 10 East 53rd Street, New York, N.Y. 10022. Published simultaneously in Canada by Fitzhenry & Whiteside Limited, Toronto.

FIRST EDITION

Designer: C. Linda Dingler

Library of Congress Cataloging in Publication Data

Jones, Monica Loose.
    Home care for the chronically ill or disabled child.

    Bibliography: p
    Includes indexes.
    1. Chronically ill children—Home care—Handbooks, manuals, etc. 2. Handicapped children—Home care—Handbooks, manuals, etc.   I. Title.
RJ380.J66   1985   649'.8   84-48171
ISBN 0-06-181433-4   85 86 87 88 89 10 9 8 7 6 5 4 3 2 1
ISBN 0-06-091173-5 (pbk.)   85 86 87 88 89 10 9 8 7 6 5 4 3 2 1

To Dr. Sey Kinsell
and all those who shared their
knowledge and wisdom,
love and compassion,
making it possible for us to care for Bronwyn at home

Contents

CONTENTS

Illustrations

Foreword

There is little doubt that the majority of chronically ill or disabled children fare better living at home than in the hospital or another institution. A loving and caring family offers an ill or disabled child an emotional environment far more stable and healthy than that found anywhere else. Indeed, warm and supportive human interaction is as important as the medicinal regimen for the chronically ill or disabled child. Yet despite this, and despite the fact that illness and disability spare no race, color, or creed—but rather strike every sphere and level of society —the importance of home care for the chronically ill or disabled child has for too long been underestimated, and home care has been a neglected area of health care.

In many areas of the United States (and the rest of the world) community resources in health care and professional help for chronically ill or disabled children are extremely limited or nonexistent. Increased public and government support is needed for planning family health care and for disseminating information on the chronically ill or disabled child. But government cannot do it alone. The battle can be won only if we wage it on a united front, through a mass collaborative effort involving official agencies, professionals, community volunteers, and parents.

Compounding the lack of resources are the glaringly large gaps in our knowledge of illness and disability. Unfortunately, little knowledge regarding improved treatment approaches for the chronically ill or disabled has accumulated through the years.

So until science and technology provide us with better management and treatment for chronically ill and disabled children, and until optimum care and management programs are perfected, parents themselves must resolve many of the fundamental problems pertaining to their child's care. In conjunction with the appropriate professionals, parents must utilize the resources at hand as fully as possible, and try to do so with hope and optimism.

Home Care for the Chronically Ill or Disabled Child makes an important contribution here, teaching parents about the daily care of an ill or disabled child, enabling them to respond to emergencies, and teaching them how to effectively carry out many necessary medical procedures. It is a comprehensive book, yet it is concise and written in a style that allows parents and professionals alike to utilize it in a practical setting without complicated preparations.

Furthermore, this book answers questions about more than daily medical care. Where do parents go and what do they do when first confronted with the fact that their child is disabled or chronically or terminally ill? The frustrations, anxieties, and dilemmas can seem overwhelming. Suddenly, the goals, hopes, and aspirations for their family change and, for many, the world seems to be crashing in around them. Monica Jones helps instill in parents a sense of confidence and hope that will greatly facilitate the task of caring for their ill or disabled child effectively and safely.

Many parents have unrealistically high expectations for home care, perhaps hoping that their child will be "cured" by love and care alone. For these parents, *Home Care for the Chronically Ill or Disabled Child* helps realistically define the special demands of caring for such a child at home. The book helps them meet these realities with endurance and acceptance, and with a firm commitment to care and protection.

A word about the child. What thoughts must pass through the mind of a disabled or ill child as he or she develops and recognizes dissimilarities to siblings and peers and faces the inability to compete with others academically, socially, or recreationally? Such a child may never be able to understand the question "Why did this happen to me?" Certainly, every child desires "normal" experiences, friends, and the satisfaction of accomplishment and success. What hope can we extend to the chronically ill or disabled child? What explanations can parents and doctors alike offer as solace? Monica Jones helps parents learn how best to help their child come to terms with his or her condition, and she demonstrates how patience and continued care will provide not only better health but also greater independence and worldly accomplishment for their ill or disabled child.

Moreover, the lessons the child learns at home are carried out into larger, outside groups, and ultimately reflect his or her social adjustment, cooperation, and friendliness toward others. This is the heritage all parents can and must provide, whether or not their child is disabled or ill. It is their testimony of parental good faith, bounded by love, encompassed by care and concern, enmeshed within the warp and woof of continued gratification as their child becomes a dependable, responsible individual. This and this alone is *every* parent's responsibility.

My congratulations to Monica Jones. *Home Care for the Chronically Ill or Disabled Child* does a masterful job of helping teach parents how they can successfully care for their child at home.

MARGARET J. GIANNINI, M.D. F.A.A.P.,
Director, Rehabilitation Research
and Development Service, Veterans Administration,
Washington, D.C.
First Director, National Institute of
Handicapped Research

Preface

Bronwyn could hardly move. Our daughter was thirteen months old when we suddenly realized that she could no longer lift her head up, roll over, or crawl. She was bright, cheerful, and alert, learning new words every day—but she obviously had been "unlearning" how to move. Why hadn't we noticed sooner? In retrospect, I don't think we were trying to ignore reality. We simply didn't know anything about normal child development, and we had no friends with infants. I do remember wondering at what age a child should be able to sit unassisted and then trying to look it up in Dr. Spock. When I failed to find the answer, I hesitated to disturb our doctor about such a minor matter and didn't search further.

But one November day in 1968, when we decided to watch precisely what Bronwyn could and couldn't do, we realized she could hardly move. We immediately called the pediatrician, only to find that he had become acutely ill and had given up his practice. His partner, however, saw us the same day. Although the two doctors had apparently discussed Bronwyn with some concern, no one had told us anything. Our new pediatrician indicated something was wrong but couldn't tell us what. So Bronwyn was given an appointment with a neurologist for diagnostic testing.

My husband, Desmond, and I were quite ignorant of all things medical, having been raised in healthy families where the strongest available drug, aspirin, was administered sparingly. My own encounters with doctors had been so limited that when I once needed a routine immunization as a teenager I fainted with fright. In college I couldn't understand why my friends wanted to go to medical school; now I wished *I* had become a doctor. Undaunted by the fact that I knew no chemistry or biology, I read all I could find on neurological illnesses and determined that Bronwyn must have Werdnig-Hoffmann's syndrome (infantile spinal muscular atrophy). This is a rare birth defect that causes rapid deterioration of the anterior horn cells of the spine so messages from the brain cannot be transmitted through the spinal cord to the muscles. The muscles atrophy through lack of use, causing paralysis and usually death in infancy.

After Bronwyn had completed medical diagnostic testing, we met with the neurologist who had the difficult job of breaking the news to us. He tactfully began by telling us what Bronwyn didn't have, starting with the mildest disorders. When he finally said it was not muscular dystrophy, I thought, "Too bad, those children live into their teens." The only disorder left was Werdnig-Hoffmann's syndrome. The doctor's diagnosis, based upon medical expertise, confirmed my own lay diagnosis, but his prognosis was only partially accurate. He thought she would die before she was two. Although she did become progressively paralyzed, to the point where she could only open and shut her eyes, talk softly, and move two fingers, Bronwyn lived happily to the age of nine and a half.

After the diagnosis our family began quickly to gain a medical education. Since the disorder is rare, no pediatrician in our town of 75,000 had ever treated a similar case. Very little information on treatment was available, partly because most children who had this birth defect died very young. The members of the medical community worked together with us on what was often a trial-and-error basis to provide the necessary medical care. The ways we dealt with problems, which were constantly arising due to changes in her condition, seemed easy *after* we had found the solutions. But there was much "muddling through" to reach them. I knew that other parents must have faced similar problems, and sometimes I wished one of them had had the time to share his or her knowledge and written a "how-to" book for parents of disabled and acutely ill children. Based upon the practical experience of parents, such a book could help answer questions such as:

- What do you do when you find your child has a problem?
- How do you cope with your feelings?
- How do you find and utilize the medical assistance you need?
- How do you care for your child and tend to his or her medical needs at home?
- How do you educate your child?
- How do you provide play and recreation for your child?
- How can the whole family come to live each day to the fullest?
- How do you cope with the last stages of terminal illness?

Although there are no definitive answers to all these questions, I hope that my experience in and research on home care will not only help you see how such a child can be cared for at home but will show how helping such a child can be a wonderful learning experience, where love, intelligence, knowledge, the help of friends and neighbors, and the growth of the family can all occur around the growth of the child.

Acknowledgments

My husband has often said that I view the whole world as a vast labor source, and he may be right. Certainly I not only asked for but received much help from parents and professionals alike, and I do want to thank all of them. The following gave generously of their time, sharing with me what they knew, and then reading and evaluating the material relating to their area of expertise: Stephen Abbott, MD; Claire Adler; Craig Bagdasar; Tom Baldwin; Louise Barcus, PT; Elizabeth Billet, RN; Mary Brooks; Pam Brooks, OTR; Tom Brooks, MA; Barbara Browne, RN; Leonard Burgess, MD; Mary Caldwell; Peter Caldwell, R.Pharm; Annette Carrel; Christina Cooper, PT; Richard Crockett; Laurie Deal-Tackett; Peg Decker; James Dow, DDS; Blair Edwards, MD; Sandi Enders, OTR; Jami Ferrer, MA; Kenneth Finkel, MD; Kay Frakes; Sanford Gerber, PhD; Marylou Gooden, MA; Thomas Gorman, MA; Louise Greene, MA; Phillip Greene, MA; Martiana Grogan, RN; Frederico Grosso, DDS; Barbara Gurga; Elton Hall, MA; Bill Hamilton, PhD; Leslie Hanson, MS; Louise Harris; John Hauschild; James Holroyd, MD; Mary Ella Isham, PT; Nandini Iyer, MA; Raghavan Iyer, PhD; Andrea Jameson; Marcy Jochim, MSW; Harri Kallio; C. Seybert Kinsell, MD; Stanley Klein, PhD; Jean Kohn, MD; Armand Kuris, PhD; Asha Lee, MD; Stephen Lee, PhD; Stephen Lemon, MD; Clif Leonard, PhD; Edwin Levine, MD; Myron Liebhaber, MD; David Medina, MD; Eileen Medina; Harris Meisel, MD; Eilis Dillon Mercier; Erin Miller, OTR; Steve Miller; Joan Mitchell, PhD; Bob Moore, RN; Donna Moore; Rose Mucci; Pauline Meyers, RN; Elizabeth Nitschke; Ruprecht Nitschke, MD; Christine Nolt; Audrey O'Neil, PhD; Lolita Parr; Anne Pasanella, PhD; Joe Pasanella, MA; Ina Pierson; Emma Plank; John Ridland, PhD; Muriel Ridland, MA; Mary Robinson, PhD; Sharron Roemer; Robert Roemer, PhD; Robert Robb, RTR; Susan Ryan; Bernard Schaefer, MSW; Helen Schultz, MD; Janet Stitch, RN; Vanessa Stitch; Diane Stowell; Darcy Sylvester; William Sylvester; Lee Thompson, R.Pharm; Maggie Trunk; LaVelle Ure, MA; William Ure, MD; Jessica Velazquez, MA; Barbara Weber, MA; Robert Henry West; Fran Wiley, MSW; Don Willey, RRT; Ruth Wilvert; Julie Yamamoto, PT; and Fred Youngblood, RRT.

I also wish to express my gratitude to those who read and evaluated every chapter of the whole book: Jeanne Dorrance; Lynn Hudson, RN; Marcy Jochim, MSW; Gerhard Loose, PhD; Maureen McKenzie, RN; and Muriel Zimmermann, PhD.

My appreciation goes to Bernice Heller, formerly of J. B. Lippincott, the medical division of Harper & Row, who saw the value of this project when I first explained it to her, and to Ann Harris, formerly of Harper & Row. At Harper's my thanks go to my editor, Carol Cohen, and to Lucy Adelman O'Brien, who worked on the manuscript with diligence and good cheer.

And finally my special thanks go to my husband, Desmond, and my son, Gareth, for their love, patience, and ability to have survived the time it took to write this book in spite of a dearth of apple pies.

HOME CARE
for the
CHRONICALLY ILL
or DISABLED CHILD

1

Learning to Accept Your Child's Condition

Most of us realize that the real world is not a place like Lake Wobegon, Minnesota,* "where all the women are strong, all the men are good-looking, and all the children are above average." Still, when we first think of having a child and then when we actually have one, most of us unconsciously assume that our child will at least be average in health, intelligence, behavior, and appearance. Therefore it comes as a shock when we realize our child has definite medical problems.

Some of us may have had nagging suspicions that something was wrong and the diagnosis just confirms them; in other cases, the "bad news" just seems to drop on us out of the blue. Our minds suddenly fill with questions such as "What will happen to our child?" "What kind of medical care will our child need?" "Can we care for our child at home?" "Why me?"

The medical problems will seem enormous if you start thinking immediately of everything that may have to be done. But if you stop and calm down and think, it should become clear that what you really have to deal with today is *today*—not things that might arise in the future. And while today your child may require a certain amount of medical care and assistance, he or she also needs your love and good cheer. This isn't always easy. When Reinhold Niebuhr wrote ". . . give us serenity to accept what cannot be changed, courage to change what should be changed, and wisdom to distinguish one from the other," he didn't add, "PS: It's

*That legendary place Garrison Keillor talks about in "A Prairie Home Companion" on American Public Radio.

easy"—because he knew it isn't.

Everyone confronts problems in life. We must each in our own way come to realize that there are certain things in life that cannot be changed but must be accepted as "given," and other things that respond not only to our efforts but to our basic attitude toward them.

Accepting your child's condition, most likely a "given," can actually be harder than administering the medical care or finding the equipment your child needs. Learning to accept what can't be changed takes time, and on certain days this may seem easier than on others. Different people are helped in different ways—by religious or philosophical beliefs, by talking with other parents who have had similar experiences, by sharing ideas and feelings with family and friends, and through professional counseling. While there is no easy way, the more you accept your child as he or she is, the more you help your child and yourself live each day to the fullest.

Your Emotional Response to Your Child's Condition

No doubt, upon learning of your child's diagnosis, your first response was not one of calm acceptance. There are several common reactions to learning of a child's disability or illness, and since they may be provoked repeatedly over the years it is worth spending a little time thinking about them and why they may occur.

Fear may have been your first reaction on learning of your child's illness or disability. But knowledge dispels fear, and the more you understand about your child's condition, the more you learn to care for your child, the less afraid you will be. When you realize that you are able to care for your child, you will no longer live in fear of the future.

Denial is another common reaction to the news of an illness or disability, especially if the condition is not visible. However, denying that your child has a problem, or spending vast amounts of time, money, and effort to find a doctor who will give you a diagnosis you like, will not make the problem go away. At a certain point you must accept the given, do what you must to live within the boundaries the condition sets, and learn to appreciate each day to the fullest.

Anger is another troublesome emotion that can prevent you from coming to terms with your child's condition. Inwardly working through your anger can be a learning process, but translating it into visible behavior can do more harm than good. Anger at your child, at the doctors, at your child's condition, or at your lot in life may be a way of shunning reality and avoiding responsibility. Anger won't change your child's condition for the better, and your foul mood will only make things worse for everyone.

Guilt too is destructive. It stems from the feeling that we could have acted differently. But we are neither omniscient nor omnipotent. You did not knowingly cause your child's illness or disability. You must believe in your honest intent to do your best and to learn from the mistakes you may make rather than feel guilty about them.

Envy is a troublesome emotion. It is tempting to compare your child with another and wish your child were different. While it might sometimes be helpful to look at another child with a similar condition, to consider his or her treatment and see if you can learn anything to apply to your child, it is useless to spend time wishing for what is not. Learn to accept your child for what he or she is, be grateful for what he or she can do, and convey your genuine love and affection to your child and those around you.

Overprotectiveness usually stems from the best of intentions. You could keep your son or daughter in a bedroom and feed your child with a sterilized spoon. Although this might protect the child from bacteria lurking in the outside world, it will do nothing to further normal growth and development. If your child has severe respiratory problems, insisting that visitors be free of colds is a reasonable precaution; not allowing your child to play with *any* children is unreasonable. No matter how mild or severe the disability, your child needs to develop the capacity for growth and to become as self-reliant as possible, and this entails as many risks as raising a "normal" child.

Helping Your Child Understand and Accept His or Her Condition

While you must come to terms with your child's condition yourself, you must also help your child come to understand and accept it.

As with all important issues, your child will surely ask you questions about his or her illness or disability. Answer questions honestly and directly. In the beginning, your child may want to know only so much and may even tune you out if you attempt a lengthy or detailed answer. So try to answer your child's early questions without amplifying them or adding information not requested. Your child will think about your answers and will more than likely come back to you with more questions, whether the following day, week, or month. Remember, honesty is vital. Giving your child an unrealistic picture of his or her condition will only lead to false hopes and disappointment. Of course, if your child's condition is progressive, there may be no need initially to give a detailed description of what the future may hold. The important thing to remember is that the information you give should help your child cope on a day-to-day basis. If you want to give your child a religious framework for understanding and coping with his or her condition, do so. But do not try to impose your own beliefs on a child old enough to have beliefs different from your own.

Especially if your child's condition is visible or disabling, it is important to explain the condition in language the child can understand and use. Not only will your explanation have meaning for your child but your child will be able to explain the condition to friends. And if your child understands the condition in this way, he or she will not be hurt by the remarks and stares he or she may encounter.

Contending with the Outside World

Be honest and realistic with your friends and relatives about your child's condition. This will make it much easier for them to accept it. The tendency to avoid the straightforward approach may be rationalized as a concern to protect your child; more likely it indicates a fear of coming to terms with the facts. Other people will quickly pick up on such feelings and may have difficulty accepting and dealing with your child if they sense that you are having trouble doing so yourself. If you are open and straightforward about your child, and if you give friends and relatives time to interact with him or her, they can come to love and accept your child as he or she is.

Do not shelter your child from the outside world. The days of isolating disabled children are over. When you take your child into the outside world, you will find that it is filled with people who are basically good, helpful, curious, and full of questions. While you may sometimes feel exasperated, especially if you are asked the same questions again and again, you can come to welcome them as exhibiting goodwill and interest. With time you will become good at fielding questions in a friendly manner, asking for and also accepting help when needed or just thanking for the offer when things are under control.

As your child gets older, he or she can be taught to answer the questions and respond to the comments. You will find that your child can speak very well for himself or herself.

Be honest and direct with other children, too. This will make it easier on your own child. Children, of course, are a little more forthright than adults in their comments and will often come straight out with "What's wrong with him?" or "Why can't she walk?" You simply have to learn to welcome such open interest and explain things as they are in language children can understand. If your child is old enough and able to speak independently, let him or her do the talking. If you listen to what your child says to other children, you may learn something about how he or she perceives the disability (and you may find that you underestimated your child's ability to understand).

Understanding helps eliminate teasing and name-calling among children. If your child accepts his or her limitations, can explain them, and can interact positively with other children, teasing should not become a problem. However, difficulties do arise, often with children who have problems that are not visible or that are sporadic in nature, like seizures. In such cases understanding is still the best approach. Explain your child's condition to these children, even invite them to your house for milk and cookies so they can see how you live. If this doesn't help, explain the situation to their parents and your child's teachers and politely enlist their help. Your child has to live in the world, and doing so begins in your own neighborhood. Again, your positive example is crucial in this effort because your acceptance of your child as he or she is will be emulated by your child, by your child's friends, and by their parents.

Learn from those who have managed in similar situations. The problems you face may seem overwhelming at times, but you only have to look around you to see the burdens of others. It will broaden your perspective. You can see how other people have succeeded in overcoming their handicaps in magazines such as *Accent on Living* and in biographies of great individuals such as Helen Keller.

Your local library should have books describing how ordinary families such as yours have managed under similar circumstances (see Appendix 3, "Suggested Reading"). When you can accept the fact that your situation isn't unique, you will be able more easily to integrate your own difficulties and suffering into the universal suffering of humanity.

PART 1

MEETING YOUR CHILD'S MEDICAL NEEDS

2
Finding and Utilizing
the Medical Help You Need

Since medicine has become so complex that it is impossible for one person to be knowledgeable about all aspects of the profession, you will probably work with doctors in several fields. You may also work with qualified individuals outside of what the American Medical Association defines as the medical profession who provide valuable assistance in areas such as chiropractic, acupuncture, massage, and nutrition. (Within these areas, however, as within the medical profession itself, be suspicious of anyone offering quick miracle cures.) Take time to consider how you choose your doctor and how you and your doctor can work together for the good of your child.

If more than one doctor is caring for your child, it is important to have a primary-care physician (probably your pediatrician) who coordinates your child's care, answering day-to-day needs and referring you to other doctors as necessary. Although consultations with specialists are invaluable, your primary-care physician considers your child's needs as a whole rather than focusing on a particular part of the body.

WHAT IS A GOOD DOCTOR?

Good doctors come in all shapes and sizes. There are, however, various factors to consider in choosing your primary-care physician.

Is the doctor compassionate? Since a doctor is a person with whom you will have much contact, you must find someone who is emotionally sup-portive and with whom you feel comfortable. It may take time and effort on both sides to establish close rapport, but it can be established with many different kinds of people. Establishing rapport, especially in a professional relationship, requires work, a willingness to learn, and mutual respect.

Is the doctor competent? This is a crucial question, probably the most difficult for a lay person to judge. Although you shouldn't be overly impressed because someone attended a big-name educational institution, hospital appointments are significant. To achieve a hospital appointment (the privilege of having one's patients admitted to the hospital) a physician must meet certain standards of competence and peer review. In a small town, all doctors may admit patients to the one or two local hospitals. But in a large city with many hospitals, a physician who may admit patients to at least one medical-school-affiliated or otherwise excellent hospital is more likely to be a good doctor.

What are the doctor's areas of interest? Different doctors, even within a particular specialty such as pediatrics, may be interested in different kinds of problems. One may be interested in short-term illnesses, while another may be interested in ongoing care and thus have much to offer children who are severely disabled or chronically ill. Try to find out if a doctor treats other children with problems similar to those of your child or if he or she spends time working with volunteer agencies or in special school programs.

How does the doctor view children? Your child may be a fascinating medical phenomenon, but any child who will have to see a doctor frequently needs a physician who will view him or her as a total person, with physical, mental, emotional, and spiritual needs. Only the rare doctor will remember your child's birthday, but any doctor should be willing to talk directly with your child and have time for a bit of humor and fun.

Is the doctor open-minded and able to listen? Your physician should be able to define problems and suggest options. Furthermore, he or she should be interested in innovative approaches and current research and should be able to interpret the information and results for you. Your doctor should regard you as an intelligent and knowledgeable parent, respecting your judgment and listening to your ideas and suggestions. If you read about a new medical treatment, your doctor should be willing not only to read the article but to contact the author directly if that is advisable. Be suspicious of any doctor who says, "I'll take care of everything!" Much better is the honest doctor who, while knowledgeable and capable, can admit that he or she doesn't know everything and is willing to learn. This is an indication that the doctor will devote thinking time to your child, trying to discover how best to help.

What is the doctor's age? An older physician will have more practical experience than a younger one, which can be very valuable with chronic disorders. Having looked down thousands of throats and listened to thousands of chests, an older physician may be able to detect small differences. Furthermore, he or she may be more confident and have developed a better bedside manner. On the other hand, a younger doctor may have more up-to-date knowledge and be very alert. Also, a younger doctor just setting up a practice is more likely to have a lighter patient load and, quite possibly, will have more time to spend treating your child and getting necessary information. You must decide, but remember that experience can be an important factor when treating chronic disorders.

Is the doctor accessible? While you may see a specialist only occasionally or at regular intervals, and can make the necessary appointment well in advance, your primary-care physician should be readily available for regular appointments, phone calls, house calls, and emergencies.

If your child is chronically ill, you will have to call your primary-care physician often. Find out what the doctor's policy is about returning phone calls. With a severely ill child, the call you place at 9:00 A.M. should be returned as soon as your doctor gets to work in the morning or, if not urgent, then before he or she goes to lunch—but not at 8:00 P.M.

If your child is acutely ill or severely disabled, occasional house calls may be necessary. Therefore, check whether the physician will make house calls. (If you live near to your pediatrician's office, he or she will probably be more willing to make a house call than if you live far away.)

Is the doctor punctual? Don't be deluded into thinking that the doctor who chronically runs late is very good; he or she may just be poorly organized. You should not regularly have to wait more than 30 minutes for an appointment. However, if your doctor is chronically late but you still feel that he or she is the best for your child, you may be willing to wait.

Is the doctor engaged in solo or group practice? If you need to contact your primary-care physician often, and if you know emergencies may arise when you need to speak to or see a doctor after office hours, you may be better off with a doctor in group practice. If your doctor is in a group practice, the other physicians should be informed about your child's condition. Should your doctor have a night off, you will be able to call another doctor who will know something about your child's medical problems.

If your doctor is in a solo practice, it will be your responsibility to be sure that the other physicians with whom your doctor share-calls are informed as to your child's condition. Ask your doctor to help you with this.

Is the doctor a member of a clinic? If all your doctors work at a clinic, they will communicate with each other about your child. But unless you live in a large metropolitan area, doctors in your locality probably know and communicate with each other anyway. Therefore, it may be best to choose each physician you need rather than feel that all your doctors should be members of the same clinic. Although all doctors at a reputable clinic have a certain level of competence, this is no guarantee that all will be the best for your child. Large clinics may also be impersonal and less able to provide the individual care and attention your child may need.

It may seem that a clinic could save you time and effort, making it possible to see two doctors in one day. However, since most doctors don't run on time, most clinics will not give you two appointments for the same day. Your child may not have the strength or attention span to see two physicians in one day anyway.

If you are insured through a health maintenance organization (HMO), you are limited to the doctors at a certain clinic, unless your child needs a specialist not on the staff. Within the clinic, you may still have a choice if there is more than one doctor per specialty, so try to find the most appropriate doctor for your child. If you feel there is a doctor in the community who could work much better with your child than the doctors in the clinic, your only choice may be to change your insurance coverage from HMO to a regular group plan. Most employers offering HMO also offer a regular plan.

What are the doctor's fees? Fees are not an indication of quality. Ask the doctor or his receptionist about them in advance. If they seem high, check with your local medical society or Medicaid office to find what charges are reasonable and customary in your area. Also, if a doctor enthusiastically and regularly promotes expensive services that you are not sure your child needs, you should be suspicious.

What are some qualities not to look for in a doctor? Irrelevant considerations that can sidetrack you in your search for the right doctor include your doctor's looks, dress, social status, address, office decor, or the size of his or her practice. Although doctors offer a service, beware if you feel you are being sold. Someone exuding self-confidence may sound impressive, but this is not necessarily an indication that he or she is a good doctor.

HOW DO YOU FIND A GOOD DOCTOR?

Having decided what you want your child's primary-care physician to be like, how do you actually find the person who fulfills your needs?

A referral from a good doctor, even one in a different field, may be the best way to find your primary-care physician.

If such a physician gives you the names of three doctors, ask what the differences among the three are. It may be that the first name is really his or her first choice, in which case contact that physician first. On the other hand, the referring physician may feel that all three are equally competent. It is perfectly acceptable to ask with whom he or she thinks you would get along best. You may want to ask who takes care of his or her children. Anyone good enough for the doctor's children should be good enough for yours. Once you have found a good primary-care physician, the rest of the team will be easy to choose because that physician will refer you to the specialists you may need.

A referral from a person engaged in health care such as a nurse or a therapist can be helpful, since such a person often knows which doctors provide good medical care and which are more interested in their golf game.

A referral from someone working with a service organization such as the Muscular Dystrophy Association of America might be helpful, since he or she may know which doctors in the community see many disabled or ill children.

A referral from another parent whose judgment you trust can be valuable. While parents may not be able to assess medical competence fully, they can give you an indication as to how their doctor is working with them and helping their child.

A referral from the chief of a medical service in a large medical-school-affiliated hospital may be helpful in a metropolitan area, particularly if only one doctor in the city deals with your child's specific disorder. However, medical-school-affiliated doctors often keep very limited office hours and therefore might not be good choices as primary-care physicians themselves.

A referral from a medical society is not much better than going to the yellow pages of the phone book. Medical societies rarely give the names of the three best doctors in a given specialty; rather, they give three names selected at random from their list.

Doctors you meet socially deserve your careful and friendly consideration. While you should not pump such a person for every bit of medical information you can get, thus making a nuisance of yourself, you can ask a few leading questions and through general conversation find out what kind of a person he or she is.

INTERVIEWING A PROSPECTIVE DOCTOR

When you have decided on a doctor, you may want to make an appointment to discuss professional services. (Expect to pay the physician for the appointment.) Begin by honestly, fully, and clearly explaining your child's needs as you see them and give information about your family and economic circumstances. It is important to be honest from the outset. Otherwise, how does the doctor learn about your family and your child's medical problems? A doctor should be honest with you in return. It is with this approach that you are most likely to begin to establish rapport.

Before your appointment, carefully consider what you want to discuss. It is very helpful to bring a list of written questions in order of importance, such as:

- Is the doctor interested in treating children with problems such as those your child has?
- Has the doctor dealt with many such cases?
- When is the doctor available? Can the doctor be reached after hours or does he or she share call? Does he or she make house calls?
- Does the doctor refer to specialists and recommend consultations?
- To which hospitals can the doctor admit patients?
- What are the doctor's fees, and how does he or she wish to be paid?

After such an appointment and before choosing your doctor, review which factors you think make a good doctor and then consider the physician in light of these criteria. In some cases a doctor may be unable to help you but may be willing to refer you to an appropriate physician.

CHANGING DOCTORS

Even after spending time and effort with a doctor, you may still not be sure a good working relationship can be established.

While there are good reasons for changing doctors, you should think carefully about why you are dissatisfied with yours. In some cases you may find that you should change your expectations rather than your doctor.

Do not change doctors simply because your child did not get an immediate diagnosis and treatment. It takes time to gain familiarity with medical problems, to know and establish rapport with a child.

Do not change doctors because yours has not cured your child. You must be realistic about your child's condition, for some conditions can't be cured and some even get worse. If you accept this, you will avoid that futile, expensive, and enervating search for the cure that doesn't exist, which is often the reason for changing doctors. No doctor can satisfy a patient who makes unrealistic demands.

There are valid reasons for changing doctors. While changing doctors should not be a hasty decision, there are reasons for doing so. If your doctor moves to an office many miles from your house, for example, or becomes seriously ill and cannot devote sufficient time to your child, you may want to find a new doctor. Finally, if you or your child simply cannot develop a good working relationship with your doctor, you should consider looking for another, equally competent physician.

Whereas your primary-care physician must be someone with whom you can work closely, you do not need to feel so close to specialists whom you see only rarely. But even the occasional office visit is important, and you may have reasons to change specialists as well.

How do you go about changing physicians? A good doctor who genuinely wants to help people is not deluded into thinking that he or she is the only one who can provide the appropriate care. Any doctor who flies into a rage or feels threatened by your changing physicians or requesting a consultation is well worth leaving. Also, don't fear that a doctor will blackball you within the medical community, because good doctors just don't do that.

Most doctors try to do their best and value constructive criticism. Therefore, if you decide to change doctors, consider politely telling your physician, verbally or in writing, why you are doing so, so he or she can better meet the needs of other patients.

Express your gratitude. If you make up your mind to change doctors, thank the first doctor for caring for your child, just as you would thank anyone who has helped you.

Have your child's records transferred. Request in writing that your child's complete medical records be sent to any new doctors, remembering to include in your note not only your child's name and address but also the name and address of the new doctor. The new physician must have your child's past medical history to read *before* your first visit.

YOUR CHILD'S APPOINTMENTS

Your child's appointments are an important part of your working relationship with your doctor.

Following are suggestions for making an appointment, waiting to see the doctor, and interacting with him or her.

Choose your appointment time wisely. When you call to make an appointment, tell the receptionist why you want to come in so the appropriate amount of time for your visit can be allotted. Also consider when you want to come in. Monday mornings are often very busy with children who became sick over the weekend; by Friday afternoon everyone is tired and wants to go home. So midweek is better for scheduled appointments.

If your child has difficulty waiting, make your appointments for early in the day, before your doctor has a chance to get behind schedule. Try asking for the first or second appointment in the morning. If you live close to the doctor, try for the second appointment so you can call from home to see if the doctor is running on schedule. If the doctor hasn't arrived in the office, ask the receptionist to call you when the doctor arrives, saving you a wait in the office. There will usually be only a few people waiting early in the afternoon as well.

The last appointment in the morning or afternoon is advantageous if the doctor tends to spend more time than allotted with you.

If you are friendly to the receptionist and explain your child's needs and problems, he or she will be better able to help you schedule your appointments.

Be on time for your appointment. If you are late, your doctor will have less time to spend with either you or the next patient. Punctuality is important in building a good working relationship. If you have to be late, call and let the office know. When you do arrive, be sure to give your name so the receptionist knows you are there.

Try to avoid exposure to germs at the doctor's office if your child is very susceptible to illness or becomes sicker than most children. If your child should avoid exposure to germs:

- Make sure your doctor (particularly one who is not your primary-care physician) is aware of the germ problem.

- Make sure the receptionist knows you want to cancel any nonurgent appointment if the doctor or the office staff have bad colds.
- Carefully consider at what time of day your child should see the doctor. If you have one of the first appointments in the morning or afternoon, the doctor is more apt to be on time, and there will be fewer patients waiting who might expose your child to illnesses.
- Wait for your turn outside or in another room, such as the library or the doctor's private office, after you have signed in with the receptionist. Do not be shy about asking for this privilege.
- Be sure you can amuse your child, if there is no alternative to sitting in the waiting room, so he or she doesn't feel the need to handle the toys with which other children have been playing.

Make waiting fun. Despite careful planning, there may be times when you simply have to wait. If you get annoyed, so will your child. Therefore, plan to have a happy time together. Consider bringing a tote bag with you so you can carry the following:

- *Food*—It is perfectly acceptable to nurse your child. If your child bottle-feeds, bring a bottle along. Shops carrying backpacking equipment sell small plastic leakproof bottles in which you can easily carry water, juice, or milk for older children. Little bits of food, such as raisins and small pieces of cheese, can take a long time for your children to eat if *you* feed them one piece at a time. They can be hidden away in different places to add the element of surprise to spice up a long, tiresome wait.
- *Extra diapers and clothes*—Your child might need them.
- *Toys*—Bring those that will take some time to play with, such as a doll, a puzzle, a workbook, or a coloring book and crayons.
- *Books*—Make sure they are ones your child will enjoy listening to or reading alone for some time. (You might even include one for yourself if your child doesn't need to be entertained.)

This may seem like a lot to carry, but the extra effort is worthwhile.

You might also amuse your child by exploring the surroundings—just be sure you are not disturbing others. Within the waiting room there may be an aquarium or a window out of which you can observe life on the street or simply the cars coming and going in the parking lot.

Rehabilitation centers and hospitals can be fun if your child does not have a contagious condition. Sometimes there are noncontagious patients you can visit who will be happy to chat with you. Some clinics and hospitals provide free juice or crackers, which can be very exciting for young children. Or you can look at the newborn babies through the viewing window of the maternity ward.

Include both parents when possible. It is helpful if both parents go to an appointment since both should understand the child's needs. The additional adult can help absorb information and ask questions as well as care for the child while the other parent takes care of business. One parent might wait in the reception room while the other amuses the child playing outside on the lawn or exploring the building. When you are seen by a doctor, both parents can participate in the medical consultation. Consider bringing along a sibling who wouldn't mind the wait, would play quietly with the disabled or ill child, and could watch and learn from what goes on without becoming a nuisance.

THE MEDICAL EXAMINATION

There is a great deal of give and take during a medical examination, which begins with a discussion between you and your doctor.

You begin by telling the doctor why you are there (this is called the *chief complaint*). The doctor may ask you questions to clarify the problem further. You may not know exactly what is wrong, but try to state the problem briefly as you perceive it. Some problems may be embarrassing or difficult to talk about, such as the fear of an organic disorder or a sexual problem, but it is important to be honest and explicit as to the real reason for your visit. Your doctor can help you only if he or she knows why you are there.

The story behind the chief complaint is known as the history of the presenting illness. Some people have difficulty organizing their thoughts in the doctor's presence and forget all that they want to say. Therefore, *before* you leave home think the problem through and make a checklist. The purpose of this is simply to remind you of things you want to discuss, so both you and your doctor can make the best use of your time. If you have extensive concerns and would like to spend more time than usual with your doctor, tell the receptionist this when you make the appointment. A checklist for a regular appointment would include such relevant details as:

- What is the problem?
- When did you first notice it?
- How did it manifest itself?
- Has it gotten better, worse, or stayed the same?
- Why do you think it occurred?
- Have you done anything about it, such as give your child medication?
- What medications does your child take regularly? (Be sure to note carefully the name of the drug, the strength, the dosage, and how much you have left. In case of doubt, bring the medication along, even if the doctor prescribed it.)

Attempt to be a careful observer and a complete recounter of events, for you are the doctor's most valuable source of information. Important background information may include:

Your child's past medical history, particularly if you are seeing the doctor for the first time. You may have been asked in the waiting room to provide information about birth history, growth and development, immunizations, etc. It is important to be as accurate as possible (drug allergies and medications are the subjects most frequently misreported). Misinformation could seriously endanger your child's health.

The family's medical, social, and occupational history. Many health problems run in families. The physician who knows the size, composition, and health of the family, the parents' occupations, the family's interests, and the living environment will have a better understanding of the child.

Your doctor's questions may be personal. Since your answers may assist in treating your child, be frank. For the doctor, this preliminary discussion before the physical examination is often as revealing as the physical examination itself.

The physical examination is performed systematically. Your doctor may ask questions while conducting the examination, not only about your child's physical condition but also about your child's emotional and mental condition. A specialist may limit the examination to aspects of his or her area of expertise. The child should be as involved as possible. Encourage your child to answer any questions he or she can. This will aid your child in assuming some responsibility for his or her own health care.

Your doctor may want you to help with the examination. At a certain age, however, many children misbehave, and the doctor may ask you to leave the room in order to proceed alone. Trust your doctor's judgment on the degree of your involvement.

In discussing any unusual findings with you after the examination, your doctor will probably not indicate things that are normal. Unless the doctor discusses a certain aspect of your child's health with you, you may assume no problems exist in that area.

DIAGNOSTIC TESTING

During the period of your child's diagnostic testing, it is easy to concentrate on the search for what is *wrong*, losing sight of what is right. If you combine the search for what is wrong with the anxiety and fear caused by ignorance of the problem or of the implications of any diagnosis, you can readily see why the period of diagnostic testing can be difficult or even traumatic. Yet if you keep sight of what is right, if you realize that a diagnosis gives you only a basis for medical treatment and nothing more, you can view this period in a more positive light.

Before diagnostic testing begins, ask any questions you have about your child's condition and the testing, but remember two things. First, the doctor doesn't know exactly what the problem is or he or she wouldn't be subjecting your child to all these tests. Second, the testing process and its results may be so complicated that you won't understand the test as well as your doctor no matter how well it is explained. Therefore, you have to respect your doctor's judgment. If your doctor says he or she doesn't know something, accept the fact and simply try to find out what his or her general opinion of the situation is. (You might ask, for example, whether the doctor thinks your child will require hospitalization or any other question of immediate interest.)

Since innumerable tests *can* be run, the following question must always be held in mind so you can decide which tests *should* be run: *Will the test provide information that will affect decisions to be made about your child's medical care?* If so, how? Sometimes both doctors and parents come to feel that the more they know the better, forgetting that a child should be subjected to testing only if it will yield truly useful information.

What to Know about Any Diagnostic Test

You should know generally how your child will be tested, for this helps dispel your own fear and makes it possible to explain the testing to your child. Discuss the following factors with your doctor before the testing begins:

- *Which test is going to be done?* Knowing the name of the test is not sufficient. If you are told it will be an EEG, for example, you need to know that stands for electroenchephalogram, which records brainwaves.
- *Why is the test being done?* This question gives a clue to the suspected medical problem. An EEG may be done to see if abnormal physical development is due to problems with a child's brain.
- *How useful will the results be in determining your child's future care?* An EEG would determine if the problem stemmed from the brain; otherwise it would come from the spinal cord or the muscle. This is crucial to know in deciding on care.
- *Are any risks involved?* Some tests are risky, in which case you must decide with your doctor if the information to be gained justifies the risk.
- *How is the test performed?* Find out in advance what is going to happen. If you understand the procedure, it is easier for everyone to work together. You may even be able to assist or at least be present, if that would help keep your child happy.
- *Who will administer the test?* This is important, especially if even routine procedures are difficult with your child. In most cases it is best to let the assigned person do the procedure. But if that per-

son is having difficulty and you or your child is becoming anxious, ask the person to get someone to assist.
- *When and where will the test be administered?* If the doctor does the testing in the office, you will have a specific appointment. If your child needs hospitalization, read pages 17–25 before any testing is done.
- *Is there any discomfort or pain involved?* Children are frightened by pain, particularly if they do not understand what is going on. However, they have a great ability to tolerate pain and discomfort if they are prepared for it. You can help your child by explaining in advance as much about what will happen as the child can understand. When and what you tell your child will depend upon the child and type of procedure anticipated. A three-year-old might best be told he or she will get an injection just before it happens. A ten-year-old might want to be told what will happen on the drive to the doctor's office. If a major procedure or hospitalization is required, preparatory education is important.
- *How much will the test cost?* While you should know how much a test will cost, you may decide in the beginning that your child should get whatever medical attention is needed and that you will find the money later. Of course, if it is extremely questionable whether an expensive test will yield any useful information, you should think carefully before proceeding.

THE DIAGNOSIS

After testing is complete, your doctor will inform you of the diagnosis, which may be tentative, based upon what he or she knows so far. The diagnosis will carry one of four prognoses:

1. Health can be restored, maintained, or improved.
2. The disease or condition may produce residual disabilities.
3. The disease or condition may offer an uncertain or dubious outlook.
4. The disease or condition may offer a grim prospect and a poor prognosis.

Your attitude is extremely important at this time. Your doctor may be able only to maintain comparative health for your child, but there are always things you can do to make your child happier and more comfortable. Ask for advice— do not demand a cure.

CONSULTATIONS

In case of a serious diagnosis calling for complicated treatment or surgery, many doctors will suggest getting a second opinion, that is, consulting another expert. Or you may request one yourself if you feel further consideration should be given to the diagnosis or treatment. Many insurance companies now pay for second opinions. Since a doctor does not usually view a second opinion as a challenge, do not feel uneasy about making such a request. If your child is given a discouraging diagnosis and it is confirmed by a second opinion, you may have to accept it realistically and work within the framework it provides. (See pages 1–3 for advice on accepting your child's condition.)

It is much harder to decide what to do if doctors *don't* agree about what is wrong with your child; in some cases, the doctors cannot even arrive at a definite diagnosis. At a certain juncture you will have to decide which doctor's advice you will follow and get on with the important task of helping your child develop to the fullest potential.

SPECIALTY CLINICS

Many associations established to aid children with particular disorders, such as muscular dystrophy, spina bifida, or hemophilia, set up specialty clinics in metropolitan areas so children with that disorder can be periodically evaluated. You may want to make an appointment at such a clinic after your child has been diagnosed, since the doctors on staff are particularly experienced in treating children like yours. If you live in a metropolitan area, the specialist may function as your child's primary-care physician, but usually the specialist will serve as a consultant, giving you and your doctor recommendations for your child's treatment. Such clinics often have health-care professionals to review your child's needs in other related areas as well.

To find out if any specialty clinics exist that can help your child, check not only with your doctor but also with any associations that you think might sponsor such clinics (see pages 284–297).

YOUR CHILD'S MEDICAL PROGRAM

Be sure you understand the instructions for the care of your child. If you don't, you cannot help your doctor care for your child. Consider the following:

- Take written notes on what you are told.
- Ask your doctor to write down any specific instructions.
- Understand the purpose of each drug or treatment.
- Ask if any special problem might arise, such as side effects of medication.
- Consider whether your child can follow the prescribed program. If you foresee difficulties, discuss them with your doctor now.
- Understand under what conditions you should call the doctor.
- Ask whether a follow-up examination is necessary and, if so, when.

Follow the instructions after agreeing upon the program. Medication for ten days means for ten days, even if outward symptoms disappear. Twice the prescribed amount does not help twice as much but may be injurious to your child's health. Daily exercises means daily excercises.

Follow the instructions even if all the reasons aren't clear to you. Naturally, if you feel the instructions are inappropriate, phone the doctor and discuss this. Also, if your doctor told you to expect your child to improve by a certain time and that does not happen, or if your child gets worse, call the doctor, for there may well be some reason why your child is not responding.

DOCTOR AND PATIENT RAPPORT

There must be rapport not only between you and your child's doctor but between the doctor and your child as well. Work to establish a friendly, cooperative relationship. If you show interest in learning about medical things and the like, your child will come to accept them as part of life. You can describe physicians as friends who are there to help. Reading books to your child about children receiving medical care can also be helpful. If you sense trouble, try to determine the cause and help your child adopt a more positive attitude. Feel free to discuss any problem with your physician. If the problem is with one doctor in particular, and if you see no way to resolve it, consider changing doctors (see pages 10–11).

Speak of doctor's appointments with warm anticipation. Allow enough time to get ready so you don't feel rushed. When you arrive at the office, give your child your full attention so he or she will have a good time before being examined (see page 12). When you meet with the doctor, involve your child as much as possible. When your child is actually examined, either you or the doctor should honestly explain what is being done and tell your child if something will hurt.

Occasionally specific problems arise, and these must be handled with care. For example, if your child cannot do certain routine procedures in a physical examination and you have developed alternative ways to accomplish these, feel free to explain them to the doctor *before* the examination. If your child is afraid of a specific, one-time procedure, such as having a mole removed, you may want to explain this to your doctor before your child's visit so your doctor will be prepared to help allay your child's fears and to proceed in the most appropriate manner.

PHONE CALLS

Learn when you should call the doctor. In the beginning this can be difficult to decide. Many parents call too often, not because of their child's need but because of their own apprehension. Remember, the doctor is very busy; weigh in your mind if you really need to speak with him or her.

If you have a pressing question about what to do or if your child is acting strangely, do call, even if you have recently spoken with the doc-

tor. If your problem arises during office hours, call and leave a message. But if it is at night or on the weekend, ask yourself whether the problem can wait until the morning or until Monday. If you foresee that your child is going to have difficulties during the night, call the doctor early in the evening to discuss what you should do if your child's condition continues to deteriorate. If it is getting late, it is better to call at 11:00 P.M. than at 3:00 A.M. If you do have to call your doctor during the night, be brief, specific, and able to provide any needed details, like your child's temperature and pulse. Be polite and grateful for your doctor's help.

Do not call your doctor at home unless specifically instructed to do so. The answering service can quickly contact the doctor.

"Can you hold?" is often the first question the receptionist or the answering service will ask. They don't always wait for an answer before placing you on hold. Therefore, if it is an emergency, be ready to yell "Emergency!" into the phone the minute you hear the first syllable of that short question.

When you leave a message for the doctor, be brief and specific, giving your name, your child's name, and your phone number. Tell why you are calling and indicate specific changes in your child's condition and when they occurred. And then tell what you have done. (Usually it is best not to give any medication, not even aspirin, until talking with the doctor, for it may hide symptoms.)

Keep your line open if the doctor is going to return your call.

Describe your child's problem carefully when you do speak to the doctor. Be as accurate and specific as possible, for the diagnosis will be based entirely upon what you tell the doctor on the phone.

3
Hospitalization

Since most children feel unhappy and vulnerable in the hospital, especially when they receive painful medical treatments, try to avoid hospitalization for your chronically ill or severely handicapped child whenever possible. Administer as much treatment and therapy as you can at home, with the guidance of your doctor and, if necessary, other health-care professionals. If hospitalization for diagnosis or treatment that cannot be done elsewhere is necessary, make the stay as short and pleasant as possible.

Hospitalization is very expensive, and your insurance may not cover all expenses. Find out about all possible financial assistance and apply now, for some may not be available retroactively (see Chapter 17).

WHEN IS HOSPITALIZATION NEEDED?

There are several reasons a child may need to be hospitalized.

Emergencies of some types require hospitalization. Discuss with your doctor which situations you should try to handle at home and which require that you take your child to the hospital. Certain emergencies may occur frequently, and you can sometimes learn to handle these at home. In such cases you may actually be able to handle the emergency faster and more efficiently than someone who has never seen your child before. (See Chapter 4 for information on preparing for emergencies.)

Diagnostic testing must sometimes be done in a hospital. Some procedures require a stay in the hospital, but others can be carried out on an outpatient basis, which means patients do not spend the night there. If you decide on outpatient procedures, make sure your insurance will cover them. Also check that the necessary medical care (especially adequate recovery facilities) is available.

Specific short-term treatment, such as most surgery, requires hospitalization.

Parental fatigue can easily occur during a period of severe illness of a chronically ill child. Then the child might be hospitalized not necessarily to get better care but because the parents need a rest if they are to provide ongoing care at home. If your child requires very specialized care and your family has a live-in helper, the helper could spend the better part of the day in the hospital caring for your child.

Long-term treatment often necessitates hospitalization. Then you have to work to make your child's stay as pleasant as possible.

During long-term hospitalization your continuing support is crucial to your child. If you can't stay with your child, give support through phone calls, tapes, letters, photographs, and visits from friends. Discuss with your doctor the possibility of picnics on the hospital grounds, weekend visits at home, or anything else you can think of to enliven the daily routine and to keep your child in contact with the outer world.

Institutionalization is called for when you don't think you can care for your child at home permanently and feel long-term institutional care is necessary. (See pages 211–212.)

TO WHICH HOSPITAL SHOULD YOUR CHILD BE TAKEN?

Your doctor is the one to help you decide which hospital is the most appropriate for your child. If your community has only one hospital with a pediatric unit, the choice is easy. But if you live in a metropolitan area, or if your child has to receive specialized care not available in your community, the choice is difficult. This is what you should consider when choosing a hospital:

Where does your doctor have admitting privileges? Discuss which of these hospitals is best equipped to meet your child's needs. If you choose a hospital where your doctor does *not* have admitting privileges, your child may have to be admitted as the patient of another doctor.

Does the hospital provide the specific medical care needed? Consider not only in which hospitals such care is given frequently enough to have personnel skilled in the areas but also which hospitals frequently treat children with similar problems, since many procedures that are routinely performed on adults are much more difficult when performed on infants and children.

Does the hospital encourage family participation in caring for the child? Your child will probably do better if you are present and can help, as appropriate, with care. Many hospitals now allow parents to spend the night with their children and some allow sibling visits during the day. Others allow parents to prepare meals for children when there are no special dietary restrictions.

Does the hospital provide a warm, emotionally supportive atmosphere for the child? Since many parents cannot stay with their child continually, a pediatric staff that treats children with genuine care is desirable. Usually a small community hospital is more personal. However, if only a large teaching hospital can provide the medical care your child needs, this overshadows concern for the child's emotions. If the medically appropriate hospital is noisy and impersonal, family and friends must provide extra love and warmth. The child-life professionals (also called child-activity or child-development workers) on the hospital staff focus on the needs of the whole child and can provide valuable support for you and your child.

Does the hospital provide parents and children with understandable information about the child's treatment and condition? The more you understand, the better you can work with your doctor to provide the best possible care.

HOW CAN YOU PREPARE FOR HOSPITALIZATION?

After you have chosen a hospital, you must lay the groundwork for a positive hospital experience. As soon as you think your child may have to be hospitalized, you should:

Learn as much as possible about your child's condition and what will happen at the hospital. Ask your doctor, hospital personnel, or other resource persons in your community any questions you have. Your doctor may be able to refer you to parent-support groups or to families who have had similar experiences. Unless you understand what will happen, you cannot adequately prepare your child for hospitalization.

Prepare your child for hospitalization. Discuss hospitalization with your child at a level he or she can understand and answer all questions in a friendly, supportive way. It is most important that you be honest. If your child will be hospitalized for a month, don't say it will be a short time. Say it will be a month, but add what kinds of interesting things will happen in the hospital and then make sure they do, like visits from you and friends, phone calls, and games you will play with your child. Be sure your child understands that he or she will come home again as soon as possible.

If your child asks what will be done to him or her, tell the truth. For example, if you say there will be no pain after surgery, your child will not only be surprised when there is but will wonder whether you can be trusted in the future. It is much better to say that there will be some pain but that, in time, he or she will feel much better. Inform those caring for your child of your explanations so they can provide continuity of psychological and emotional care.

Toys, such as doctor kits and hospital games, can help a child become familiar with the medical world. Most public libraries have children's books about hospitalization. Many large hospitals with pediatric units also have such books, but it is best to begin with such reading material *before* your child is hospitalized (see Appendix 3, "Suggested Reading").

Visit the hospital before your child is admitted. Many hospitals have orientation tours. If not, phone the pediatric unit and ask if your child could be shown around briefly. As a last resort, take your child to the hospital during visiting hours, let him or her look through the glass door to the pediatric unit, and then conclude your visit with a positive experience like looking at the newborn babies, taking a trip to the gift shop, or eating a snack in the hospital cafeteria. Often you can take care of at least some of the paper work necessary for admission on such a visit.

Pack your child's suitcase. This should be done in a matter-of-fact way the day before departure. Doing it a week ahead leads to unnecessary anticipation, whereas a last-minute effort results in frayed nerves. If possible, your child should help pack, choosing what to take along. His or her choices of toys or clothing may seem outlandish, but familiar objects can be very important to a child. Although you can try to help make sensible decisions, you can always take home the things that the child doesn't use and bring the things that he or she wants later. If the hospital is out of town, just put the items your child doesn't want to take now but may need later in another suitcase without making an issue of it.

Tell the hospital staff about your child. Some hospitals request written information about your

child's daily habits. If not, write down any information you think might aid the nursing staff. Include your child's daily schedule, sleeping and eating habits (including favorite foods), special vocabulary or sign language if your child has limited speech. It is important to inform the staff of any known fears, especially if these resulted from past traumatic experiences in hospitals. All this information will aid the hospital staff in understanding and helping your child.

HOW ARE HOSPITALS ORGANIZED?

Once you know how a hospital is organized, you can work with the appropriate personnel, and you will know to whom you should address your questions.

The administrative staff consists of a *board*, which makes policy decisions to be carried out by *the hospital administrator* with the help of a staff comprising *nurses, pharmacists, physical and occupational therapists, child-life specialists, dieticians, cooks, the housekeeping staff, maintenance people,* and so on.

The nursing staff will have the most contact with your child.

The *director of nursing* has the ultimate responsibility for the nursing functions of the hospital and works with *nursing supervisors*, who take charge of the day-to-day operation of one or more wards. Some hospitals now have *nursing coordinators* (also called *head nurses*), with responsibility for the 24-hour-a-day operation, ward policies, and staff supervision of a specific nursing unit. This nurse is usually there for the day shift, from 7:00 A.M. to 3:00 P.M.; *a charge nurse* is responsible for each of the other shifts, 3:00 P.M. to 11:00 P.M. (evenings) and 11:00 P.M. to 7:00 A.M. (nights). Some hospitals (particularly those with nurse shortages) are now experimenting with other work hours. *Registered nurses* decide what kind of nursing is needed for each of their patients and arrange that such care is provided. An RN considers nursing problems, analyzes them, and comes up with nursing action. For example, if a patient's legs are swollen, the RN can make sure they are elevated. An RN is not, however, responsible for diagnosing the medical root of a problem or initiating a medical procedure to alleviate it. *Licensed vocational* (or *practical*) *nurses* provide nursing care but are not trained in in-depth problem-solving. *Attendants* and *orderlies* have on-the-job training in basic patient care and, theoretically, do nothing more sophisticated than giving baths, getting patients in and out of bed, etc., under the supervision of a registered nurse. Nevertheless, they are often the ones most involved in nurturing care. It is necessary to work with all of these persons in caring for your child.

The medical staff consists of physicians, dentists, podiatrists, and others who make medical diagnoses, decide on treatment, order the necessary tests and procedures, and follow the progress of the patient. The amount and kind of staffing will depend upon the size and function of the hospital. A large teaching hospital in a metropolitan area is probably the most complex. If you understand the chain of command there, you can apply the pattern to any hospital simply by omitting the positions that don't exist. The physicians who care for patients in the hospital are called *attending physicians* and have admitting privileges to the hospital. *Residents* are physicians who are taking additional training beyond their MD degrees. They are called *junior residents* until their last year of training, when they are called *senior* or *chief residents*. *Fourth-year medical students* may also have limited privileges within a hospital.

All of the residents and medical students are supervised by the *director of medical education.*

Typically, the admitting history and physical examination are done by a medical student, a junior resident, and the attending physician. Perhaps the senior resident will check the patient too.

In this system, as orders are written into the patient's chart, each entry is checked by the writer's superior to evaluate the order and catch any error.

Although your child may be treated by a whole team of doctors, there is usually one primary-care physician at the hospital who is responsible for your child's care. This doctor will probably not spend the whole day in the unit. In a very small hospital, there may not be any permanent doctors on the staff. Nurses provide the care and contact your regular physician in case of need.

HOSPITAL ADMISSION

The following advice may facilitate hospital admission.

Confirm your child's admission date and time by phone the day before you go to the hospital. There is nothing worse than arriving at the hospital with the letter giving the admission date and finding that no one is expecting you. It can also be difficult if you arrive before a room is ready for your child. (Be prepared in case you do have to wait; see pages 11–12 for advice on waiting with your child.)

Bring your spouse or a friend so one can care for your child while the other tends to formalities. You may find your initial encounter with the hospital world a bit overwhelming; your companion can lend moral support, help absorb information, and ask questions.

Arrange for a direct admission if necessary. If your child is very ill or in pain, ask your doctor if your child can be admitted directly to the floor, bypassing the preliminary paperwork and lab tests. Then when your child is settled in the hospital room you can go back to the admitting office to complete the paperwork. Such "direct admission" must be requested by the physician. If this is not possible, sometimes one adult will be allowed to take the patient to the room while the other one does the paper work.

Read all papers carefully before signing anything. Most of the forms will be routine, but you should know to what you are committing yourself.

Although you may be asked to sign a blanket release form, this is not legally binding. You will be asked to sign a release form for each separate surgical or other major procedure. You should discuss these forms carefully with your doctor so you understand what is going to be done. You may even want to write the following on the bottom of the form: "Please discuss any procedure with parents before proceeding" or "I want all procedures to be done on my child to be discussed with me before they are performed."

The receptionist or secretary may insist that you sign papers immediately. If you are pressured to sign before you understand the papers, or if you need more information, you may have to insist upon seeing the doctor.

THE HOSPITAL ROUTINE

You should understand how the hospital routine will affect your child and try to lend a helping hand.

Room assignment is made according to your child's diagnosis and a variety of other factors:

- What is your child's age?
- What is your child's general condition: critical, fair, good?
- Is your child's illness contagious?
- Should your child be protected from contagious diseases because of planned surgery or a generally weakened condition?
- Should your child be put in a single room (which can be handy if you want to spend the night but boring for a child in the long run), in a double room, or in a ward? You may not have a choice. If you do, check what rates your insurance or Medicaid pays for each type of accommodation, for this may influence your choice of placement.

You should understand the reason for your child's room assignment. For example, if your child is put in a "clean room," a room in which no other patient has a contagious disease, this is because it is important that your child avoid exposure to germs. Therefore you should not allow visitors with colds or walk your child up and down the hall where exposure to germs is inevitable.

If you think your child's room assignment is inappropriate, talk to your doctor.

The daily housekeeping routine includes room cleaning, ice-water delivery, and so on. Naturally, the staff can't do everything for your convenience, but if you find something particularly disruptive to your child's well-being (like the delivery of ice water at 5:00 A.M.), politely request a change in the routine. If it is simply a "housekeeping" chore, it is sometimes easiest to say you would be happy to do the job yourself. The more you can help the busy staff, the better the care will be. Of course, there may be instances when the change you request depends upon health care professionals. In that case, if no one lower in the hierarchy responds to your request, you may have to ask your doctor to add instructions to your child's chart.

The nurturing routine includes the physical care such as bathing, dressing, toileting, and feeding that you would provide for your child at home. Anything you can do to help your child in these areas will make it possible for the nurses to provide more medical attention. Also, you can do some of the essentials in a personalized way and even add a few extras. For example, you may be able to help your son fix his hair and brush his teeth before the nurses come to give him a bath. Depending on your child's condition, you may help with the bath or give it yourself. You may meet a nurse who is hostile and delights in exposing your nursing incompetence. Don't take offense at such a thoughtless nurse who will be in the minority. Just stick to your desire to be involved and helpful. Remember not to talk with the nurses too much, for they don't have the time. Ask how you can help or if you can do this or that. You will find that the time passes more quickly and that you feel better if you keep busy.

You may also want to take responsibility if you notice a snag in the nurturing routine. For example, if a snack is late one afternoon, do not simply complain. Indicate politely that you know the nurses are busy and that you would be delighted to help or to get it yourself. This way you avoid annoying the nurses by complaining, and you save pushing the call button for more crucial needs.

As with housekeeping, if there is a continuing problem with the nurturing routine that you can't resolve by appealing upward through the nursing hierarchy, ask the doctor to place instructions on your child's chart.

VISITING YOUR CHILD IN THE HOSPITAL

If a long hospitalization for your child is anticipated and you have other children at home, you can't be in the hospital all the time. A younger child may cry when you leave; tell the child and the nursing staff when you will return, so the child can look forward to your next visit. (And of course make sure you come when you said you would.) A teenager may actually want to establish his or her own relationships and not always want you around. Try to determine your child's needs as an individual.

When you visit your child, your active involvement with him or her is important. If your child is extremely sick or not completely conscious, physical contact like hand-holding can be important. Hearing familiar voices may also help your child's mental orientation, especially if he or she is semiconscious or comatose. If you find it difficult to carry on a monologue with your child, you might want to read books out loud in the room so your child can hear your voice and know you are there. A healthier child will be happy to play with you. If you or your friends want to bring presents, bring them one at a time. Choose gifts that can be used more than once like books, construction toys, craft kits, and art and writing materials with which children can express their thoughts and feelings. Through play, your child may come to share more about his or her hospital experiences with you. If your child starts to talk about those experiences, listen and help your child express his or her feelings rather than interject your own.

Check with the nursing staff before you bring food or gum because it may interfere with diagnostic testing or the special diet of your child (or of a friend with whom he or she shares).

Throughout this period of hospitalization, remember that you know your son or daughter better than the doctor does. Therefore, your observations about your child's condition can be helpful. You may not only be able to assess how your child is doing generally but may also help in judging specifics—for example, if he or she needs pain medication. If you see significant changes or think something is going wrong,

bring this to the attention of a doctor or a nurse. Complications can occur, especially if your child is receiving complex medical care, and you may be the first to notice the early signs or symptoms.

While at the beginning of your child's hospitalization he or she may need you to be there as much as possible, as the end of the stay approaches do not feel compelled to stay with your child all the time. It is important that you get rested, see to the needs of other family members, and get your household organized so you will be ready for your child's homecoming.

Most children are grateful if a parent spends at least the first night with them. Many hospitals encourage parents to sleep in the room with their children. Even if it is officially against the rules, many hospitals will find ways to work around such rules and regulations. If you are polite and persistent, you will probably be allowed to stay.

Even if your child is a teenager, your cheerful presence and calm, helping hand can mean much, especially in the middle of the night. If, at that age, you ask if your child wants you to stay and he or she replies "You don't have to," your child may well mean "Please do!" Try to discern what your child really prefers.

DEALING WITH EMOTIONAL PROBLEMS

You must make your child realize that in spite of his or her condition he or she must try to be as cheerful, friendly, and polite as possible.

You may love your child enough to tolerate rude behavior with a smile. A nurse will have to tolerate it too, smile or no, but the nurse also has the option of becoming as scarce as possible. The eternal bell-ringer does not get the call button answered faster; rather, he or she becomes like the little boy who cried wolf.

You influence your child's attitude by setting an example. Offer the nurse a cheery hello, ask how he or she is doing, and share something interesting that you and your child have been doing. Do not moan and groan about the hospital, your child's miserable condition, and how you don't see how anyone in the family will survive the ordeal. Remember, your child's response to the situation is largely conditioned by yours.

Sometimes hospitalization causes a child temporarily to alter his or her behavior or regress somewhat. If you think your child is developing severe psychological problems, discuss this with a member of the staff such as the doctor, the child-life worker, or the psychologist.

LEARNING FROM THE HOSPITAL STAFF

It is important to know how to obtain from the hospital staff the information and knowledge you need.

Write down your questions as they occur to you. When you start asking questions in the hospital, you may be bombarded with words and concepts you never heard of. Carry a pencil and notebook and write down what you have been told. Ask questions about what you don't understand. If a medical term slips by you, ask the doctor to spell it or write it down for you. A good medical dictionary is indispensable.

You may decide to read up on your child's medical problem yourself, but remember that unless you are a trained health-care professional you may have difficulty understanding everything correctly. Furthermore, in areas where there have been rapid advances, information may become outdated. (For example, some cancer patients have a much better prognosis today than literature that is five years old would indicate.) Also, medical literature may give a very factual and terse description of your child's disorder which may sound very discouraging. Therefore, while you may want to do reading on your own, your primary-care doctor is the best qualified to answer specific questions about your child's medical condition and clarify points relating to information you have read or heard. You will have to ask when he or she is usually "on the floor" and can talk to you. You may find yourself firing your questions at the doctor in a busy corridor, the infants' ward, or wherever. Move along with your questions, one by one, writing down anything you don't think you will correctly retain. (Some patients have tape-recorded such medical discussions for future reference.

Doctors, however, may balk at being taped.) If you don't understand something, ask for clarification.

After your discussion, go over what you have learned, look up the words you don't fully understand, and write out more questions for the next time you see the doctor. Knowledge will come slowly, partly because you are trying to get a complex medical education very rapidly and partly because your doctor may not yet have fully diagnosed your child's problem.

If you need more time than the doctor can provide on the floor, make an appointment for an office visit.

You may be tempted to learn more about your child's condition by speaking with other parents or by eavesdropping on conversations between members of the medical staff. While the information you gain may be useful, it may also be distorted or incorrect. If you want to know something, ask your doctor directly.

Among the rest of the hospital staff, different people can help educate you in different areas. Nurses often have handy tips on nurturing care. Therapists may be more knowledgeable than doctors in the practical aspects of giving physical or respiratory therapy at home. Pharmacists can help in understanding the dosages, effects, and side effects of medication. Dieticians can help with nutrition.

Social workers are knowledgeable about the financial resources available in your community.

If your child is being hospitalized for the first time, it is important to have a social worker help you determine what your insurance will actually cover and whether any assistance is available to help you with your share of the cost. (How to pay for medical help you need is more fully discussed in Chapter 17.) Make an appointment to see a social worker. If you do not know what specific questions to ask, simply inquire generally what resources are available. A social worker can also help you find other resource persons in the community to assist you once your child comes home. And he or she can provide family counseling, which you may well appreciate.

Child-life professionals, on the staffs of more and more hospitals, are child advocates who work with the children through play, music, and art therapy to help them understand and accept what is happening.

They do not administer medical treatment but can provide significant emotional support, like explaining medical procedures and accompanying the child to the operating room. Child-life professionals often function as liaison persons to the medical staff and have an important role to play in assisting both child and parents.

DIAGNOSTIC TESTING

Diagnostic testing is more fully discussed in Chapter 2, but if your child is hospitalized for testing, consider the following.

If the proposed test seems risky or questionable, and you are unsure whether to proceed, you can ask that your child be released and take him or her home until you and your doctors come to a decision about what to do. (For help in deciding whether or not to proceed with a test, see pages 13–14.) Of course this is relevant only if the situation is not an emergency requiring immediate attention.

If you are proceeding with diagnostic testing, it is very important to find out *when* it will be done. Some procedures may be carried out only at certain times of the day or on certain days of the week. So if a test is scheduled for a specific date and time and is late, rather than simply wait, ask whether or not the test will be performed that day.

SURGERY

Surgery is a major event. Anesthesia itself is extremely hard on the body, especially for very weak children. Furthermore, although your surgeon has thoroughly studied the problem, he or she can only guess at what the operation will disclose. Acute abdominal pain in the right lower quadrant is likely to be appendicitis, but it may turn out to be something else. And whereas certain operations have very high success rates, other operations meet only limited success. Therefore, you will have to consider carefully what should be done, when, and by whom.

Aside from elective surgery, surgeries fall into three categories—emergencies, which must be performed immediately; urgent surgeries, which must be done in the near future; and those that can wait. Emergencies are in one sense the easiest on your nerves because you don't have time to fret and fume.

Surgeries of the second type are those that can wait but not for long. Some types of cancer are cases in point. Here you have time to get a second opinion, though excessive delay can be harmful.

With operations that can wait, you can choose *when* the operation should be done and may take into account your child's age, present state of health, and any recent disruptive emotional experience such as a birth or death in the family or a divorce. Your decision about surgery is more difficult if experts give you conflicting advice on what to do. If you find that the experts disagree, try to find the answers to two questions: what do they disagree about, and what are the reasons for the disagreement?

This information is necessary for you to make a decision. You may want to consult with your primary-care physician or ask yet another specialist to interpret the case and help you understand the issue so you can make an intelligent decision. Sometimes your decision may not be which procedure to perform but whether to perform a procedure at all. If your child is near the end of his or her life or is unlikely to improve, a painful procedure such as surgery, which only temporarily improves the situation, may not be appropriate, especially if it compromises the quality of your child's life.

If, after considering all the options, you feel that surgery should be done, learn as much as you can about the procedure and honestly prepare your child for it.

Your child should understand to the best of his or her ability what is going to happen, step by step. (See pages 18–19 for advice on preparing your child for hospitalization and surgery.) When the actual day for the operation arrives, try to be with your child *before* he or she is taken to the operating room. If possible, stay with your child until he or she is anesthetized and be there again when he or she wakes up, for your presence will be very reassuring.

GOING HOME

You and your child will probably be delighted when you are told that he or she can go home. To facilitate the transfer from hospital to home, try to take care of the following matters *before* your child is released from the hospital.

Arrange for the payment of the bill. If you have not yet seen a social worker about resources to help you pay your share of the cost (see pages 228–241), you may want to now.

Take home most of your child's personal items before the day of release. This doesn't mean that Teddy and other favorites shouldn't spend the last night with your child, but if there is an accumulation of flowers, gifts, toys, and so on, it is helpful to take most of these home in advance. Then on the day of release you can concentrate on getting your child home.

Obtain any necessary medications. Sometimes the hospital will provide medication. If not, get the prescriptions filled at your local pharmacy. (See page 45 on how to find a pharmacist with whom you think you can establish a good working relationship.)

Discuss follow-up care with your doctor. Be sure to get *written instructions* about medication and treatment. Do not rely on your memory.

Arrange for any necessary home treatment by health-care professionals such as nurses or therapists. The hospital social worker can help you here.

Obtain any special equipment and supplies your child will need at home. Borrow, rent, or buy these now. Check with the health-care professionals involved in your child's care as to whether your community has loan closets from which you could borrow items you will need only for a short time. (Often the Visiting Nurses Association and service organizations have loan closets.) If you need to rent or buy items, professionals should be able to advise you as to which supply house to contact. (See page 79 for basic guidelines.)

Arrange the first few days at home so you have time to get used to caring for your child. You may want to ask a relative, friend, or baby-sitter to help with your other children. You may want to cook dinners ahead or ask a friend to bring in a meal. Try to think of ways to simplify your life for the first few days while you get used to, and adept at, providing home medical care.

Devise a daily record chart so you can record your child's progress and medical treatment (see pages 37–38).

Arrange for a home teacher. Home and hospital teachers are more fully discussed on pages 199–201. Contact your child's school directly or have the hospital teacher help you make the appropriate arrangements. Try to have school begin as soon as your child gets home. You may wonder if your child is strong enough, but home/hospital teachers are good at assessing the strength of a child and usually have alternative activities in case the child is not feeling well. That hour of school also gives you an hour to fix dinner, take a bath, make the beds, or even take a nap.

Arrange for transportation home at least the day before release if not sooner, especially if you need an ambulance or assistance from a friend.

Once at home, your child may feel at liberty to relax and behavior may regress a bit. But if you're prepared for this, it is easier to balance the amount of firmness and laxity needed.

4

Providing Medical Care at Home

If you can manage your child's daily medical care, as well as minor emergencies that may arise, without calling your doctor all the time, this will benefit all involved—your child, your doctor, and you.

The first step in learning to care for your child at home is to let your doctor know you are willing to assume as much responsibility as possible. Once your doctor understands that you are willing to learn, he or she will be willing to teach you.

How You Learn What You Need to Know

To learn you must listen to what you are told, ask appropriate questions, and follow through on what you have learned. Since your doctor does not have the time to provide a complete lecture course on home medical care, your questions determine what he or she explains to you.

Ask questions that will yield useful information, beginning with basic questions to gain the general information you need. Then ask any specifics. For example, if your child becomes ill, you should learn generally why he or she has become ill and what you should do. If your child needs to be on continuous antibiotics and you have to keep changing them, you may specifically want to learn about the range and scope of antiobiotics used for children. With that information you and your doctor can work together to change the antibiotic as necessary. Or if you learn which side effects to watch for with a new prescription and ask whether you

will have to watch for any interaction between the three drugs your child is now taking, you are asking questions that help you and your doctor to work together.

Keep asking questions—write them down if it will help you to remember them.

Be sensitive to your doctor's reluctance to explain everything in detail. Your doctor may presently lack the time to do so or may rightly feel you don't really need that much information at this time. However, if you really think you need to know something, explain why.

Reflect upon the reasons for your questions. You may find that some of your questions are not truly aimed at finding out specific information but stem from other motives. For example, your questions may actually spring from fear and anxiety and the hope that more information may dispel your very real concerns about your child's well-being. Or your questions may derive from concern about your doctor's ability to provide appropriate care and the desire to maintain total control of the situation (which in the case of complicated medical problems is impossible). These two examples are not given for the purpose of discouraging you from asking questions but to indicate that it is important occasionally to reflect upon why you are asking questions, so if there is an underlying problem you can discuss it with your doctor.

Avoid asking questions in which criticism is implicit. It is one thing to ask for information like "What side effects should I watch for with this medication?" or, if you have been reading about the particular drug, to ask specifically, "Do we have to be concerned about gastric bleeding if Mike uses prednisone?" It is quite another thing to say, "Why didn't you tell me gastric bleeding can be caused by prednisone?" In some cases one part of your question (and perhaps the tone of your voice as well) implies criticism. If you say, "Mary had the same problem and her doctor didn't treat her this way," you are questioning the treatment but in a negative way. Neither you nor your doctor may know if Mary's condition is exactly like your son's, and even in the unlikely event that it is there may be a number of ways to treat the same disease. Similarly, a question such as "Why aren't we using ———— I read about on my child?" not only questions the treatment but implies that the doctor is not up on the latest information.

Think not only about what you are saying but the way you are saying it. When your questions to your doctor move from requesting information to implying criticism, you may hit a sore spot, putting your doctor on the defensive; the conversation then becomes a confrontation rather than an effort at cooperation.

Carry through on what you have learned to do. True cooperation requires effort on both sides. When your doctor teaches you what you need or want to learn, you in turn have to make the effort to implement his or her recommendations.

Keep Your Child's Needs in Perspective

In providing medical care, you must think not only of your son's or daughter's physical needs but of your child's emotional and psychological needs as well.

If you focus only on the physical, or let your child do so, you are forgetting about the rest of the human being. This is not only limiting but can also be depressing, since you are looking at what doesn't work rather than at what does.

Furthermore, since you know your child as a human being much better than any health professional does, you are in many ways the best observer of how your child feels and acts. This

knowledge is crucial to providing the best care for your child at home.

Include your child as an active member of the family. Treat your child as normally as possible.

For starters this means keeping your child "in the middle of the action" whenever possible and not off in a bedroom somewhere. Bedrooms are for sleeping or resting, and pajamas are clothing in which you sleep. The living room, dining room, kitchen, den, and backyard are where you and your child, dressed in clothes, should spend most of the day. You may have to make adjustments in your living areas, like using a sheet to turn the couch into a bed or even putting a hospital bed into the living room if your child needs to spend much time lying down. But this can be done, and if your house doesn't look like everyone else's, that's fine. You need to see your child as an integral part of the family, and you can arrange your household so he or she is.

Give your child jobs and responsibilities; involve your child in normal childhood activities and encourage him or her to become as independent as possible. This will help keep the illness in perspective as just one part of life.

Teach your child to be courteous and thoughtful at all times. Your child's condition from day to day will influence not only what your child can and can't do and how he or she feels but also how your child acts. On bad days, it is best to avoid unnecessary confrontations and to make life as pleasant as possible. But always insist that your child maintain a level of proper behavior. Grouching, hitting, swearing, and the like should be unacceptable.

Your example in all this is crucial. If you are grouchy when you are tired, or panic-stricken when medical emergencies arise, or willing to wait on your child hand and foot and give in to every whim, you aren't doing yourself, your child, or your family a favor. This isn't to say that we don't all have good and bad days, but we do have to strive for normalcy. If you are experiencing strong emotions and are unable to set a positive example for your child, discuss this with your doctor and consider professional help.

HOW DO YOU KNOW IF YOUR CHILD IS SICK?

A child who smiles and plays happily is probably not very sick. Still, if you think your child may be sick, consider the following.

Is your child acting differently? This is something you can often judge better than your doctor because you are with your child so much more. However, you may be less apt to notice gradual changes, such as progressive changes in your child's physical or mental condition. Therefore, it is good periodically to write down information in a notebook. This will help you notice gradual changes and enable you to tell your doctors when any change occurred.

Do not rely upon friends or relatives to tell you about changes or that something is wrong. They may not notice changes in your child's condition, or they may be hesitant to point them out to you.

If you do notice a change, do not assume that it is directly associated with your child's condition and that nothing can be done.

Patterns within the day vary, of course, for most people have up and down periods. For example, fevers generally go up late in the afternoon, and some children are tired at the same time every day. Still, if you have taken such variations into account and you notice significant changes in your child's behavior even within one day, call your doctor and describe the situation as accurately as possible. (See page 16 for information on talking to your doctor over the phone.)

Does your child look different? Here the gradual changes are tricky to detect. If your child has a progressive condition, what you think is just a manifestation of his or her condition may actually be a different medical problem that needs treatment. Again, keeping a notebook or diary can help you notice any gradual changes.

Although your doctor will tell you of specific things to watch for with your own child, there are certain general signs to keep in mind:

- *Flushed red complexion* may indicate that your child is running a fever.

- *Pale, gray, or blue complexion* can mean your child is not getting enough oxygen and is having trouble with his or her heart or lungs. If your child is blue, call the doctor *immediately*.
- *Puffiness* may mean your child's body is retaining fluids and the kidneys or urinary system aren't working properly.
- *A wilted look* can result from dehydration or lack of sufficient body fluid. This is a hazard if your child is too weak to eat or drink, has been vomiting, or has had diarrhea. The first indication is a very low urine output (few wet diapers or infrequent trips to the bathroom). Your child's mouth may seem dry and you will note an absence of tears if your child cries.
- *Rashes* may indicate skin disorders, infectious childhood diseases (like chicken pox or measles), or drug or food reactions.

Is your child running a fever? A fever is a sign that something is wrong, but it doesn't tell you what.

The most common causes of persistent fevers in children are colds, sore throats, earaches, diarrhea, urinary infections, contagious childhood illnesses, and occasionally pneumonia, appendicitis, and meningitis. If your child has medical problems, a fever may also indicate a problem relating to his or her specific condition. Ask your doctor for guidelines as to when you should contact him or her.

As common viral infections can result in anything from a normal to a very high temperature, temperature alone is *not* a reliable indicator of the seriousness of your child's condition.

Management of temperature should be governed primarily by the child's need for comfort, except if your child has febrile seizures, in which case careful temperature control is essential to prevent seizures from occurring. (See pages 31–32 for advice on fever control.)

Don't panic if your child runs a fever. Try to remember the adage "What goes up must come down." Take the appropriate medical steps to control the fever (see pages 31–32) but also try to maintain an attitude and vocabulary that keep things in perspective. You might tell your child that he or she is cooking cookies or anything else that may prevent alarm.

How do you know if your child has a fever? The easiest way to tell if your child has a fever is to compare his or her skin temperature with your own by touch (providing you are healthy and not running a fever yourself). The excessive use of thermometers isn't necessary, and you can get hooked on numbers. The touch method gives you a rough idea: if your child feels hot, you and your doctor may want to know how hot. If you need only an approximate reading, you can use a heat-sensitive strip, which you just lay across your child's forehead or stomach.

If you need a more accurate reading, measure your child's temperature rectally or orally. Although we say normal body temperature is 98.6°F, every part of the body has a different temperature. A rectal temperature will not only be higher than an oral one but the thermometer will rise to within a degree of where it is going to stop within the first thirty seconds. It can take one and a half to two minutes to register the correct oral temperature, by placing the thermometer under the tongue. In addition, an oral temperature reading can be influenced by the way your child breathes, whether he or she keeps his or her mouth shut when the thermometer is in, and whether your child has recently eaten hot or cold food.

If you think your child may bite the thermometer or may not keep his or her mouth shut, a rectal thermometer is the better choice.

When should you call your doctor about a fever? It is important to remember that childhood fevers come on more rapidly and may rise much higher than with adults, even with a minor virus. The younger the child, the more serious the situation can be. Consult your doctor immediately if your child has a fever and is under four months of age; if your child's temperature reaches 104° and won't come down; or if your child's fever continues for more than three days.

You must decide with your doctor if there are other circumstances in which you should call, since it may depend on your child's condition. If your child is chronically ill and any infection could cause serious difficulties, your doctor may want to hear from you as soon as your child starts running a fever. When you report your child's temperature, tell your doctor not only how and at what time of day you took the temperature but also what your child had

been doing, since all these factors can affect temperature.

What is your child's pulse? Pulse rates change with activity and physical condition. When your child moves about quickly, his or her heart beats faster. When your child is ill, his or her pulse can be much faster, or it can slow down.

It is helpful to know your child's normal pulse rate and determine with your doctor at what point above and below normal your doctor wishes to be notified.

It is easiest to feel an infant's pulse on the brachial artery, which runs down the inside of the arm between the shoulder and the elbow. On older children you can feel it on the inside of the wrist by sliding your fingers off the tendon leading toward the thumb down toward the little finger. On a skinny weak child you can see the heart beating beneath the ribs.

Your child may find it uncomfortable if you use a large cortoid artery in the neck for taking a pulse.

When you take your child's pulse, count the beats for 15 seconds and multiply by four to get the pulse per minute. If your child has an irregular pulse, your doctor may wish you to count for a longer period of time.

Although pulse rate is important, don't panic just because it goes up. A child can survive long periods of elevated pulse rate that an adult cannot tolerate.

A very irregular or weak pulse could mean that the heart is not pumping normally or that there is internal bleeding; no pulse could mean that the heart is not pumping at all or that there may be damage to the particular artery you are feeling. Pulse can be a valuable indicator of your child's condition.

What is your child's rate of respiration? How rapidly and in what way your child is breathing can tell you something about how well his or her lungs are functioning. Infants breathe 50–60 times a minute. Within a year this will slow to 25–35, although an active one-year-old may have a respiratory rate as high as 45. For a child between the ages of one and five, a rate of over 40 when at rest is of concern; for a child over six, a rate of over 30 breaths per minute is of concern. Respiration changes are quite common in children during sleep, and these should never be a cause of alarm unless they are associated with other signs and symptoms suggesting illness.

To check your child's breathing rate, just place your hand on the upper chest with your thumb extending up to the collar bone and count each time you feel the complete cycle of the rise and fall of the chest. Also check to see if your child's breathing is regular and whether he or she seems to be having any difficulty. If the breaths are quick and shallow, irregular, or take great effort, and particularly if there is grunting, groaning, or crowing respiration, your child is having trouble breathing.

Fever and respiratory illnesses such as pneumonia can elevate the respiratory rate. So can aspirin overdoses, diabetes, metabolic disturbances following diarrhea, and any number of other things that might relate to your child's specific condition. Therefore, if your child's breathing is slower or faster or sounds different than normal, call your doctor.

Are there more subtle signs of illness? There are three additional clues that suggest your child may be sick. If you think your child may be sick, ask yourself the following questions.

1. Is my child "wilted" (inactive, unresponsive, and weak)?
2. Does my child look and act the way he or she usually does when I look at him or her?
3. Above all, does my child smile?

Your doctor may also tell you of special conditions to look for while caring for your child. What is of no consequence with one child may be serious with another. For example, a cold and its possible complications can be life-threatening for a child with chronic respiratory problems, whereas for a hemophiliac a cold is not a cause for alarm. Discuss with your doctor what your child's major medical problems are, how to recognize them in the early stages, and what you should do if they occur. You need to learn what you can handle yourself and when you should ask for help. You can do that only if you can recognize problem situations.

If your child's condition is ever-changing, you may have to constantly reevaluate when you need help. You and your doctor may agree that you should not give any medication, including aspirin or other nonprescription drugs, without consulting the doctor first, since these may hide symptoms. On the other hand, if certain problems or emergencies arise often, your doctor may want you to take certain steps immediately, even before you can contact him or her.

PREVENTING AND TREATING COMMON CHILDHOOD ILLNESSES

Try to Keep Your Child Away from Germs

The first step in dealing with illness has to be prevention.

Some children can handle colds without any difficulty and shouldn't be overprotected. But other children, especially those with impaired immune systems or chronic disabilities involving the respiratory tract, can become quite ill even from what begins as a simple cold. If your son or daughter has such problems, develop a sensible routine to avoid contracting an illness.

Keep your house as germfree as possible. Let only healthy people come into the house. Remind friends and playmates that if they have colds they are not welcome. If they forget and arrive coughing and sneezing, you simply have to ask them to leave. Of course, if someone in the family gets sick, you can only try to keep them away from your ill child. Since cold germs are potent 24 hours before you feel symptoms, isolation is not possible for the entire time germs are viable. Try to keep sick siblings away from your child; if you get sick, try to go to bed and get some rest.

Make everyone who comes into the house wash their hands. Your hands touch things when you're out and about, and when you come home and touch things in the house you spread the germs you picked up. When friends visit, simply hand them soap and a towel in the kitchen if the bathroom is upstairs so you don't make a big thing of it. What you do touch before you wash your hands on entering the house is, of course, the door handle, so you might get in the habit of giving it an occasional scrub.

When you go visiting, check in advance that everyone in the household is healthy. This may cramp your social style, but if a cold can make your child very ill for a week or two, it just isn't worth it to visit friends who have colds, even for an hour or two. Also, ask your doctor's receptionist to call you before your appointment if someone in the office has a bad cold so you can change your appointment.

Limit your visits to indoor public places when there is much illness in your community. You know when the cold and flu season has hit. If you don't know the current disease rate in town, your pharmacist or doctor can easily tell you. At these times you may not want to take your child to indoor places such as stores or theaters. Doctors' offices are one of the worst places for picking up viruses.

There is no point in becoming fanatical about germs. Your child is bound to meet a germ some day and get sick, even if you take precautions. Just do your best within reasonable limits.

The Common Cold

The common cold accounts for about 85 percent of childhood illnesses. It usually affects the whole person, causing swollen mucous membranes, a runny nose, a sore throat, and so on.

A cold is caused by a virus, and since you can't treat viruses, you can't do much about a cold except relieve the symptoms and prevent complications, often called "secondary infections." Because these complications, such as bronchitis, pneumonia, or an ear infection, may be dangerous for your child, you may have to treat his or her common cold differently than you would that of a "normal" child.

Little children get colds frequently, perhaps because their immune systems are not fully developed. You may be able to cut down on colds in children under about six by limiting their exposure to other people and their germs. If a cold (and its potential complications) is a major health threat to your child, you may have to consider keeping all of your children out of school as long as possible, perhaps until they are five or six. Nine-year-olds get half as many colds as six-year-olds, and a 12-year-old is apt to be laid up only half as much as a nine-year-old; so there may be hope as your child gets older.

Medication for colds should be discussed with your doctor. Do not give your child any drug (prescription or nonprescription, including aspirin) without consulting your doctor first.

Viral Infections Such as the Flu

The other recurrent illness that affects young and old alike throughout the year is the flu. Like a cold, the flu is viral and therefore cannot be treated except symptomatically. However, secondary bacterial infections are more common in flu and will respond to antiobiotics. Although the flu is common, you should take it seriously.

HANDLING COMMON CONDITIONS

There are certain steps you should take in case of any illness.

Control high fevers. Most children can tolerate high fevers. Only about one in 20 is genetically prone to seizures with high fevers, called febrile seizures. While a febrile seizure may look frightening, it is not serious in most children and does not result in seizures later in life unless your child has a specific nervous abnormality which is disclosed through the febrile seizure.

Nevertheless, high fever in children can be troublesome. While your doctor may request you to try to bring down a fever, do not assume that the reduction will cure your child. In general, fever is a symptom and not a cause of illness. (Slight elevations may even be beneficial in aiding the body to fight off an infection.)

Determine with your doctor what you should do in case of fever, and follow his or her instructions. Find out what your doctor considers to be a danger level, at which point you should call. Fevers will become easier to control as your child gets older, when the temperature-regulatory center matures and he or she gets rid of baby fat that keeps excessive heat in during illness.

You can control your child's fever through a variety of methods, often used in combination.

Utilize your child's own natural bodily processes to bring the fever down:

- Dress your child in light clothing with maybe a sheet for comfort, so the body can give off excess heat.
- Turn on a fan or a cool-mist vaporizer if you have one, if this makes your child feel better.
- Wipe your child's body with a cool damp cloth. Do not use cold water or alcohol, as these will cause the temperature to drop too rapidly and cause the skin to get cold. Your child can't lose much heat through cold skin. Inhaling alcohol vapors can also be dangerous, especially in a poorly ventilated room.
- Give your child a bath in room-temperature water (again, not cold) and let your child play there, if you think this would help.
- Pay attention to the most important signal of all—your child's comfort. If what you do feels good to your child, it is probably the right thing to do. If your child starts shivering and the teeth chatter, the body has cooled too quickly and is trying to warm itself. In that case, your efforts are getting you nowhere.

Have your child drink lots of extra liquids, since the body will lose liquid through perspiration. Obviously, hot drinks can further elevate the temperature, whereas cold drinks may help lower it. If your child is nauseated or has a very sore throat, colder drinks may be more soothing (or feel less uncomfortable).

Give medication only in the way your doctor prescribed. This includes aspirin and acitominophens such as Tylenol, both of which are commonly used for fever control. Be careful about the dosage. Many of us are rather nonchalant about aspirin because it is available without a prescription. But it is a potent drug; had it been discovered today, it would probably be available only by prescription. The aspirin bottle gives "suggested dosage," but your doctor considers your child's age, weight, and general condition when deciding how much and how often aspirin should be given to your child. Follow your doctor's recommendations and *don't think that more is better.* If your child is very sick and running a high fever, you have to be careful about how much aspirin you give, especially if your child's fluid intake is low. If your child is very sick and unresponsive, you may have trouble knowing if the unresponsiveness is the result of the illness or the effect of all the medication taken. So if you give aspirin, keep a record and write down how much your child gets and when. Since one out of five childhood poisonings is caused by aspirin, be careful to keep even baby aspirin out of the reach of children at all times.

Give sufficient liquids to prevent your child from becoming dehydrated. Determine with your doctor how much liquid your child should drink per day. Then keep careful track of your child's actual liquid consumption. With nursing babies you can monitor this by wet diapers, with older children by keeping track of how much liquid they drink and also, if appropriate, how often they urinate. Children can dehydrate very quickly, and this can be serious. (See page 28 for symptoms of dehydration.) If you aren't getting enough liquid into your child in the way he or she usually consumes it—breast, bottle, cup—see pages 163 and 167–168 for alternative methods of giving liquids and discuss with your doctor how you should proceed.

Establish a rest time. This doesn't mean you should just put your child away in the bedroom. Usually, quiet play around the house or yard is fine—just try to prevent overexertion.

It is hard to draw an arbitrary line on the basis that x amount of illness warrants y minutes of nap or rest time. It is much easier just to have a nap or quiet time every day, even when your child is healthy. You and your child need time to get out of each other's hair and relax anyway.

Vomiting

Vomiting can occur in connection with a wide variety of conditions, ranging from a cold to appendicitis to accidental poisoning. Although a very serious condition may be quite unlikely, you should monitor any vomiting carefully.

The type of vomiting can sometimes tell you and your doctor something about your child's condition. Is your child just regurgitating a little, vomiting small amounts calmly, vomiting frequently, vomiting in response to coughing up and then choking on mucus, or is there projectile vomiting? What are the contents—undigested food, bile, or bloody matter? Does your child have any other symptoms, such as fever, stomach cramps, sleepiness?

Although vomiting is common, you should discuss with your doctor what to do in case your child vomits. Obviously, your child's condition or treatment may also cause vomiting. For example, your doctor might tell you to expect vomiting after chemotherapy. But even if you have discussed your child's vomiting with your doctor, if it continues for a long time or your child complains, gets exhausted, or acts differently than usual, you should call your doctor.

While most children vomit with ease and have no problems, vomiting can be a real hazard for those few children with neurological problems that make aspiration (taking of vomitus into the lungs) likely, or for children who are sedated and not functioning normally. Therefore learn if your child has a condition with which vomiting is a potential emergency and discuss with your doctor now what you should do if your child ever even feels nauseated. (Obviously, if your child is too young or unable to speak, you will have to intuit this.) If your child might aspirate, see pages 66–68 for important information.

Discuss with your doctor whether you should take any of the following steps if your child feels nauseated.

- Position your child properly (fig. 4-1). Have your child lie on his or her side on a wedge-shaped pillow head down at the edge of the bed or table. If you don't have a pillow, quickly put anything at hand (books, bricks, wood) under one end of the bed or table so your child will be lying head down.
- Give your child antinausea medication if it has been prescribed. Distract your child if possible while the medication is working. (Try reading or television.)
- Call your doctor.
- Be sure your child's head is down and turned to one side to prevent aspiration if your child starts to vomit. If you don't have time to get a pot for your child to vomit into or to cover the floor with newspapers, don't worry about the mess. You can always clean it up afterward.

If vomiting is imminent and you have learned how to do postural drainage (see pages 64–66), your child is less apt to aspirate if he or she is not just tilted but hanging upside down. However, do not try to move your child once he or she starts to vomit, since your child may easily aspirate. So if your child has started to vomit, just keep the head down with the face turned to one side.

- Call for help if your child does aspirate. A child who turns blue or has trouble breathing after vomiting has probably aspirated. *Call your doctor or paramedics immediately.*
- Prevent dehydration. This is a more common problem than aspiration with most children. Therefore, if vomiting continues, call your doctor and ask how you should replace the fluids your child is losing. If you are told to feed your child, discuss with your

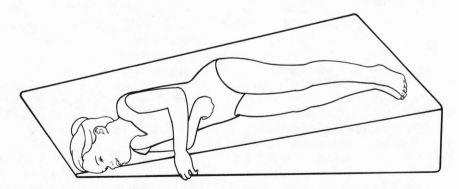

Figure 4-1   Positioning child on wedge-shaped pillow for nausea.

doctor exactly how this should be done. Generally, you should let the stomach rest a bit and then begin with only very small amounts of clear liquid. If you try to put in too much too fast, your child may well begin vomiting all over again.

If you are unable to give sufficient fluids by mouth, ask your doctor for alternative ways of giving fluids. (See page 28 for symptoms of dehydration.)

Diarrhea

Diarrhea can also be associated with a variety of conditions or circumstances, from gastroenteritis (stomach flu) to the medication your child is taking. (Antiobiotics, by killing some of the bacteria normally found throughout the body, can cause diarrhea.) If your child has diarrhea, try to figure out why and, after briefly organizing your thoughts, call your doctor. Don't give your child over-the-counter preparations used by adults to control diarrhea, for these may not be safe or effective. And medication can mask symptoms, making it more difficult for your doctor to see what is really wrong. Dehydration is a hazard of diarrhea as well as vomiting. Read pages 28, 32, and 33–34 for symptoms and prevention of dehydration.

Diet for Vomiting and Diarrhea

Diet is important if your child is vomiting or has diarrhea, for if you feed your child too much of the wrong thing too quickly your child won't get better and may get worse. Discuss with your doctor what you should do. Usually you begin with small feedings of clear liquid. Small is more important with vomiting and small really means that: perhaps only a teaspoon at a time every ten minutes, slowly working up to a tablespoon. Clear juices such as apple juice often work better than water. Some children prefer soft drinks or Kool-Aid. Iced fruit bars or popsicles may also be effective. Then you can gradually add clear gelatin desserts. When your child tolerates this, you can move to easily digestible foods. In the case of diarrhea these should also be constipating, like the "brat" diet: b=bananas, r=rice, a=applesauce, t=toast. Milk and fat are often hard to digest, but yogurt is sometimes tolerated and the

acidpholis bacteria in yogurt may be helpful. (Your child must consume natural yogurt; the sweetened, flavored kinds are often pasteurized, which kills the acidpholis bacteria.)

Try to get your child back onto a normal diet as quickly as your doctor thinks it is appropriate; for example chronic diarrhea can result from maintaining your child on large amounts of apple juice. Fiber is important to reduce the amount of water passed in bowel movements, and the "brat" diet does not contain much fiber.

Common Contagious Childhood Illnesses

The common contagious childhood illnesses are mumps, measles, rubella (German measles), roseola, and chicken pox. Your child should be immunized against mumps, measles, and rubella, unless your doctor feels your child might not be able to tolerate immunization or unless you object to it on religious grounds.

Usually, there are no complications with common childhood diseases. However, a child whose immune system is not functioning normally because of his or her disorder or because of medication can become seriously ill with one of the common diseases. Also, contagious childhood illnesses may get more severe the older your child gets and can cause complications in a teenager or an adult. Therefore, if your child has a normal life expectancy, decide with your doctor whether you should intentionally expose your child to these diseases by a certain age.

Seizures

Your child will probably never have a seizure unless he or she is among the 5 percent of children between the ages of one and four who have febrile seizures when they run a high temperature, or unless he or she has a central-nervous-system disorder such as epilepsy. Although a seizure may look very frightening, it is usually not dangerous or life-threatening and will usually stop in a few minutes, whether any treatment is given or not.

A seizure occurs when the electrical impulses that the brain normally gives off are massively increased and disorganized, causing abnormal brain function. It can happen spontaneously or can be triggered by fever, poison, infections (meningitis), or even by a breath-holding spell.

Seizures can vary in severity, but you will probably recognize one if it happens. Some children become stiff and roll their heads backward; others rhythmically jerk their arms and legs; some have staring spells and suddenly collapse.

If your child has a seizure, try to stay calm. Don't be alarmed if your child's breathing seems momentarily irregular or seems briefly to stop.

If your child should have a seizure, take the following steps:

- Don't try to restrain or revive your child.
- Don't move your child unless the area is clearly dangerous, like the middle of a busy street or in the bath tub.
- Remove hazards such as hard, sharp, or hot objects that could cause injury if your child falls or knocks against them.
- Loosen tight clothing and glasses, if your child wears them.
- Put something soft under your child's head.
- Help keep your child's airway open by gently turning your child onto his or her side, so any fluid in the mouth can drain safely. If your child vomits, clear the mouth after the seizure ends. Never try to force your child's mouth open and jam in an object, for this can do more harm than good.
- If your child has a fever, when the convulsion ends begin with fever-lowering procedures outlined on pages 31–32.
- Be calm and reassuring. When your child starts to regain consciousness, he or she may not know what has happened, may feel disoriented, or may be embarrassed. A child will do much better if confronted with smiling faces rather than worried, panic-stricken ones. If your child seems confused or sleepy, let him or her rest.

Try to observe what happens during your child's seizure and how long it lasts so you can report this to your doctor.

If your child has not had a seizure before, call your doctor and discuss the situation with him or her. If your child has recurrent seizures due to epilepsy or some other central-nervous-system disorder, plan with your doctor how to proceed. Probably you won't have to call your doctor unless your child has one attack after another without regaining consciousness or if the seizure lasts longer than ten minutes. In such a case your child may need medical attention.

If your child has a seizure for the first time, your doctor will try to determine its cause through a thorough medical examination and perhaps other testing. You may want your doctor to prescribe medication so your child never has a seizure again. If your doctor feels it was a febrile seizure and doesn't think your child will have one again, he or she may not feel that medication should be taken daily to prevent something that may never happen again. You may have to make the choice of whether you can handle the occasional seizure or whether the thought of another seizure is such a source of anxiety that you'd rather have your child take a drug like phenobarbital daily.

If your child has recurring seizures, you can assure your child (and your family and friends) that he or she is in good company with such people as Julius Caesar, Alexander the Great, and Napoleon. It is important to be honest and let your child's friends and teachers know that your child may have a seizure. Then they won't be surprised if one does occur and will know how to help.

Pain

Children often cope with pain differently than adults. Whereas adults often withdraw and go to bed, many children cope with pain by keeping themselves busy, even to the point of appearing hyperactive. However, children may also become sad, depressed, and withdrawn. Sometimes this is the only way a child can react to the pain. Particularly when the onset of pain is gradual and then the pain continues, a child may not know how badly it hurts or if anything can be done about it.

You can probably get your son or daughter to tell you how and where it hurts. Your child may not explain this as adults do, who can use over 160 words in the English language to communicate pain. But you can learn from your child if you listen. Sam once said, "My leg feels like a lemon." Upon further questioning, he explained he meant it hurt like when he had sucked on a lemon drop, keeping it in one spot against the inside of his cheek for too long. You will, of course, have to be even more intuitive with a younger or nonverbal child.

If you are trying to determine where the pain is, have your child point to that place on his or her own body or on a doll. Or draw an outline of your child's body and ask him or her to color in where it hurts. Or you can get more complex by asking your child to choose four colors and then indicate in different colors where it doesn't hurt at all, where it hurts a little, where it hurts quite a bit, and where it hurts a lot. This will, of course, give you much more specific information. If you keep the drawing and then have your child color in another figure when needed, you may see trends as to where and how great the pain is. But since pain radiates, the site of the discomfort may not always be the site of the problem.

How much pain a child feels can be influenced by his or her emotional state. A child who feels scared, lonely, abandoned, or depressed will feel more pain than one who is happy and playing with friends and loved ones. Also, a child may feel more pain at night when he or she is tired and there is less distraction than during the day.

Drugs of varying strength can be prescribed for pain. If your child is in acute pain, strong narcotic painkillers may be appropriate. With your doctor, measure the possible complications of a strong drug against the emotional trauma of a child who is in great pain due to surgery or terminal illness. Unrelieved pain may also sometimes make physiological problems worse. If, for example, a child is unwilling to breath deeply after surgery because of pain, respiratory complications are more apt to occur.

It is unfair to tell a child who complains of pain that it doesn't really hurt. If you sense that your child is complaining of pain just to get attention, it is more important to recognize and meet your child's needs for attention than to say that nothing hurts or to reprimand your child for lying. If your child is actually experiencing pain, you may lose your credibility by trying to talk him or her out of it. It is often best to admit that pain may exist, take any appropriate measures to relieve it, and then try to draw your child's attention to something else.

If your child has a condition causing chronic pain, you may want to discuss with your doctor methods of pain control utilizing mental and physical exercises rather than drugs.

HOME MEDICAL RECORDS

A written daily record of your child's medical condition, to which you and your doctor can refer, is useful.

Use notebooks, so you can keep all the information together for present and future reference. What you include depends upon your child's specific problem, but you should consider including some or all of the following information on each page:

- Your child's name.
- The date: Include the year, for if your child needs long-term care, this will be helpful for future reference.
- Day of the week: If you make a mistake in writing down the correct date, you can double-check by looking at the day of the week. The day of the week can also help remind you if you have any special obligations that day.
- Doctor's orders: Be sure to write in any instructions the doctor gives you. If the doctor makes a house call, have him or her write on the chart specifically what needs to be done.
- Medications: Make a complete list of medications, including the dosage, how often the medication is to be given, and any special instructions. Then leave space to fill in the actual times given.
- Therapy treatments: List these along with any special remarks you may have.
- Evaluation of condition: Your observations may relate to your child's specific medical complaints; however, you may also want to include general notes about how your child slept, ate, played, and so on. If you find there are specific factors you want to make notes about daily, you can include these as separate headings on your sheet.
- Liquid intake, urination, bowel movement, temperature, pulse, and respiration are items you may want to include, depending on your child's condition. Of course, use your common sense here, since measuring urine output and pulse daily, for example, may not be appropriate if your child is healthy but very important during severe illness.

Your daily care chart might look like that in figure 4-2.

DAILY CARE CHART

For _____   Date _____

Day Month Year (Day of week)

MEDICATION	DOSAGE	TIMES	EFFECTS

TREATMENT:

EVALUATION OF CONDITION:

Liquid intake (volume in ounces) _____
Urination (volume in ounces) _____
Bowel movement (consistency) _____
Temperature _____
Pulse _____
Respiration _____

DOCTOR'S ORDERS:

Figure 4-2   Daily care chart.

An hourly chart like that in figure 4-3 is useful if your child is very sick and you need more detailed information.

Begin by carefully planning one chart and having seven to ten copies photocopied so you can try them out. After using your chart for a few days, you will see what changes you want to make before photocopying enough sheets to last a month or more.

A medication history chart is valuable if you want to consolidate this information into a single chart. A medication history chart might look like that in figure 4-4.

A medical portfolio containing a record of your child's diagnoses and treatment is very im-portant to have with you whenever you travel or change doctors. If a new doctor has to treat your child, you can provide the background informa-tion the doctor needs. Discuss making such a portfolio with your doctor, as it is not difficult for him or her to photocopy the relevant informa-tion for you.

MEDICAL ALERT BRACELETS

A medical alert bracelet, which your child can wear all the time, can be very helpful if your child has a medical condition that cannot be eas-ily seen, such as diabetes, severe allergies, or epilepsy. If you buy such a bracelet (or necklace) through an international foundation such as Medic Alert Foundation (P.O. Box 1109, Tur-

HOURLY CARE CHART

For _____ Date _____

Day Month Year (Day of week)

	TEMP.	PULSE	BLOOD PRESS.	MEDICATION (DRUG & DOSAGE)	FOOD (% OF NORMAL)	URINE VOL.	BM (CONSIS-TENCY)	OTHER TREATMENTS	HOW IS CHILD DOING?
Midnight									
1									
2									
3									
4									
5									
6									
7									
8									
9									
10									
11									
Noon									
1									
2									
3									
4									
5									
6									
7									
8									
9									
10									
11									

Figure 4-3 Hourly care chart.

DRUG	DATE STARTED	DATE STOPPED	DOSAGE	COMMENTS
Erythomycin	9/3/84	9/26/84	5cc 4× per day	Bronchitis cleared up, but diarrhea for a week

Figure 4-4   Medication history chart.

lock, CA 95381), it will inscribe your child's medical problem, file number, and the telephone number of the foundation so the person aiding your child can immediately get vital information, such as the address and phone number of you or your doctor.

If your child has no medical problem that may need emergency attention but is nonverbal, it's a good idea to get a bracelet engraved with your child's name, address, and phone number, so if he or she wanders off the person finding your child can locate you.

EMERGENCIES

It is important to be as prepared for emergencies as possible. If you can recognize emergencies and have thought through what you should do, you will be better able to handle them.

What Is an Emergency?

There are three conditions which are always emergencies, for which you must act immediately:

Breathing difficulty can be caused by a blocked airway, blocked lungs, or by nervous-system failure. Since the brain suffers damage if it is deprived of oxygen for more than four minutes, you should know how to help your child immediately yourself, even if you also call for help.

A *blocked airway* can be caused by an object, food, or secretions. Check with your doctor as to how you should proceed should this occur with your child.

If you suspect your infant is choking on an object, look in, but never poke your finger deeply into the mouth, for you can easily push the object in even farther. With an older child, carefully check with your finger.

Children who have great difficulty swallowing often choke on food or their own secretions. If your child has this problem, make sure you can always quickly pick up your child and hang him or her upside down over your knee: gravity will probably help whatever your child is choking on to come out. This is more fully described in Chapter 6 in the discussion of postural drainage (see pages 64–66). If you need to do this frequently you will probably learn to do it while standing, propping up one leg if possible so your child can hang over it. Such positioning isn't optimal but may be necessary. Needless to say, a child who chokes frequently should only be left in the care of a person who knows how to get the child breathing again and feels confident in being able to handle the emergency.

Blocked lungs cannot be quickly unblocked. However, if you suspect aspiration, begin postural drainage and suction in that position (see pages 66–68).

Nervous-system failure requires immediate attention. If you have tried to clear the airway and your child is still not breathing, then you must breathe for your child, using mouth-to-mouth breathing. If, in addition, your child's heart is not beating, you must do total cardiopulmonary resuscitation (CPR).

CPR classes are available at minimal cost in most communities. Since you actually practice the procedures in class, often on dummies, you become much more skilled than you would from just reading about how to do CPR in a book. CPR classes are especially valuable for parents of children who may need such emergency treatment.

Disorientation is the second emergency situation. This can be caused by diminished oxygen due to breathing difficulty, by shock, fever, and illness, or drug side effects or overdose. Since disorientation is a sign that something is wrong and could be getting worse, contact your doctor immediately.

Limpness of your child's body is an emergency situation that can be caused by unconsciousness, dehydration, or severe illness. If your child becomes limp, something is wrong. Get help.

Discuss with your doctor what to do if any of these three situations occurs. In addition, there may be emergencies related to your child's specific disorder. Find out from your doctor what these might be and what you should do if they occur. It is important to think through with your doctor what should be done in an emergency. He or she may wish to teach you any necessary emergency procedures; may give you written materials to study; or may suggest you take a course, such as a CPR class. Some situations you have to learn to treat (at least initially) at home; in other instances going to the hospital might be more appropriate.

With a terminally ill child, what looks like an emergency may be a signal of the beginning of the end. In that case, it may be appropriate just to do your best at home. This is fully discussed in Chapter 18.

Learn When and Whom You Should Call for Help

Determine with your doctor at what point you will need help and whom you should call. There are a few options as to whom to call.

Your doctor may want to be contacted in an emergency. Ask what to do if an emergency happens at night or when the doctor is not on call. Should you call the answering service or call him or her at home? If the doctor's partners are to take over, make sure they know of your child's condition.

The paramedics or ambulance service (or the fire department in some communities) are equipped to handle certain emergencies. Discuss with your doctor whom you should contact in case of need.

The emergency room at the hospital might be the place to take your child. Discuss with your doctor not only which situations might warrant emergency-room treatment but also to which

hospital you should take your child. One hospital in your community might be better equipped to handle the type of emergency your child may experience than another. Make sure you know the way there and what to do when you arrive. Also consider how you should get your child to the hospital. Should you call an ambulance, drive yourself, have a friend drive you, or call a taxi?

Friends or neighbors may also be willing to be on call and come over if you don't think you can manage alone in an emergency.

Decide whether to live close to the services you need. If you are often in dire need, it may be reasonable or necessary to move closer to the doctor and hospital so you can quickly get help if needed.

Keep emergency information posted on or by the phone. Put a list of important information on the wall or tape it directly to your phone, if it will fit. Such a list should not only be clear enough for yourself but also for anyone else who might be watching your child. Relevant information might include names and phone numbers of people to contact (with alternates listed if necessary), what procedures should be started immediately at home, and, briefly, how to do them.

After you write out this information, you might want to go over it with your doctor, to make sure it is clear and complete. When you go out, leave a number where you can be reached.

The sicker or more disabled your child is, the more apt you are to have emergencies. But this should not deter you from caring for your child at home. When you question your ability to care for your child at home, you are questioning whether your child would be better off at home or in a hospital or institution. Strictly from the standpoint of medical expertise you might feel that a professional could provide better "technical" medical care; but if you think of your whole child, with his or her physical, mental, emotional, and spiritual needs, you will likely feel that you as a parent can provide better "soul" care. The quality of your child's life at home, with the love and comfort you provide, probably outweighs the value of trying to prevent emergencies by having your child hospitalized or institutionalized.

5
Medication

Giving medication is both a science and an art. It is a science in that we understand a great deal about how medications act upon the body; it is an art in that even for the most knowledgeable physician there are constant surprises as to how medications actually work, so a physician must use both intuition and common sense. To doctors medications are commonly known as drugs, for technically a drug is any substance used as a medicine. Therefore in this chapter we shall speak of medications as drugs. We do not mean by drugs what are commonly termed "street drugs." Here a drug is any substance used to treat disease or injury.

Your doctor combines knowledge of medication with trust in your ability to carry out his or her instructions and to observe carefully the effects. You must combine your faith in your doctor's medical expertise and your ability to learn about medication with your understanding of your child, so you can accurately report to the doctor how the medication affects your child. Your pharmacist, who not only dispenses medication but also has been educated in the chemical composition and effects of drugs, may also be helpful.

In our society we often think every illness should be treated with a drug. Yet while drugs can sometimes be helpful, sometimes giving medication is the wrong thing to do. Therefore, before choosing a drug, your doctor has to decide if drug therapy is indicated. If your doctor decides against medication, accept the decision and don't push. Drugs alone do not cure disease. Rather they help the body help itself. Medication can be applied locally, as with eye, ear, or nose drops, skin creams, and ointments; it can be inhaled, as in the treatment of respiratory disorders or for general anesthesia; it can be given rectally in suppository form either for treatment of local conditions (such as hemorrhoids) or to treat systemic conditions (such as asthma); and it can be injected into the vein (intravenously), into the muscle (intramuscularly), or just beneath the skin (subcutaneously). The most common form of administration is oral.

Drugs can be very potent. The correct dosage of the active ingredient in a drug can be as little as one millionth of a gram, too minute a quantity to be given alone. So although drugs are prescribed by their active ingredient, what the pharmacist gives you consists not only of the drug but fillers, dyes, flavoring, and other additives. In certain circumstances, such as allergies, the type of additives used may be very important.

Liquid medications contain the active chemical(s) in a liquid called a suspending agent, designed to keep the concentration consistent throughout the mixture. Since some chemicals will separate from the suspending agent, it is very important to shake liquid drugs thoroughly before use; otherwise, the concentration of the drug in the delivered dose can steadily increase as you get closer to the bottom of the bottle.

Should You Buy Generic or Brand-Name Medication?

The generic name of a drug describes the kind of drug, let us say aspirin. The brand name is the trademark, for instance, Bayer. You may have bought plain-wrapper, generic items in the supermarket. If so, you probably found that for some items there was little difference between the generic and the brand-name product, while for others the brand-name product was definitely preferable. Obviously the manufacturer of the generic product is able to sell the product less expensively by cutting out advertising costs, by using less expensive packaging, less expensive ingredients, and less expensive manufacturing procedures. In some cases this affects the quality of the product significantly and in others it doesn't. A pharmaceutical manufacturer makes the same types of decisions, which may affect the quality or the price of the drug.

As with supermarket items, the difference between a generic and a brand-name drug may sometimes be insignificant and at other times substantial. If you buy generics, you are trusting your pharmacist to give you a sufficiently effective drug. When your doctor writes a prescription, ask him whether the generic drug would be as effective as the brand-name drug, and follow his or her advice.

How Do Drugs Act?

Genetics, or your child's own physical makeup, will affect the way the drug acts. Individuals vary as much in their reactions to medication as they do in appearance. You can see this, for example, in the different ways people react to the mild drug caffeine.

Furthermore, not only do people react differently to the same drug but a single individual may have a variety of reactions to the same drug. Food in the stomach, heavy exertion, extreme heat or cold, exposure to sunlight, as well as our physical, mental, and emotional condition, can all influence the way we react to a given drug. Therefore it is important to follow any instructions your doctor gives you as to whether to take a drug before or after meals, etc.

The intended effect of a drug is the change you want to occur within the body. This sometimes occurs only in the presence of disease or another abnormality. For example, aspirin may reduce a high temperature, but it will not lower a normal one.

Side effects can occur with any drug. The more potent the drug, the greater the risk. Reading the manufacturer's literature about the possible adverse reactions of a drug your child is taking can be frightening, for manufacturers usually list everything they can think of that might happen. This is more to cover themselves legally than to present a realistic picture. It is important to remember that all those things don't happen to every patient. While it is sensible to have your doctor and pharmacist tell you of the possible side effects to watch for so appropriate steps can be taken if they do occur, remember that your doctor wouldn't have prescribed the drug unless he or she was quite sure it would help your child.

If your child starts taking a new drug, you may think that any new symptom is a side effect. But it may not be. Any assumed drug reaction must be carefully evaluated, since it can be serious if a doctor decides, because of a misinterpretation of events, that an important and valuable drug has to be avoided.

Predictable avoidable side effects may occur. For example, three similar drugs, chemical cousins you might say, which can be used to prevent motion sickness—Dramamine (dimenhydrinate), Marezine (cyclizine), and Bonine (meclizine)—are all apt to cause drowsiness. Since Dramamine is the *most* apt to do so, if you want your child to stay alert you would use Marezine or Bonine. Bonine is effective for much longer than Marezine, but it is not recommended for children under 12. So if your child is under 12 you would use Marezine. In this case, because a variety of drugs is available to prevent motion sickness, you can give your child the drug that is least apt to have the predictable side effect of drowsiness.

Treatable side effects may be unavoidable if you can find no medication without side effects. For example, some broad-spectrum antibiotics kill off the helpful as well as the harmful bacteria in the intestinal system, altering what is called the "intestinal flora." When this change occurs, the patient is apt to experience diarrhea, which is usually treatable.

Unpreventable untreatable side effects can sometimes be anticipated. For example, chemotherapy is very apt to cause a person's hair to fall out, yet most people are willing to take chemotherapy anyway with the hope of overcoming their cancer.

Some strong drugs are known to cause severe adverse reactions. With some experimental drugs, safe and therapeutic dosages and possible side effects have not been clearly established. If the use of medication such as "phase II" drugs for the aggressive treatment of cancer is recommended, you must decide whether the side effects are worth the possible remission or cure.

Long-term side effects are those that do not appear until after the drug has been used for some time or even after the drug has been discontinued. Drugs are tested for safety before they are put on the market, but until the side effects of a new drug become better known a doctor may favor an older drug over the new one.

Drug interactions can occur when two or more drugs are taken together. There is always the possibility that such an interaction can cause an increased, decreased, or entirely new effect from what would occur if each drug were taken separately.

This is why, before prescribing a new drug, your doctor will consider what drugs your child is presently taking. If your doctor does not ask you what your child is taking now, politely review with him or her your child's prescription and nonprescription drugs, vitamin and mineral supplements, and any unusual dietary habits before accepting a new prescription. It is crucial to review this information.

Also, ask your pharmacist to double-check for drug interactions before filling any prescription. If you buy from only one pharmacy, which keeps records for each client, your pharmacist should make such a check without your even requesting it.

Allergic reactions are not rare, especially if someone has hay fever or other allergies. Most allergic reactions to drugs take the form of a rash, hives, itching, localized swelling, wheezing, or difficulty breathing. A severe allergic reaction can cause anaphylactic shock, which is quite dangerous. This is most apt to occur with injectable medication. Therefore, your doctor may inject new medication and have you wait for 15–30 minutes in the waiting room to make sure no anaphylactic reaction occurs, for this would have to be treated immediately. Once your doctor knows that your child will tolerate a medication, he or she may want you to give any further injections at home.

Especially in the case of mild drug reactions, it may be difficult to distinguish an allergic reaction from a side effect. If you suspect your child might be having an allergic reaction to a drug, discuss this with your doctor.

Many allergic reactions are temporary, self-limiting, and don't necessarily occur every time the drug is taken. Thus sometimes the benefits of a drug outweigh the disadvantages of taking it.

If your doctor determines that your child has had a serious allergic reaction, also tell your pharmacist, who should note this information on your child's prescription record. If you know from past experience that your child is allergic to certain drugs, be sure to remind your doctor of this whenever he or she prescribes new medication.

Drug addiction, either physical or emotional, can occur even with children, especially if they are taking tranquilizers, sedatives, or analgesics (painkillers). If you think this is a potential problem, discuss it with your doctor. However, drugs affect children differently than adults. For example, phenobarbital in normal doses can be taken for extended periods by children with no indication that it will cause later addiction.

Emotional side effects are not uncommon. It is, of course, difficult, if not impossible, to decide whether changes in mood are determined by your child's physical illness, mental state, or the medication. But a drug may cause extreme sensitivity, nervousness, irritability, or other mood changes. If your child needs the drug you will learn that at such times you just have to handle your child with kid gloves.

What Should You Do If You Suspect Accidental Drug Poisoning?

If you suspect that any of your children has eaten medication (or any other poisonous substance), call your doctor, hospital emergency room, or poison-control center right away to find out what you should do. If your child is having trouble breathing or is unconscious, you will need help immediately and must proceed as your doctor has recommended for emergencies (see pages 39–40). However, if your child is still acting normally, your doctor may want you to take steps at home either to neutralize the medication in the stomach or to induce vomiting. Be sure you know which of these you should do, for the course of action will be determined by the chemical composition of the drug your child has taken.

Never assume that you should do nothing, since the effects of some poisons may not even begin to show up for two or three days, at which point it may be too late to do anything at all.

In most drug poisonings, your doctor will want you to induce vomiting to get the medication out of your child's stomach. Always have a supply of Ipecac Syrup on hand to induce vomiting. Keep twice as much on hand as recommended: if a wriggly uncooperative child spits out the first spoonful, you will have enough for a second dose. Your doctor may also want you to have activated charcoal on hand, which can be given after vomiting to neutralize any residual poison left in the stomach. However, particularly with infants, do not give anything (including Ipecac) without calling your doctor first.

Why Is the Correct Dosage So Important?

Your doctor determines the dosage, or how much of the drug your child should take, on the basis of your child's age, weight, and general condition. Accuracy is of the essence. Consider, for example, that a tiny amount of a tranquilizer might make you a bit groggy, a medium dose could put you to sleep, a large dose could make you unconscious, and an overdose could kill you. *Follow your doctor's instructions carefully.* Never think if a little helps, more will help more. It won't, and may even cause bad side effects.

The frequency of the dosage must be carefully planned so the desired amount of the drug remains in the bloodstream at all times. Sometimes one large "loading dose" is given (often in the form of an injection), followed by smaller maintenance doses so a sufficient amount of the drug is available for effective medical treatment 24 hours a day.

In figure 5-1, curve *b* shows how, ideally, the drug in the bloodstream remains at a therapeutic level at all times. If the medication is given too frequently, or if the body does not eliminate the drug as fast as anticipated, the level of the drug in the blood can rise, causing drug toxicity, as seen in curve *a*. This can be very serious and is sometimes hard to distinguish from the symptoms of the illness itself. Most drugs in common use have wide safety margins.

If the maintenance doses are not given often enough or are too small, the amount of the drug in the blood falls to an ineffective level, as shown in curve *c*. While you should give your child his or her medication regularly, if for some reason you miss a dose, consult with your doctor as to whether it would be better to increase the next dose or just to give the prescribed amount.

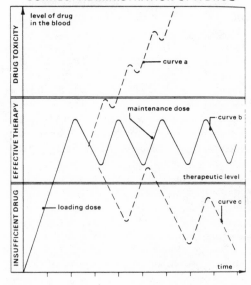

Figure 5-1   Correct administration of a drug.

The length of time that your child takes a drug is also carefully planned. The drug must be taken long enough to have the desired effect yet no longer than necessary. Through learning and experience, your doctor will know how long your child should take the medication or at what point you should report to your doctor so he or she can determine whether to continue the medication. One frequent error parents make is not giving medication for the entire prescribed period. They think that once the visible signs of illness start to disappear the child is healthy. But this is not always the case. For example, if your child is taking antibiotics for a respiratory infection and feels better after several days, there may still be microorganisms in the lungs that have been subdued by the drug treatment but not yet killed. If you stop the medication, they will flourish and your child will become ill again. But these microorganisms have built up resistance to the drug, so when your child is sick again it will not be as effective.

Follow your doctor's instructions carefully. Strict adherence to the prescribed dosage schedule is especially important with drugs that are very potent and consequently have very narrow margins of safety.

YOUR PHARMACIST

Your pharmacist can be a crucial member of your health-care team. Your pharmacist knows about the chemical composition of the drugs and how they theoretically work. Choose your pharmacist with care. Some items to consider might be:

Is the pharmacist willing to work with you? Although your doctor can tell you everything you need to know about drugs, it is good to have another person to help give you the medication education you need. Your pharmacist is often more accessible by phone than the doctor and, if you want to know something, you can call and ask. If you have a long question, say so and ask if the pharmacist has time now or would rather call you back. This kind of simple courtesy will help you develop a good relationship with the pharmacist. Your pharmacist can not only answer questions about how drugs work but can also answer questions like "Does this drug come in butterscotch flavor?"

Does the pharmacist carry the drugs your child may need? Most pharmacies carry commonly used drugs, but severely ill children may need special items that only a few pharmacies carry. Generally, a pharmacy that concentrates on medications carries a larger line of drugs and is more informed about them than a corner drug store, which also has a soda fountain and sells cosmetics, candy, and so on.

Does the pharmacist keep patient records? While all pharmacies must keep a record of prescriptions they fill by prescription number, you want a pharmacy that has a patient record in which all prescriptions filled for that individual are recorded. Your pharmacist can then keep track of the medication your child is taking, and watch with your doctor for correct dosages and possible drug interactions. Buy from one pharmacy only, so your child's record is complete.

Will the pharmacist set up a charge account for you? A charge account simplifies your finances because you have to pay only once a month and you get a written record of your purchases, which helps you keep your accounting for your insurance and the IRS straight.

Does the pharmacy deliver? If your child is very ill, or might become very ill, a delivery service is more than a convenience. It is a necessity.

How Do You Best Work with Your Pharmacist?

To develop a good working relationship with your pharmacist, in addition to common telephone courtesy mentioned above, you should understand how a pharmacy works. When the pharmacist receives an order, he or she checks your record, fills the prescription, and has it delivered as soon as possible. Anything you can do to facilitate this process helps. So consider the following:

Call early in the day. If you need something by evening, don't call at five minutes to five. Place your order as soon as you know you need something, so the pharmacist can fill your prescription when there is time between the clients who come into the store and wait until their prescriptions are ready. If your pharmacist has an answering machine, you can even place your order in the evening or early morning before the store opens.

Place fewer but larger orders. Try to order enough of the medication and supplies to last a reasonable length of time. (Many medications are cheaper in larger amounts.) Check your total supplies before calling, so you can put in a complete order that can be filled at one time. Even if a pharmacy delivers, you really shouldn't expect more deliveries than necessary.

Keep extras of regularly used items on hand, if they have a sufficiently long shelf life. This not only saves you the worry of running out of something, it also saves your pharmacist the extra trip to your home five minutes before closing time.

WHAT YOU NEED TO KNOW AND DO WHEN YOU GET YOUR CHILD'S MEDICATION

Know the name of the drug. If you know the name of the drug, you can check to make sure the pharmacist has delivered the right drug, and can also find out more about the medication if you so desire.

Know why the drug is prescribed and what are its anticipated benefits. If you know this, you can tell your doctor if the drug is working or not.

Know how your child should take the drug. Make sure you know how much medication your child should take, when he or she should take it, and whether he or she should or should not eat or drink anything at the same time.

Know of any possible side effects. There probably won't be any, but since there may be, it's better if you can recognize them in their early stages.

Know of any possible drug interactions. As we've said before, make sure your doctor and

pharmacist both know all the medications your child is taking and warn you of any possible interactions.

Check the expiration date on the bottle. All medications have this on the label. Occasionally your bottle may be past the expiration date. Check with your pharmacist to see if this was an oversight or intentional. Many medications are perfectly good for some time beyond their expiration date, but only your pharmacist knows for sure.

Write important information down. The prescription label will give you some information. However, if you need more than the name of the drug and how often to take it, ask your doctor to write down the information you need. Or write it down yourself and have your doctor check what you have written. Don't rely on your memory. Whereas verbal instructions can be forgotten or muddled, accurate written ones can be referred to in the future.

Keep the medication clearly labeled in the original container, for you never know when someone else may have to administer it. If your doctor has adjusted the dosage of the medication in phone consultation, note that on the label. If you need only a small amount of the medication for a trip, ask your pharmacist to make up a small amount of the medication or ask him or her to label some smaller bottles for you so together you can *carefully* transfer some medication. In an emergency, the less confusion regarding medications the better. An envelope with assorted colored pills can be a disaster in an emergency room. Sending your child off alone on a trip or to camp with inadequately labeled bottles or envelopes containing pills is, of course, equally foolhardy.

Check for any special storage instructions. Proper storage of medication is crucial to the drug's effectiveness. Drugs are often unstable and can be affected by moisture, heat, cold, or sunlight. For example, some liquid antibiotics will be effective for two weeks if stored in the refrigerator, for three days if kept at room temperature, and even less if left in the sunlight.

Your pharmacist should tell you where and how long a drug can be stored until it is no longer effective.

You must find a safe place for storage. A child-resistant cap should be your first security measure. If the medication should be refrigerated, keep it near the back, out of reach of little hands. High kitchen cabinets are usually less accessible (and also cooler and dryer) than your bathroom medicine cabinet. If you have to store something really potent or poisonous, make it impossible for children to reach, perhaps in a place to which even you have difficulty getting. It does, of course, help to explain to your children that medication is not candy and is never to be taken without your supervision. But you can't rely on your child's good judgment: keep temptation away by storing medications out of reach. If you are really worried that your child will get into the medication, get a drug safe designed to keep drugs away from children.

GIVING MEDICATION AT HOME

Take great care when you give your child medication. Give medication in a matter-of-fact way, as if it never occurred to you that your child wouldn't take it. If you apologize, rationalize, or even act a bit unsure of yourself, your child may figure it is worth a try to fight or to spit or to do most anything else to avoid consuming the stuff. While older children should need no cajoling, threats, or bribery (taking medication may be nasty, but it is a fact of life), younger children, with whom you can't reason so effectively, may require a bit of ingenuity.

Never lie about the taste. Your child has to trust you, and you must never risk betraying that trust by lying. You can try to mask the taste by mixing it with food. Your child still might not like it very much, but might be willing to eat it. Try applesauce or ice cream, but *use only a little.* If you mix up a whole cup of ice cream, your child may not be willing to eat that much, especially if it tastes strong. If you mix medication in small amounts of liquids, don't try milk. Your child knows what milk is supposed to taste like and will become suspicious if it tastes funny. A strongly flavored juice which your child doesn't drink often, such as cranberry, might work. There may be some foods to avoid with certain drugs. However, in general it is more important to get the medication into the child. Ask your doctor for advice.

In the rare event that the medication actually tastes good, never say it's candy, or your child may look for the opportunity to eat or drink the entire prescription at one time.

Giving Liquid Medication

There are three steps to giving liquid medication: measuring the drug, pouring the measured amount into the container you will use to administer the drug, and feeding the drug to your child.

Measuring the drug. Accuracy is essential. Never use a household teaspoon. Your doctor wouldn't write a prescription for one to three pills before each meal, but the dosage may be only that accurate if you simply use a teaspoon from your kitchen drawer. Also, with an ordinary teaspoon, it is easy for you to spill accidentally, or for your child to spill intentionally as he or she pushes it away or wriggles about.

Special devices that can be used to give your child the right amount of medication are shown in figure 5-2.

A hollow graduated measuring spoon looks like a test tube with a spoonlike curved lip at the opening. After you have filled one, you can stand it upright in a glass while you position your child. Some of these spoons even come with little legs of their own. Such spoons are inexpensive and most pharmacies carry them.

A dose syringe is a plastic syringe with a curved end, designed for giving medication. It comes with a special top for the medicine bottle, so you can withdraw medicine right out of the bottle into the syringe without having to pour it into a measuring cup first. This special lid seals so tightly that you can shake the bottle with it in place. The dose syringe is ideal for children under two. It is reusable.

An ordinary disposable plastic syringe can also be used.

A 10-cc glass, metal-tip, non-Luer-lock syringe is a fairly expensive and breakable item

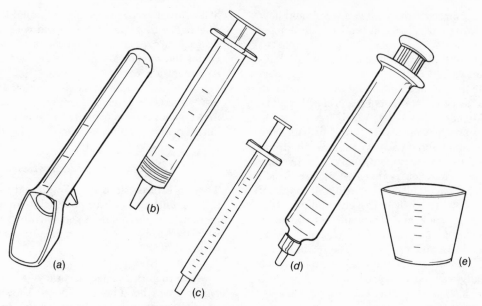

Figure 5-2   Medication measuring devices: *(a)* hollow graduated measuring spoon; *(b)* dose syringe; *(c)* disposable plastic syringe; *(d)* 10-cc glass, metal-tip, non-Luer-lock syringe; *(e)* plastic medication cup.

that may have to be special-ordered by your pharmacist. But if you are using one for feeding (see pages 167–168), you'll find it ideal for giving medication.

Plastic medication cups, as used in the hospital, give an accurate measurement and are good for use with a glass syringe or if your child is cooperative enough and able to drink the measured portion. Usually your doctor or nurse can get you a few of these.

Pouring the medication into the desired container.

1. Reread the label to check for the correct dosage. If your child can read or understand what you are saying, review this information with him or her so your child knows how much he or she should take and assumes as much responsibility as possible. (Your child may even alert whoever is administering the medication to a mistake one day.)
2. Wash your hands.
3. Shake the bottle well to mix the contents.
4. Uncap the bottle. Place the cap upside down on a clean surface.

5. Pour the medicine. Hold the bottle with the label facing up, so spilled liquid won't obscure any printed information.
6. Check the dosage you have poured. If you have poured too much, it is better to pour the excess into the sink. If you return it to the bottle, you may contaminate the whole bottle.
7. Wipe the bottle lip with a damp tissue or paper towel if necessary before replacing the cap.

Feeding the medication to your child. If you know your child will simply sit or lie still and open his or her mouth you have no problem. But if you doubt it, or know your child will not be willing, remember that threats, bribes, or brute force are all undesirable. It is easiest just to position your child so he or she is most apt to cooperate.

Hold your child on your lap or lift him or her onto a kitchen counter so your child is about as high as you are. As illustrated in figure 5-3, clamp your child's right arm against your body, hold the left arm with your left forearm. Now you have your left hand free to control your child's head and your right hand free to give the medication. Once your child realizes that taking the medication is the only alternative, he or she is apt to comply. This method also works well for nose drops or clearing out the nostrils with a rubber syringe.

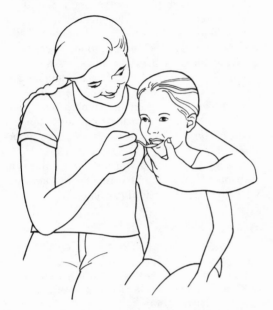

Figure 5-3   Holding child to administer medication.

If you are giving your child the medication with a syringe, squirt it between the cheek and the teeth. That way your child won't choke if you squirt too hard and fast. Also, he or she will taste it a little less. Some children like to hold their nose, since they think that cutting the smell helps cut the taste.

Regardless of your method of giving medication, be sure to have water or juice ready as a chaser so your child can immediately wash away the taste. Particularly if taking medication is a frequent occurrence, it is better that your child gets used to taking the medication with liquid chasers rather than relying on candy.

Praise your child for any cooperation. If cooperation wasn't superlative, but still was better than last time, you should give praise for the improvement.

Giving liquid medication to infants is slightly different. Any oral medication your doctor prescribes is to be given with a dropper in very small doses. First, get a bib or clean diaper ready to put under your child's chin and perhaps have another diaper for your shoulder. Next, measure the medication. Then hold your child in your lap. Immobilize your baby's arms if necessary, as described for older children above. If your child won't open his or her mouth, try gently squeezing the cheeks so your fingers push the jaws apart. Then drop in the medication.

Giving Tablets and Capsules

For the older child who can swallow well, premeasured medication in capsule or tablet form is great.

Tablets come in both coated and uncoated form. Coated tablets usually have no taste. Don't break up or ask your child to chew any hard-coated tablet without checking with your pharmacist; breaking the coating may prevent the medication from being properly absorbed and the interior may taste nasty. Usually, coated tablets should not be taken with milk or antacids, since they will disintegrate prematurely.

Uncoated tablets can taste nasty. Such tablets can be crushed to make them easier to take. However, you should check with your pharmacist to make sure the drug's action won't be affected by mixing the medication with liquid or food.

Capsules enclose powders, granules, oils, or other liquids in a thin shell, usually made of gelatin. Soft uncoated capsules can be opened. But if you want to do so, check with your pharmacist to be sure that the drug's effectiveness won't be changed by mixing it with food or water.

Prolonged-action or repeat-action capsules should never be opened, for if the contents of these capsules are absorbed all at once you increase the risk of an overdose.

Help your child learn to swallow tablets and capsules. First, have your child swallow some water. Then put the tablet or capsule far back on the tongue. Have your child tip his or her head forward and swallow a large mouthful of water.

Do not have your child throw the head back when swallowing, for he or she may aspirate.

You may also try placing the tablet under the child's tongue, since the tongue will automatically flip the pill up and back when the child swallows. Regardless of the method, in the beginning your child may have to try a number of times, each time with a new mouthful of water. However, success will come soon.

Giving Medication by Injection

While in most cases it is possible for your doctor to give your child the necessary injections, it is often difficult to coordinate your doctor's schedule with your own. This is especially true if your child needs daily injections. You can learn to give your son or daughter an injection if this would make it easier to care for your child. It is a step-by-step process and really not that hard.

If you and your doctor think you can learn to give your child injections, your doctor will teach you how best to do so. He or she may have you practice injecting water into an orange before giving your child an injection.

In case your doctor doesn't give you written instructions, the steps outlined below may be helpful. Remember, *never* give your child an injection unless your doctor (or the health-care professional your doctor has designated) has given you instructions and has actually supervised you giving injections.

As with oral medication, injections must be given in as matter-of-fact a manner as possible. Distraction may help with very apprehensive or uncooperative children. If you add a little humor and spirit to the proceedings, it will help decrease your child's anxiety.

Let your child have as much control over the situation as possible. Although your child won't have any choice about getting the injection at a particular time of day, he or she can perhaps choose the room, help you get the supplies ready, and so on. Your child may also help you step by step, giving verbal instructions as to what you should do next, or your child may help decide where he or she should receive the injection.

Discuss with your child exactly what is going to happen. If he or she asks you whether it will hurt, be honest and say that it may (or really will, depending upon the medication you are using). But remind your child that cooperation will be most helpful. If your child flexes a muscle it will cause pain.

Work out with your doctor where the injections should be given. The smaller or skinnier your child is, the fewer will be the possible sites for injection. Choose your injection site carefully to avoid major nerves and blood vessels. Also avoid any area with wounds, inflammation, hair, or birthmarks. If your child needs frequent injections, you may want to establish with your doctor's help a pattern for rotating the placement of the injections. If necessary, make yourself a chart.

Injections can be given just below the skin (subcutaneously), into the muscle (intramuscularly), or into the vein (intravenously).

Subcutaneous injections.

1. Wash your hands.
2. Get needles of the prescribed length and thickness. (If you will be using many needles, they are cheaper if you buy them in large quantities from your pharmacist.)
3. Mix the medication. If it is in liquid form, simply shake well. If you have been given powder and a diluent (such as a small bottle of sterile water) separately, proceed as follows (fig. 5-4):
   a. Wipe the stopper of both tops with a prepackaged sterile swab or a piece of cotton dipped in isopropyl alcohol, which is 91 proof and a more effective antiseptic than ethyl (rubbing) alcohol, which is only 70 proof.
   b. Inject an equal amount of air into the bottle before you draw out the diluent in order to avoid creating a vacuum in the bottle, which could make it difficult to withdraw the medication. If, for example, you wish to withdraw 2 cc of diluent, first pull the plunger on an empty sterile syringe up to 2 cc, insert the needle through the rubber cap of the diluent bottle, and push the plunger down, thereby injecting 2 cc of air into the diluent bottle.
   c. Draw up the recommended amount of diluent into the needle and syringe.
   d. Inject the diluent into the medication bottle.
   e. Shake the bottle well. Remember also to shake the bottle well before each use.
4. Squirt air equal to the needed amount of medication into the bottle.

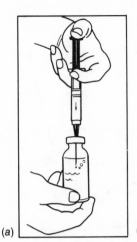 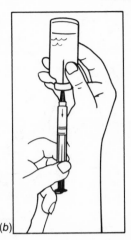 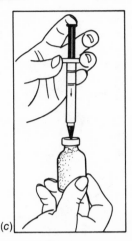 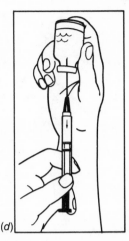

(a)   (b)   (c)   (d)

Figure 5-4 Mixing medicine and diluent for injection: (a) injecting air into the vial of diluent; (b) drawing out the diluent; (c) injecting the diluent into the medication bottle; (d) drawing out the medication.

5. Draw out a little more than the needed amount of medication, holding the medication above the syringe. Now tap the syringe, enabling any air bubbles to rise toward the needle. When you squirt out the extra amount of medication to get the prescribed amount, you will also squirt out any trapped air.

6. Change needles at this point if your doctor has so recommended. Then there is no danger of using a contaminated needle, the outside of the needle doesn't have medication on it (which can sting), and the injection will be given with the sharpest possible needle. Ask your doctor whether you should change needles.

7. Rub the site for the injection with a sterile swab or cotton with isopropyl alcohol. Allow the alcohol to evaporate so you don't push some of the alcohol into the tissue, causing pain.

8. Squeeze the skin firmly together to elevate the subcutaneous tissue.

9. Quickly insert the needle to the desired length. The needle hurts while it is moving but not once in place.

10. Draw back on the plunger (not the needle) a little. If you draw out blood, you may have punctured a vein. Take the needle all the way out, replace it with a new one, and try again. If no blood appears, continue to the next step.

11. Steady the needle and inject the medication. Inject it slowly or quickly, according to your doctor's instructions. (If you inject the medication quickly, you get it over with fast. But injecting

slowly gives the medication time to be absorbed into the tissue and this may hurt less.)

12. Pull the needle out fast.

13. Rub the site with a sterile swab or cotton with isopropyl alcohol and gently apply pressure to help seal the punctured tissue and to prevent the medication from leaking out. If your child tends to develop hematomas, apply pressure for a couple of minutes. Gentle rubbing can help increase circulation and thus the absorption of the medication. However, with a few very caustic medications, which produce a burning sensation, rubbing would not be indicated. So ask your doctor or pharmacist if there are any special instructions in this regard.

Intramuscular injections provide much more rapid absorption than subcutaneous injections, as more blood flows to the muscles. Sometimes a doctor will begin treatment with an intramuscular injection to get a high blood level of the medication and then have your child continue to take the medication orally. However, if your child is vomiting, unable to swallow, uncooperative, or unconscious, continuing with injections may be indicated. (Also, some medication is available only in injectable form.) Since the needle for intramuscular injections is longer than that for subcutaneous injections, there are fewer available sites where you don't risk hitting blood ves-

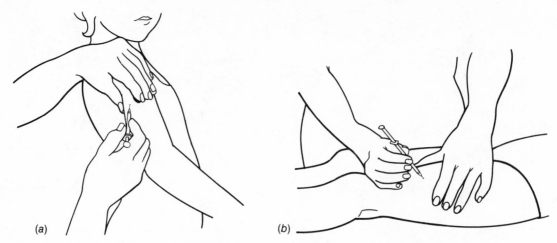

Figure 5-5   Placement of needle for *(a)* subcutaneous injection and *(b)* intramuscular injection.

sels, nerves, or bone. It is most important to discuss with your doctor which sites you should use, particularly if your child is small or skinny, for such a child will have fewer areas with muscle thick enough to take an intramuscular injection.

The procedure for giving intramuscular injections is almost the same as for subcutaneous injections (fig. 5-5). You will, of course, use a longer, stronger needle and when you first insert the needle with that quick, dartlike thrust, you will feel some resistance. But since the pain occurs when the needle moves through the tissue, you should insert the needle as quickly as possible.

After inserting the needle be sure to pull back gently on the plunger to confirm correct needle placement: if blood appears in the syringe, you may have punctured the vein. If so, take the needle out and apply pressure to stop the bleeding and to minimize bruising. Before trying again, your doctor will probably want you to replace the needle and perhaps even the medication if there is a fair amount of blood in the syringe.

Intravenous injections are absorbed the most quickly of all, as the medication is given directly into the blood stream. Your doctor may give intravenous injections in emergency, life-threatening situations.

Only children with certain disorders, such as hemophiliacs, will regularly need intravenous

injections. If your child needs such injections, discuss with your doctor whether you can learn to do this at home.

Your doctor may have trouble finding your child's vein when giving an intravenous injection, especially if your child is severely ill. This is by no means a sign of incompetence.

If your child is hospitalized with intravenous feeding (IV), the doctor will usually prescribe that your child's medication be added to the IV so your child doesn't need injections. In a family committed to home care, a seriously ill child may on occasion be given intravenous feeding as an outpatient in the emergency room. Even on an outpatient basis medication can be added to the IV. So if you take your child into the emergency room, review with your doctor what your child is taking in order to determine if any of these medications could be added to the IV.

Giving Medication
by Suppository or Enema

If your child is vomiting, unconscious, or unable to swallow, your doctor may want to give medication in the form of suppositories or enemas.

A suppository is a solid medication, usually shaped like a bullet. The medication is mixed with a firm base, such as cocoa butter, that melts at body temperature so the resulting liquid medication is absorbed by the blood vessels lining the rectum. The procedure for administering a rectal suppository is as follows:

1. Have your child urinate and have a bowel movement if possible, if your doctor recommends this.
2. Clip the nail on your index finger (or little finger in the case of a small child) as short as possible. Wash your hands. (Some people prefer wearing a plastic glove or finger cot; however your clean finger will work just fine.)
3. Lubricate your finger and your child's anus with a little water-based lubricant such as K-Y Jelly. Unwrap the suppository and gently push it into the anus, following it in with your finger up to about your first finger joint, so that you are sure it is in past the strong sphincter muscles that close off the anus. Be careful that the suppository is placed next to the rectal wall so it can be absorbed. If it is buried in bowel movement, it cannot be absorbed.
4. Keep the suppository in until it is dissolved. (Ask your doctor or pharmacist how long this takes.) Do your best to keep your child mentally distracted with stories, songs, games, TV, or anything else that works, for he or she may soon begin to complain about needing to go to the toilet. Put this off as long as possible. With some children it may help to tape their buttocks together with nonallergenic tape. (Masking tape will also work, if that is all you have.)
5. Watch to see if any unabsorbed portion of the suppository comes out when your child finally does go to the toilet. If the suppository contains strong medication, such as a sedative, and some of the unabsorbed suppository is expelled, it may be unwise to give your child a whole new suppository, for you could overdose your child. Discuss with your doctor what you should do if this occurs. Sometimes you may check the size of the unabsorbed portion and then insert another piece of approximately that size. At other times you may simply fish the unabsorbed portion out of the toilet, wash it off with cold water (it would melt in hot), and then reinsert the unabsorbed portion.
6. Wash your hands when you are done.

An enema is an anal injection of liquid. There are two types of enemas. The most commonly known is the nonretention enema, which is expelled after about ten minutes and is given to cleanse the lower bowel. There is also a retention enema, which should stay in the patient for at least ten minutes or until absorbed. If your child is very ill and not taking much liquid by mouth, a retention enema of rectal fluids may supply enough liquid to prevent dehydration and the need for intravenous feeding. Some medications can be given rectally. Take the following steps to give an enema.

1. Have your child try to urinate and have a bowel movement.
2. Have your child lie on the left side, for the colon inside the body is shaped as shown in figure 5-6.

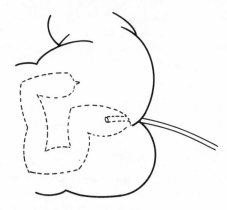

Figure 5-6   Position of colon in body.

3. Lubricate the anus and the tip of whatever you are using, such as a catheter or an enema bottle, with K-Y Jelly.
4. Squirt the liquid in slowly, for then it is more apt to stay in and be absorbed. Squirting a large amount at one time can also cause discomfort.
5. Hold the buttocks together or put pressure on the anus if this will help. Distract your child and try to have him or her hold off using the toilet as long as possible.
6. Wash your hands when you are done.

Giving Medications for the Skin, Eye, Ear, and Nose

These drugs are applied directly to the site of the problem. Although there are fewer side effects and allergic reactions to these than to medication taken internally, you should still take care to measure how much medication you are giving. As with all other types of drugs, more is not better and may actually be harmful.

Skin medications should be applied as frequently as directed.

1. Wash your hands.
2. Spread the medication in a thin even layer, taking care not to get it near your child's (or your own) eyes or lips.
3. Wash your hands.

Eye medications come in either liquid or ointment form. Never use anything for the eyes that is not specifically labeled "ophthalmic," for only such drugs are sterile and made with a special nonirritating base suitable for the eye's sensitive tissues. It is easiest to apply eye medication while your child is lying down.

Drops:

1. Wash your hands.
2. Ask your child to look up and focus on a specific object.
3. Place your index finger on your child's cheekbone and gently pull down on the skin, exposing the inside of the bottom eye lid (the conjunctival sac).
4. Gently drop the medication into the conjunctival sac at the nose end of the eye without letting the dropper touch the eye.
5. Release the lid and let your child blink. Try to

keep your child from rubbing his or her eyes, as this may rub the medication out.
6. Wash your hands.

Ointments are given as drops until actually placing the medication in the eye. Squeeze a ⅛-inch string of ointment into the conjunctival sac at the nose end of the eye. Gently bring the tube against the lower lid margin to detach the ointment.

1. Release the lower lid and ask your child to close his or her eyes briefly so the medication can spread and be absorbed.
2. Gently wipe away any excess.
3. Wash your hands after applying medication.

Ear medication comes in drop form.

1. Wash your hands.
2. Warm the bottle for about two minutes in your hand if the medication has been refrigerated.
3. Straighten the ear canal of a young child by *gently* pulling the lower part of the ear down and back (fig. 5-7). As a child grows, the shape of the ear canal changes, so by the time your child is five to seven years old, your doctor will want you to modify the procedure and pull the upper part of the ear up and back. Be very careful when you pull on the ear, for if the ear canal is inflamed, pulling will hurt.
4. Taking care not to touch the ear, slowly let the

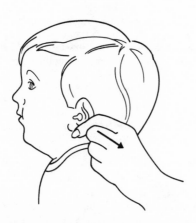
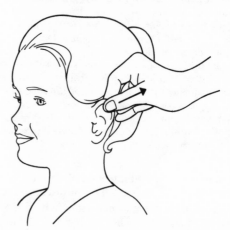

Figure 5-7   Administering eardrops: note that ear is pulled down and back on infant; up and back on older child.

medication run down one side of the ear canal so the air can escape up the other side. The drops do good only if they dribble all the way down the ear canal to the ear drum. If air gets trapped beneath the drops, it will keep the solution from penetrating any farther. If you think you have trapped air in the ear, you can give the ear and ear canal a gentle squeeze and wiggle, but if your child's ear is really tender this will be quite unpleasant. Therefore it is much easier always to give the drops very carefully.

5. Try to keep your child lying on his or her side for about ten minutes so the medication has a chance to be absorbed.

Nasal medication can be given in drops or as a spray.

Nose drops are administered differently for different conditions.

For sinus conditions, have your child lie on his or her back with shoulders elevated so the head tips way back. Again there are two methods: slowly drop the medication in, taking care that the end of the dropper doesn't touch the nostril, or put the dropper well into the nose. Ask your doctor which is preferable. A minute or two after giving the medication have your child roll his or her head and shoulders to one side briefly and then repeat on the other side.

For nasal congestion, have your child sit upright with head tipped back. Hold the dropper so it is parallel to the floor. This way, the medication will flow to the back of your child's nose and slowly be absorbed by the membranes. If you tilt the dropper so it is pointing toward the floor, the medication will simply flow down the nostril into the throat.

Atomized nasal sprays come with specific directions as to how they are to be given. This will vary with the type of medication and where it is supposed to end up—in the nose or in the lungs. Follow the directions carefully, as this will greatly influence the drug's effectiveness. Use only as often as indicated; overuse can cause problems.

6

Respiratory Therapy

An increasing number of children are being given respiratory therapy at home rather than in the hospital. Most children who need respiratory therapy, even if for several hours every day or all day long, do better at home than in a hospital or an institution.

There are several factors to consider with any home respiratory therapy program.

- The child and parent should know what needs to be done and why.
- The child should follow the prescribed treatment regularly.
- The home treatment program should be supervised by a professional.
- The child should continue the complete prescribed program until told to stop or change.
- Respiratory therapy can relieve many problems, even if a cure is not possible.

While it is impossible for anyone except your doctor to suggest what is best for your child, it is helpful if you understand how the respiratory system works and some of the basic principles of respiratory therapy so you can work with your doctor and respiratory therapist to develop and administer the appropriate treatment program for your child. Your child should also understand as much as possible, for this will aid him or her in accepting and following through on what is prescribed.

HOW DOES YOUR RESPIRATORY SYSTEM WORK?

The airways look something like an upside-down tree, with the trachea as the trunk and the bronchi as the large branches leading to the right and left lungs, where the bronchioles form the smaller branches (fig. 6-1). At the end of the bronchioles are microscopic balloonlike structures called alveoli, which look something like bunches of grapes. Each separate alveolus is covered with a network of tiny blood vessels called capillaries. On inhalation, oxygen passes through the bronchial tree to the aveoli, where it diffuses into the capillaries and is carried by the blood throughout the body. As the oxygen diffuses into the capillaries, carbon dioxide (a body waste) comes into the alveoli and is then exhaled.

Human beings take oxygen from the air into their bodies through inhalation, or inspiration, and release carbon dioxide into the air through exhalation, or expiration. This process is controlled by a group of cells in the brain, called the respiratory center, which sends signals causing us to inhale and exhale.

When we inhale, the diaphragm contracts and the ribs rise, creating a slight continuing vacuum causing air to flow into the lungs from the atmosphere. The nose warms, moistens, and filters this incoming air. The epiglottis, a flag valve, acts as a safety door, closing over the larynx when we swallow and opening when we breathe. After passing the larynx, the air flows through the windpipe or trachea into the large breathing tubes (bronchi), then to the smaller breathing tubes (bronchioles), and finally into the air sacs (alveoli). The mucous membrane that lines these passages helps to further warm and humidify the air. The sticky mucus lining also traps any small foreign material such as dust or bacteria.

Some cells within the lungs secrete mucus,

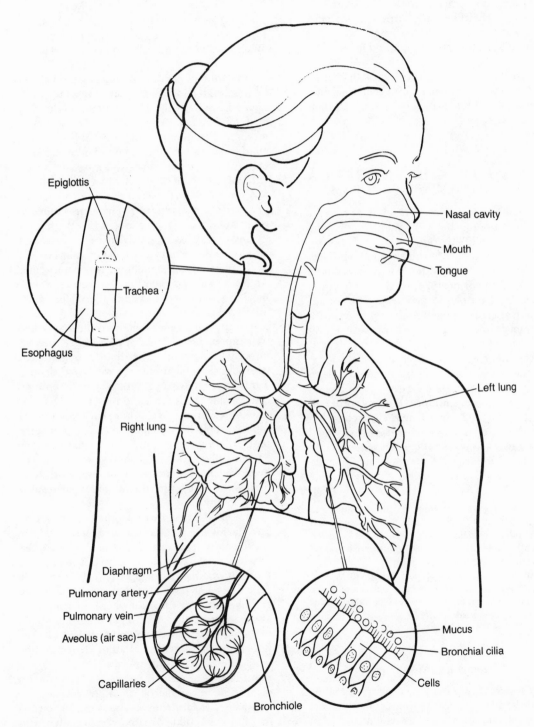

Figure 6-1   The respiratory system.

which lines the bronchial tubes. There are also microscopic hairlike structures called cilia, which wave rhythmically, moving the mucous blanket toward the trachea, helping to clear the airways.

On exhalation, the diaphragm and other respiratory muscles relax. This allows the normal elastic recoil of the lungs and they return to their original shape.

WHAT ARE THE COMPONENTS OF A RESPIRATORY CARE PROGRAM?

When your physician orders respiratory care for your child at home, he or she should discuss the goals of your child's therapy with you. There are a number of health-care professionals who may actually teach you how to provide this home care. Even if your doctor specializes in respiratory diseases, he or she may have you consult with nurses specializing in respiratory care, with respiratory therapists, or with physical therapists. Here we shall speak only of the doctor, with the understanding that he or she may designate one of these allied health professionals to assist you with your child's care.

Any effective respiratory therapy program must be designed for effective bronchial hygiene, the use of various techniques to help keep the airways clear of secretions. To achieve good bronchial hygiene, your program may include many, if not all, of the following:

- Conditioning and moistening the airways and secretions with medication, fluid intake, and breathing moist air.
- Breathing techniques to help clear the airways and control the pattern of breathing.
- Postural drainage with percussion and vibration to help loosen and move secretions out of the lungs.
- Suctioning to remove secretions when the child is unable to cough adequately.

Conditioning and Moistening the Airways and Secretions

The goal of the first part of the program is to thin secretions, dilate the airways, and get any necessary medication to where it is needed.

Adequate fluid intake is necessary to keep the secretions thin. Your doctor will tell you how much fluid your child should consume daily.

Inhalation of moist air is important. If you live in a humid climate, the air might be moist enough. But if you use a heater or air conditioner, or if you live in a dry climate, you may need to increase the amount of moisture in the air your child breathes by using room humidifiers or one of the machines that can deliver moist air, with or without medication, directly to your child.

A room humidifier, a large-volume nebulizer, or an ultrasonic nebulizer may be prescribed. A room humidifier may be used when the humidity in a small room needs to be increased. A large-volume nebulizer may be used if the child needs moisture throughout the respiratory tract. An ultrasonic nebulizer may be used to provide moisture particles of a smaller size, which can be inhaled deeply into the lungs.

If your child needs a large-volume or ultrasonic nebulizer all night, it pays to get the mist directly to the child rather than throughout the bedroom. This means having your child sleep in a mist canopy (croup tent), which is commercially available. If for some reason you have to use an oxygen tent, *be sure to cut a hole in the top* so carbon dioxide and heat can rise out of the tent. Although tent stands are available, if you have modified your child's bed you may find you need to make a stand and your own tents. If so, discuss the best way to do this with your respiratory therapist.

Your child will get wet sleeping in a mist canopy during the night. You may wrap a cloth (such as a diaper) around his or her head, fastened in front with a diaper clip. Cover the blankets with a sheet to keep them dry. You will probably want to change that sheet before you go to bed at night and also whenever your child awakes during the night. Your child may need extra heat in the room at night because of dampness from the nebulizer. Rather than heat the whole house all night, use an energy-efficient room heater to provide the necessary heat. An electric heater, which heats a coil of water, is relatively safe, dustfree, and noiseless (so you can monitor your child's breathing, especially via an intercom). However, if you are using oxygen in your child's room, the oxygen source must be at least ten feet from the open flame or possible source of electric sparks (such as might be given off by a room heater).

When using a nebulizer (either large-volume or ultrasonic), the hose to the canopy must be securely positioned inside the canopy. While this is quite easily done with commercial mist canopies, if you make your own canopy it is best to cut out not just one but three slits through the top of the canopy, so the hose can go into the canopy, out, and then in again and thus be secure through the night (fig. 6-2). The hose must be easily removed for daily cleaning.

Some water will always condense in the hose. This is called "rain-out," and there is always some danger of bacteria collecting there. If the nebulizing chamber is placed higher than the canopy opening, the rain-out will drip onto your child. If the nebulizing chamber is lower, the rain-out runs back into the chamber. If the hose is level between the nebulizing chamber and the canopy opening or the hose has a dip in it, the rain-out will collect there, stopping the flow of mist. Therefore, your doctor may suggest using what is called a *T-adapter* with a drainage bag. By intentionally putting a dip and T-adapter into your hosing, any rain-out will drain into this bag, which must be emptied and cleaned daily.

The nebulizing chamber must be filled with liquid to the level indicated in the user's manual whenever the machine is running, for the unit will burn out if the chamber ever runs dry. When using a continuous system, upon attaching the supply bottle to the machine make sure there are no air bubbles in the tubing, for they will block the flow of water. Check to see if the water has flowed into the nebulizing chamber itself.

With an ultrasonic nebulizer also be sure that the specified amount of water is in the coupling chamber.

It is important to let the canopy dry every day,

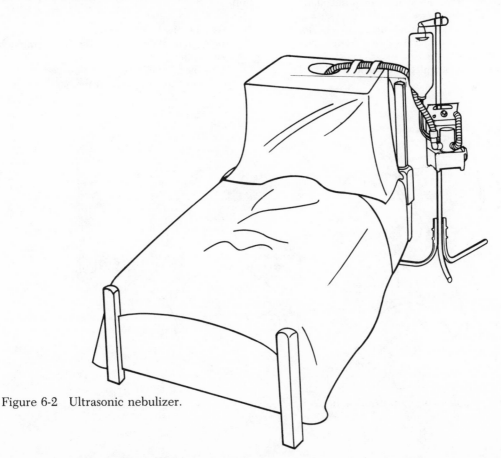

Figure 6-2　Ultrasonic nebulizer.

since the organisms you try to eliminate thrive and multiply rapidly in the damp. Open the canopy and put it in the sunlight. Periodically take it outside, hang it on the wash line, hose it off, and leave it to dry. The ultraviolet rays of the sun are a useful disinfectant. If you don't have much sunshine and dry weather, you may need two canopies—if one is not dry you will have another to use.

Medications can be administered directly into the airways by use of a number of small devices.

Small-volume (updraft) nebulizers have a jet assembly that creates small medication particles that can be inhaled into the lungs. This unit can be powered by oxygen, compressed air, or an electric air compressor designed for this purpose (fig. 6-3). Follow these steps when giving small-volume nebulizer therapy:

1. Get your child seated comfortably.
2. Fill the nebulizer through the main orifice with the prescribed amount of medication and diluting solution when necessary. Measure the medication very carefully. Most of these drugs are so potent that adverse side effects are always possible, especially with overdoses.
3. Position the mouthpiece between your child's teeth.

4. Turn on the compressor or other source of power.
5. Have your child inhale deeply and pause after inhalation.
6. Have your child exhale slowly.

Repeat this procedure until all the prescribed medication is nebulized. Periodically tap the side of the nebulizer so medication that has collected on the sides will run down into the bottom of the nebulizer to be nebulized. If the machine does not produce mist, make sure it is assembled correctly.

Encourage your child to cough periodically in order to clear the airways of any secretions.

A metered-dose device (MDD) is a very convenient, easy-to-handle device for inhalation of medications (fig. 6-4). The device consists of a small cartridge containing various types of medicine, chiefly bronchodilators or steroids, and a mouthpiece for dispensing the drug. The advantages of this type of aerosol therapy are its portability and minimal care as well as its quick action.

1. Assemble the MDD for use.
2. Have your child exhale completely through pursed lips.
3. Place the open end of the mouthpiece into your child's mouth past the front teeth.

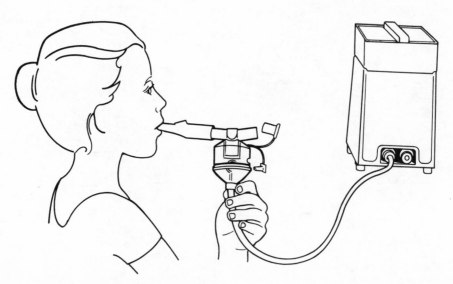

Figure 6-3 Small-volume (updraft) nebulizer.

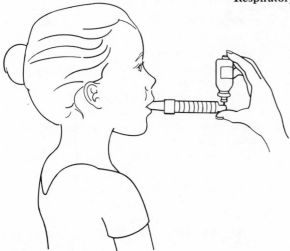

Figure 6-4 Positioning metered dose device in child's mouth.

4. Have your child keep his or her lips slightly open. This allows more air to be inhaled through the mouth to aid in carrying the medication deeper into the airways. Your doctor may want you to use a device such as a spacer tube or an aerosol chamber, which can be placed between the MDD and the mouth. This facilitates slower inhalation of the medicine and helps ensure that the medication does not just remain in the mouth but actually penetrates the airways. Also, since coordination may be difficult, such a device eliminates the chances of exhaling the medication when the child should be inhaling. You can buy an aerosol chamber or a spacer tube. You can also make your own spacer tube out of a six-inch length of corrugated plastic aerosol tubing onto which the MDD and the mouthpiece will fit. An empty toilet-paper tube will also work in a pinch.

5. Have your child exhale slowly, using pursed lips.

6. Have your child take a slow deep breath. As he or she starts to inhale, press down firmly on the cartridge to release the medication.

7. Have your child hold his or her breath for a few seconds (your doctor will tell you how long) to allow the medication to settle on the surface of the airways. This will prevent your child from exhaling the medication.

8. Have your child exhale slowly, using pursed lips.

9. Repeat only as prescribed. Your doctor may recommend waiting as long as ten minutes if multiple puffs are recommended.

10. Have your child rinse his or her mouth and swallow water after treatments so the medication does not stay in the mouth, if your doctor recommends this.

11. *Wash the mouthpiece* after each use. Store the mouthpiece in a clean plastic bag when it is dry to keep it free from dust and dirt.

Periodically check the amount of medication in your MDD so you can order refills before you run out. An easy way to estimate how much medication is left inside is to place the cartridge in a container of water and observe its position as it floats (fig. 6-5).

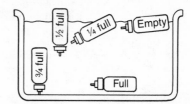

Figure 6-5 Estimating amount of medication remaining in nebulizer by floating cartridge in water.

Spin-inhalers, also called whirlybird inhalation devices, are used to deliver Intal (cromalyn sodium) to asthma patients (fig. 6-6). They only deliver medication and in the following way:

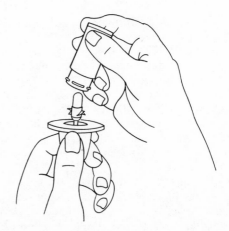

Figure 6-6 Opening spin-inhaler mouthpiece to reveal propeller.

1. Unwrap one capsule.
2. Hold the device with the mouthpiece on the bottom. Slide the sleeve to the top.
3. Open the mouthpiece by unscrewing its tip counterclockwise. Inside is a small propeller.
4. Press the colored end of the medication capsule into the center of the propeller. Avoid overhandling the capsule, since it may soften.
5. Screw the device securely back together, holding it with the mouthpiece at the bottom.
6. Slide the outer sleeve all the way down and then slide it up again to puncture the capsule. Make sure the device is secure.
7. Have your child exhale as much air as possible.
8. Have your child tip his or her head back slightly, place the mouthpiece in the child's mouth, and have the child close his or her lips around it.
9. Have your child inhale one deep, rapid breath.
10. Remove the spin inhaler and have your child hold his or her breath for several seconds. (Your child should never exhale through the mouthpiece.)
11. Now have your child exhale as much as possible.
12. Repeat this inhaling and exhaling procedure until all the medication in the device is gone.
13. Discard the empty medication capsule. Wash the device thoroughly, as often as recommended by your doctor. Make sure it is completely dry before reassembling it.

Saline solution is an integral component of nebulizer therapy. You may have to make up your own solutions of saline and water for your child.

If your child sleeps with the nebulizer running all night, he or she will inhale so much liquid that you will want to use a solution close in composition to your child's own body fluids. Since these are salty, any liquid your child inhales should have some salt in it.

You can buy sterile "normal saline" solution, which is .9 percent sodium chloride (salt). However, since children absorb and retain more salt than adults, this solution is too strong for a child, and your doctor will recommend what strength you should use.

Rather than buy commercial normal saline and mix it with sterile distilled water, it is much cheaper to make your own solution out of sodium-chloride tablets and distilled water. First you need to determine with your doctor what strength saline you need and how much liquid

you need. Then work out with your pharmacist how many sodium-chloride tablets (which normally come in one-gram size) you will need to add to the water to make a solution of the desired strength. Although some people recommend regular table salt, you will get a more accurate measurement using sodium-chloride tablets, which aren't very expensive. Use sterile distilled water. Regular water may contain bacteria and sediments that will jam the nebulizer. Either buy bottled distilled water, which you can usually get delivered, or purchase a water distiller, which is cheaper if you anticipate long-term use. Both should be covered by your insurance if you submit your claim with sufficient support information.

Here is how to make the solution:

1. Get a pot large enough to hold water.
2. Fill the pot with the desired amount of distilled water. It's hard to mark the inside of the pot, but with time you should be able to estimate accurately how high to fill the pot; an absolutely precise measurement is not necessary.
3. Bring the water to a boil.
4. Add the sodium tablets and stir until dissolved while the water continues to boil. Do not add the tablets to the cold water: the salt will eat through the bottom of your pot.
5. Replace the lid and simmer the water for ten minutes to kill all microorganisms. An electric stove with a slowly cooling burner should stay hot enough for ten minutes if you simply turn it off.
6. Let the water cool. As long as it stays covered in the pot it should be sterile for a few hours. Get in the habit of boiling the water every morning so it is really cool by evening, when you need to fill a nighttime nebulizer. Hot or warm water in the ultrasonic nebulizer can overheat the element and require costly repair.
7. Pour the boiled water into a sterile bottle using a sterile funnel when you are ready to use it.

Breathing Retraining

Breathing retraining may include diaphragmatic pursed-lip breathing and controlled coughing to aid in controlling the pattern of breathing and in clearing the airways of secretions.

Pursed-lip breathing helps decrease the work of breathing and improve ventilation. With pursed-lip breathing, the lips provide resistance to exhaled air, thus maintaining a higher pressure in the airways and keeping the airways open longer so more air can get out. Try this yourself before teaching your child:

1. Inhale through your nose with your mouth closed.
2. Exhale slowly through your mouth with your lips pursed. Make your exhalation at least twice as long as your inhalation (for example, two seconds in, four seconds out). Pretend you are whistling.

Pursed-lip breathing is a basic technique used with all other breathing exercises. When your child becomes short of breath, it should be practiced along with diaphragmatic breathing.

Diaphragmatic breathing also helps reduce the work of breathing. Normally the diaphragm does about 80 percent of the work in breathing, but in some lung diseases the diaphragm flattens and the upper chest muscles try to take over. Since these muscles require more oxygen to do the diaphragm's work, it may be helpful for your child to learn how consciously to do diaphragmatic breathing and decrease the use of the upper chest muscles, thereby minimizing the work of breathing (fig. 6-7).

1. Place one hand on your chest, the other on your abdomen to check movement. You should feel the most movement in the hand placed on the abdomen.
2. Inhale slowly and deeply through the nose and feel your abdomen rise.
3. Exhale slowly through pursed lips and feel your abdomen fall.
4. Repeat ten times at a rate slightly slower than slow respiration.

Try this in sitting and standing positions also.

Controlled-coughing technique is used to remove excess secretions so the airways remain open and your child can move air in and out of the lungs effectively. If the excess secretions are not removed, shortness of breath can worsen and the risk of infection increases. And if the secretions irritate nerve endings, this can cause

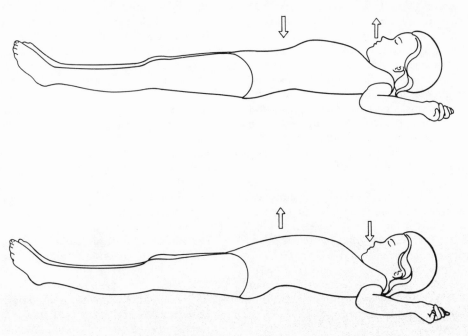

Figure 6-7   Diaphragmatic breathing: exhalation *(top)* and inhalation *(bottom)*.

involuntary coughing and fatigue. Controlled coughing can help your child conserve energy and oxygen. Follow these steps to learn this technique yourself before working with your child on it:

1. Take in a slow, deep breath through the nose, breathing diaphragmatically. (Building up the volume of air behind the secretions helps propel them toward the mouth.)
2. Hold your breath for two seconds.
3. Cough twice with your mouth slightly open. The first cough loosens and the second cough moves the secretions.
4. Exhale completely through pursed lips.
5. Pause.
6. Inhale again by sniffing gently through the nose, for a deep inhalation after coughing may cause the secretions to slide farther back into the bronchial tree.

Postural Drainage, Percussion, and Vibration

Postural drainage involves positioning your child to get secretions out of the bronchial tree. As you saw in figure 6-1, the respiratory tract looks like an upside-down tree. While the upper lobes drain quite nicely when you sit or stand, the lower lobes stay filled unless you stand on your head or at least lie head-down. Your doctor might suggest placing blocks under the foot end of your child's bed to facilitate drainage at night. That way the main part of the lung drains at night while the upper lobes drain in the day. In addition, your doctor may want your child to spend a given amount of time lying in a variety of positions to help drain various areas (fig. 6-8). This may differ depending upon which lobes are most affected, but basically you want your child to spend time tilted chest-down on each side, as well as on the back and front. Encourage your child to use controlled coughing in each position.

Often your doctor will want your child to do postural drainage when getting up in the morning to drain the secretions that filled the lower lobes at night, before lunch and dinner, and again before going to bed to make for better sleep. Postural drainage is best done before or at least two hours after meals.

Your doctor will specify at what angle you should tilt your child. A small child can lie in the trough your legs form when you sit in a chair with your legs outstretched. With a larger child, a short-term solution may be simply to use a bed pillow. Or you could use a wedge-shaped pillow or tilt one end of the bed.

The final position in the sequence should always be chest-down, with your child as close to standing on the head as possible. A larger, heavier child can lie with the legs on a chair, bed, or table and the chest and head hanging down toward the floor. You can let a small child hang over your knee, supporting the forehead with your hand. If your hand and arm get tired, you may find it easier to let your child rest the head on the floor. As the secretions drain into the mouth, he or she can say "mmm" so you can lift the forehead, enabling your child to spit. Your child's body will have to get used to this "hanging," but with time he or she will become accustomed to it.

If your child has chronic respiratory problems requiring postural drainage, a system that would position him or her comfortably and correctly would be an excellent investment. Postural drainage pillows are more comfortable than tilt tables. (The first set of such pillows designed also in pediatric sizes is the Pulmo-Pillo—New Life Designs, 32 West Anapamu Street, Santa Barbara, CA 93101). Remember, you have to find a way for both you and your child to be comfortable, for only then will you do postural drainage regularly for the prescribed amount of time.

You will need something for your child to spit onto or into when the secretions start coming out. Metal or plastic basins have to be washed and paper cups require a good aim. Newspaper is quite absorbent, and you can adjust the amount you put on the floor to the amount of secretions your child is bringing up. If your child is bringing up copious amounts of very runny secretions, a couple of tissues on the newspaper will keep the secretions from running off the paper.

Tissues are handy to wipe your child's mouth. (If your child often needs to be quickly turned upside down and hung, you may need boxes located throughout the house.) When you are done with the postural drainage, carefully fold

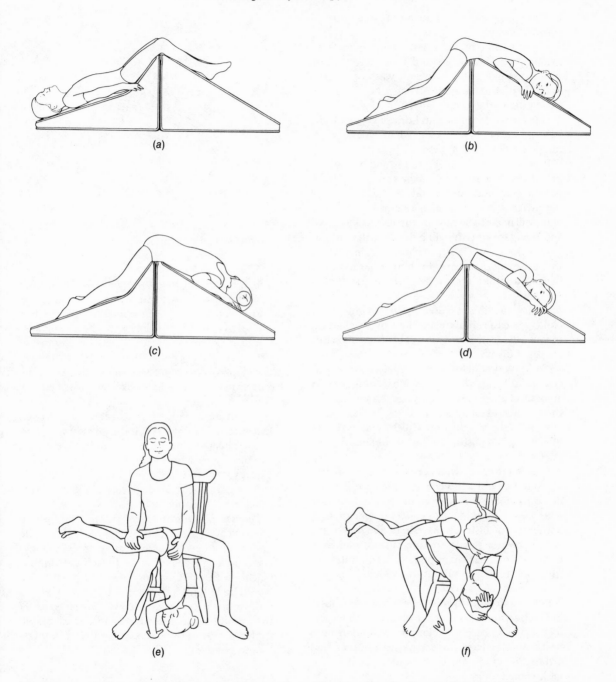

Figure 6-8 Basic postural-drainage positions: *(a)* lie on back to drain both anterior lower lobes; *(b)* lie on stomach to drain both posterior lower lobes; *(c)* lie on right side to drain left ingular segment; *(d)* lie on left side to drain right middle lobe; *(e)* most extreme position for draining lower lobes; *(f)* position for coughing up sputum.

up the newspaper with any used tissues in it and throw it away.

The bacteria in secretions can continue to multiply on the tissues and newspaper, so be sure to use plastic liners in your wastepaper baskets. Tie up the plastic trash bags and take them out to the garbage bin daily.

If you have to do postural drainage regularly, you will find that your child's hair will get very tangled unless it is short or in braids.

If your child has no gag reflex and has severe breathing difficulties, he or she can easily choke not only on foods and liquids but also on his or her own secretions. In such an emergency, your child will need to be quickly turned upside down and hung, for gravity will help clear the air passage. If your child is apt to choke it is important that everyone who cares for him or her learns to hang your child; otherwise, if he or she chokes the adult may not be able to get your child breathing again. In addition to hanging your child, you can remove secretions by mechanical means called suction. This will be discussed later on pages 66–68.

Notify your doctor if your child's secretions change in color, volume, or odor. An increased amount of thin, clear, runny secretions may be the first sign of an infection. Thick, yellow secretions indicate an infection. If your child spits up blood, stop the postural drainage and notify your doctor.

Your doctor may want to run a sputum culture if you think your child is becoming ill or if his or her condition is not responding to treatment. If your doctor wants you to collect a specimen at home, ask for instructions. (He or she may want you to keep a sterile sputum-culture cup or a mucus-specimen trap at home.) Refrigerate any specimen until you take it to the lab.

Percussion and vibration are often prescribed in conjunction with postural drainage to loosen secretions. Since percussion and vibration may be contraindicated for certain respiratory disorders, never do these without first checking with your doctor.

Percussion is performed by clapping with cupped hands (or using percussion cups) on the rib cage (fig. 6-9). Usually it is done for one to two minutes in each postural-drainage position.

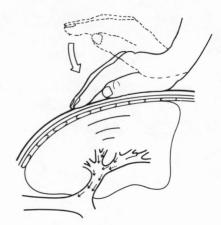

Figure 6-9   Percussion.

It is important to get proper instruction from your doctor on how to perform percussion safely and effectively. If percussion is too gentle, it is ineffective. If it is too hard or in the wrong area it can do damage. Never percuss the spine or breast bone. Also, if your daughter's breasts have developed, never percuss these. If percussion causes pain, stop and consult your physician before proceeding.

Vibration is done after secretions have been loosened within the respiratory system by percussion in order to help move secretions through the airway to where they can be coughed up. This procedure is done only while your child is exhaling through pursed lips. Again, get instructions from your doctor.

Percussor/vibrator machines may be recommended if you are having trouble getting the knack of percussion and vibration or if your child is learning to give himself or herself treatments. Check with your doctor whether a percussor would be helpful for your child, and if so, which type your doctor recommends. The strength of the vibration and percussion and the adaptability for use for independent therapy are all factors to consider.

Suctioning

Suctioning is performed to remove secretions or foreign matter from the airways if your child's cough is too weak to expectorate (expel) these.

Suctioning may be performed at home on children with tracheostomies or severe respiratory problems. Some children who have a weak cough or poor gag reflex due to neuromuscular disorders may also require suctioning.

If your child has had a tracheostomy, your doctor will explain and demonstrate the suctioning procedure for you. It is safe to do at home if done correctly, but be sure your doctor actually supervises you suctioning your child before you try to do it by yourself. Since your child will probably not like the procedure and may well gag, scream, or yell, you'll feel more confident if you really know what you are doing. Your hospital should provide written instruction on suctioning with a tracheostomy, but you may also want to get the free manual, *Tracheostomy Care*, or buy the *Tracheostomy Care Manual*. Both of these are listed in Appendix 3, "Suggested Reading."

Suction machines are generally electric powered (fig. 6-10). For versatility, some are designed to operate from alternative power

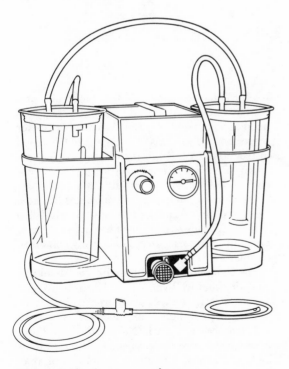

Figure 6-10   Suction machine.

sources. For example, Laerdal makes a unit that can be powered from an internal 12-volt rechargeable nickel-cadmium battery pack, any other 10–12-volt DC power source, or a car battery via the cigarette lighter. You can also get an adapter for travel abroad. Some machines come with wet-cell batteries, but these are more awkward when traveling. There are also foot-pump suction machines. If your child's life depends upon frequent suctioning, notify your electrical utility company so it can alert you in case of a planned outage or in case of power failure; also discuss with your doctor whether you should have a suction machine that will operate off alternative power sources or where you should go in case of a power outage. It is important for any child requiring frequent suctioning to have a backup suction machine in case your primary unit breaks down. Some families prefer having one portable unit for traveling.

Some communities have loan closets of medical equipment. Your Visiting Nurses Association, the Lung Association, or the respiratory therapy department at your hospital should know if any suction machines are available for loan. While a loaner may not always be the latest model, it might be sufficient for a child who needs only occasional suctioning or as a backup machine for the child who needs frequent suctioning.

A 60-cc irrigation syringe with a whistle-tip catheter can be used on a child in a pinch. Such a syringe is easy to carry with you at all times and can be used, for example, if your child suddenly needs suctioning in the supermarket or when you are going for a walk.

The location of your suction machine is very important, for you will need to have it readily available if your child needs suctioning. If your child has a tracheostomy, you may need a portable suction machine with you at all times. Other children may need suctioning only when sleeping or eating, so the suction machine may be kept in the bedroom or in a kitchen cupboard where it can be quickly reached and connected.

In an emergency such as severe aspiration, getting the machine working quickly is more important than having everything sterile, although it is, of course, best to keep a sterile catheter connected to the machine at all times. While you may usually suction your child while he or she is lying down, in case of severe aspiration it may be helpful to have your child hang over your knee or the end of the table (as described under "Postural Drainage" on page 64). This requires one person to hold the child and another to lie on the floor and suction, but combining the effects of gravity and suctioning works well.

Suctioning through a tracheostomy. If your child has had a tracheostomy, you should have been instructed on trach care and suctioning before your child left the hospital. We will just remind you here that suctioning is a sterile procedure and that cleanliness is essential.

The suctioning procedure will be performed only after you have gotten specific instructions from your doctor, watched him or her do the procedure, and then had him or her watch you suction. Your doctor will tell you whether to use the nose or mouth. The procedure should be performed as quickly as possible to prevent complications. While the doctor may give you written instructions, the following will provide you with a general outline, and you should note any special steps necessary for your child.

1. Plug in the machine.
2. Wash your hands.
3. Connect a sterile catheter of the size and type your doctor prescribed to the suction tubing.
4. Check the machine setting and turn the machine on.
5. Hyperoxygenate your child if prescribed by your doctor.
6. Dip the end of the catheter into some sterile water. (Tap water can be used in an emergency, such as severe aspiration, but since it is not sterile it should not be used for routine suctioning.)
7. Draw a little water through the tubing.
8. Insert the tube into the tracheostomy, mouth, or nose to the prescribed depth.
9. Slowly pull the catheter out, twisting it gently around while lifting your finger on and off the control valve of the catheter so you have intermittent suction. Never pull the catheter straight out with constant suction, because if the tube gets caught against the wall of the trachea it will pull membrane off the inner wall. When suctioning with a tracheostomy, remember to pull the catheter out slightly after meeting resistance, since you don't want to apply suction to the corina.
10. Draw some sterile water through the tube to clear secretions and repeat the procedure as necessary.

Remember, when you suction you place a foreign object directly into a body cavity, bypassing the normal defense mechanisms. This means that, unless your equipment is sterile, you may be putting germs into your child's body. The deeper you suction, the more careful you must be about keeping the equipment sterile. Suctioning equipment, like all respiratory equipment, should be disinfected daily or after each use if not used regularly.

Suctioning should be done only when necessary. It is best to first attempt to remove secretions by following your child's prescribed respiratory therapy program, which may include postural drainage and percussion.

OXYGEN THERAPY

Oxygen Sources

If your child becomes so ill that he or she can't get enough oxygen from the air, your child may need supplemental oxygen. When your doctor prescribes oxygen, make sure you get detailed instructions. Ask your doctor to write these down, or do so yourself and have your doctor check what you have written.

Oxygen is a relatively safe gas, but if it is concentrated or compressed it must be handled with care. While oxygen itself will not explode or burst into flames, it can aid in igniting combustible materials.

The room in which you use oxygen should be cool, dry, and well ventilated. Keep the oxygen approximately ten feet away from any heaters, radiators, pilot lights, or electrical apparatus that may cause a spark. Never store combustible material near the oxygen. Your hands must be free of any oil, grease, or petroleum product—such as Vaseline—before handling oxygen cylinders and oxygen equipment.

Obviously, no one should smoke, strike a match, or use a cigarette lighter in the same room. You may want to put "Caution: Oxygen in Use" signs (free from your local oxygen distributor) on the doors of the room you use for respiratory therapy so no one will smoke in there.

Compressed oxygen is 100-percent oxygen (O^2) in green cylinders, large and small. Some hospitals still use these cylinders in the rooms; other hospitals have oxygen piped into wall units from a central supply. Compressed oxygen is excellent if you want a supply of oxygen for emergencies or if your child uses oxygen infrequently. If your child uses oxygen continuously, an oxygen concentrator or liquid O^2 is cheaper and less trouble.

If you opt for cylinder oxygen, you will need cylinders and a stand to support a cylinder once in place. Cylinders should never be left free-standing, as they may tip and fall. The oxygen is under high pressure, and should a cylinder fall and the valve break off, the rapid elimination of the contents would turn the cylinder into a dangerous rocket. Small portable cylinders come with a wheeled stand or carrying case and can be moved about with ease.

Prepare a large cylinder for use as follows (fig. 6-11):

1. Unscrew the cap to expose the handle or knob.
2. "Crack" (open) the cylinder by slowly turning the handle or knob counterclockwise until you hear a loud rush of air. (Since your child may be frightened by such a sound, either have him in another room or warn your child before you do it.) Then quickly turn the knob clockwise to shut it off again. Do this before you attach the regulator, for this procedure keeps dust particles from getting into the regulator.
3. Connect the regulator and flowmeter to the cylinder outlet valve by fastening the regulator nut to the threaded connector on the cylinder.
4. Tighten the connection with a cylinder wrench. (Cylinder wrenches are made of special materials which will not create sparks.)
5. Attach the humidification bottle containing sterile water. (Large cylinder oxygen should always be humidifed before use for other than emergencies since it is 100 percent moisturefree and can cause dryness of the nasal and sinus cavities.)
6. Turn on the cylinder valve when you are ready to give the oxygen. To start the flow, adjust the flowmeter to the prescribed amount of oxygen. The flowmeter indicates the oxygen flow rate in liters per minute. Follow the specific directions your doctor has given you, for an overdose or un-

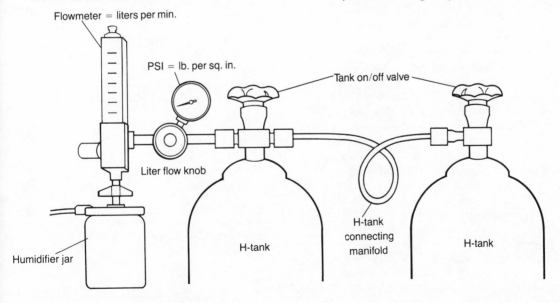

Figure 6-11 Compressed oxygen.

derdose of oxygen can cause serious complications.

7. Ask your oxygen delivery service for an oxygen cylinder capacity and flow chart (or have them explain the one in Appendix 1—pages 267–268— to you). Then you can calculate how long it will take for your child to use up a cylinder of oxygen and can judge when you will have to change cylinders and how much oxygen you need to keep on hand. If your child is dependent upon this oxygen, be sure you have a sufficient supply at home. Your supplier should have a 24-hour emergency service.

Small portable oxygen units can be used if your child needs oxygen when he or she goes out. You may also want to take such a unit along when you are traveling if you think your child may need oxygen.

Liquid oxygen is 100-percent oxygen cooled to 270°F below zero. Because it is so cold, it is much more dense than compressed oxygen, and one small container of liquid oxygen can hold approximately as much as three large green cylinders. You can refill portable containers from the storage tank.

Since the flowmeter and gauge are attached to the unit, all you have to do is attach the humidifier, which makes this system much easier to use than compressed oxygen. Obtain detailed instructions from your oxygen supplier.

An oxygen concentrator separates the oxygen from room air, thus supplying up to 96-percent oxygen, depending upon the flow rate. A concentrator may be appropriate if your child needs continuous oxygen therapy. As the flow rate goes up, the oxygen concentration decreases, so be sure the concentrator can deliver the oxygen concentration your child needs. As with cylinders and liquid oxygen, a concentrator needs a humidifier to add moisture to the oxygen. A concentrator is reasonably quiet and somewhat less "medical" looking than cylinders. Choose a concentrator with an alarm, so that you will know if the power fails. If your child is dependent upon this oxygen supply, you will need a backup supply of cylinder oxygen in case of power failure. Oxygen concentrators have a set of filters that routinely need to be changed; otherwise very little maintenance is required.

Liquid oxygen and oxygen concentrators are generally not cost-effective until your oxygen consumption is two liters per minute or greater on a 24-hour basis. The exception to this is the individual requiring a great deal of portable oxygen, since small portable oxygen cylinders are the most expensive way to purchase oxygen. Check with your insurance company about reimbursement.

Oxygen Delivery Systems

Nasal cannulas are now commonly used for infants and children, since the nasal prongs can be shaped to fit the facial contour and the oxygen flows directly and continuously into the airway (fig. 6-12). Ask your doctor which specific model would be best for your child. Although a cannula cannot deliver oxygen concentrations much above 40 percent, this is high enough for most home use. While using a cannula your child will still have some freedom of movement and be able to eat and talk.

The following steps should enable you to position a cannula correctly:

1. Place the nasal prongs in the nostrils. If they do not fit well, bend to shape.
2. Attach the cannula to your child's head. With some cannulas you position the tubing over and behind the ear and then secure a sliding adjuster under

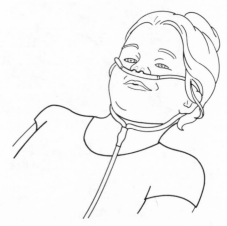

Figure 6-12   Nasal cannula.

the chin. Others have an elastic strap that fits around the patient's head.

3. Use 2-in.-square gauze pads to protect the cheek, behind the ears, or wherever needed if you see skin breakdown or your child complains of irritation from the tube rubbing.

4. Remove the cannula every eight hours and clean it with a moist cloth. At that time you may also want to wipe your child's mouth and nose. If these seem dry, your doctor may suggest a glycerine lotion (but not a petroleum-base product like Vaseline); make sure the lotion does not block the cannula openings.

The cannula should be cleaned every three days (see pages 73–74 for cleaning procedure). After extended use the cannula can become stiff and discolored and needs to be replaced.

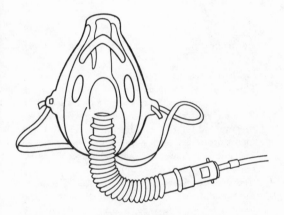

Figure 6-13   Venturi mask.

An **oxygen mask with a reservoir bag or a venturi mask** can be used when a high concentration of oxygen is needed (fig. 6-13). If your child needs a mask, your doctor will recommend a specific type and give you instructions for use. However, most alert patients prefer the cannula, since it is more comfortable and does not interfere with eating and speaking.

A **tracheostomy mask or T-tube** may be necessary if your child has a trach tube in place and needs supplemental oxygen or moisture. Your doctor will tell you which to use and how to use it.

Aids to Ventilation

Ventilation is the movement of air into and out of the lungs. Your child may need occasional or continuous assistance in moving the air.

An **intermittent positive pressure breathing (IPPB) machine** (fig. 6-14) may be prescribed to aid or improve your child's ventilation. An IPBB can also be used to deliver nebulized medication and/or oxygen during treatment. You can learn to use an IPPB machine safely at home if you take the necessary safety precautions:

• Have your doctor explain to you how the machine works and what pressure setting you should use. Be sure you understand what your doctor tells you and have him or her write out the instructions for you. This is *very* important, because if the setting is too low the treatment won't do much good; if it is too high, your child will be unable to exhale and turn the pressure off and may suffer lung damage. (Simply stated, when your child starts to inhale, the machine is triggered to deliver air until the pressure you have preset on the machine is reached. At that point, the flow stops, allowing for exhalation.) Check the setting every time before using the machine, especially if little hands are about that might like to turn dials.

• Make sure the mouthpiece fits correctly, for your child will be able to activate the machine only if he or she can make a good seal. Bennett Seal mouthpieces are effective with many children. If your child cannot use a mouthpiece, you will need a face mask. The masks made by IPPB manufacturers generally do not fit as comfortably as anesthesia masks, which you can purchase from your medical supplier. If you don't know what size your child needs and your supplier doesn't have samples, ask the head respiratory therapist at your local hospital to let you bring your child in so the two of you can determine which mask fits best.

• Attach the mask or mouthpiece with its strap, which fits around your child's head. Your child must be able to pull the mask off if necessary or to signal you immediately (which means you must be next to him or her ring the whole treatment). If your child can't pull the mask off, he or she may not want it strapped on the face, even if you are there. In that case, lay your child down. (Chest-down on a wedge-shaped pillow may be best for a child who has great difficulty swallowing secretions.) Then

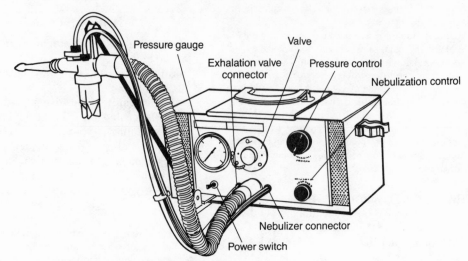

Figure 6-14   Intermittent positive pressure breathing machine.

simply hold the mask on your child's face with your hand. Make sure your child knows how to signal you (probably with a simple "mmmm") if he or she wants you to pull the mask off. It is important to respond immediately to your child's signal, for if the machine malfunctions and continues to force air when your child starts to exhale, the excess pressure can be harmful. If your child signals, remove the mask immediately, turn off the machine (so it doesn't nebulize that premeasured medication into the room), and find out what he or she wants. If the secretions are loosening, he or she may have to cough or spit up secretions. Try to have your child just turn the head to one side and spit on a tissue, for if you do postural drainage some of the medication may come out before it has had time to work. If your child feels too chokey, you may have to do postural drainage briefly or suction out the secretions.

- Nebulize all the medication for the prescribed length of time. Periodically tap the nebulizing chamber during the treatment so all of the medication still in the cup runs to the bottom to be nebulized. If the medication is used up before the end of the prescribed length of treatment, do *not* add more medication. But do continue the treatment for as long as has been prescribed. Check with your doctor to see whether you should continue the treatment without medication, or whether you should add some saline to the cup.
- Do percussion and vibration and then postural drainage if recommended.

The procedure for using an IPPB is as follows:

1. Wash your hands.
2. Measure out the medication, if your doctor has prescribed it, into the nebulizing chamber.
3. Position your child comfortably, as your doctor recommends. (Most children have IPPB treatments sitting up, because the lungs expand best in this position; however, some children are positioned lying down.)
4. Check the pressure setting.
5. Turn on the machine, and then position the mouthpiece or mask. Encourage your child to breath in the way your doctor has recommended.

A ventilator is a machine that can mechanically breathe for your child. Such mechanical ventilation has traditionally been used in hospital settings for children who cannot adequately breathe by themselves. However, in some cases it is now possible to care for such ventilator-dependent children at home.

However, if your child has a progressive condition and now has difficulty in breathing unassisted, you and your doctor may have to discuss whether long-term ventilatory support would improve the quality of your child's life or simply extend it. (See Chapter 18 for a discussion of this problem.)

If you decide upon home ventilation, there are

numerous types of ventilators available. Your doctor will have to determine which would be best for your child and will have to instruct you in its use.

CLEANING YOUR EQUIPMENT

Proper and routine cleaning of respiratory equipment is crucial to remove any left-over medicine or germs, and to prevent the establishment of disease-producing microorganisms (pathogens), all of which can be inhaled directly into the lungs when your child next uses the equipment. Many children get recurrent respiratory infections from improperly cleaned machines. Cleaning is very easy, if a bit tedious. Your doctor may recommend that you clean the machine after each treatment, in which case do so. However, all mist-producing equipment should be thoroughly cleaned at least once a day. Your doctor will recommend which cleaning method is best for your child's equipment. Soap and water are probably not strong enough. The usual cleaning solution recommended for use at home is a mild solution of acetic acid. Made by mixing one part of white vinegar with one part of tap water, this prevents the growth of pathogens more effectively than a weaker solution. If you need a large quantity of cleaning solution (as for an ultrasonic nebulizer), you can make the acetic-acid solution more cheaply by using glacial acetic acid, sold for developing film at photographic equipment stores, and diluting this with water. While white vinegar is only 5-percent acetic acid, glacial acetic is 99 proof, so it must be diluted for use. Any undiluted portion must be stored carefully out of reach of children and should be handled only when wearing rubber gloves. (Most chemical cleaning preparations you buy are also in concentrated form, so the same safety precautions would apply.)

To make a 5-percent solution with glacial acetic acid you need five parts acid to every 99 parts of water, or one part acid to every 19 parts water. If, for example, your container holds 20 cups of liquid when filled within about three inches of the top (you need to leave room for the machine parts), you would need to use one cup of acetic acid and 19 cups of water; if your pot

will hold over two gallons, or 32 cups, you would use one and a half cups of acetic acid and 28½ cups of water. After you make your first batch, draw a line with indelible marker on the container to indicate how far you should fill it with water after adding the acetic acid, which you have measured in a measuring cup. Since acetic acid is colorless, add a few drops of food coloring to the cleaning solution so everyone knows it is cleaning solution and not water.

Your doctor may recommend a commercially made cleaning solution, which you probably will have to dilute as you did the acetic acid. Most of these cleaning solutions have to be rinsed off the equipment after cleaning.

The cleaning procedure is not difficult if you proceed step by step:

1. Gather the following items:
   a. The manufacturer's diagram of how the machine parts fit together. If you do not have one, make a sketch yourself so you will be able to reassemble the parts once you have taken them apart.
   b. The cleaning solution (determined in consultation with your doctor).
   c. A plastic container with a lid in which to store the solution.
   d. A pot in which you can boil and sterilize your rinse water. (If your child uses an ultrasonic nebulizer and you make your own saline, you can make a little more saline in this pot and use it for rinse water.)
   e. A funnel for pouring liquids.
   f. A nail brush and a long-handled bottle brush for scrubbing.
   g. Rubber gloves to protect your hands. (The thin, lined type allow a better sense of feel than the thicker heavy-duty type.)
   h. A plastic colander in which to place rinsed parts.
   i. A line on which to hang the tubing to dry. You might string a line high over the sink so the tubes can drip into the sink (and probably over the counter as well).
2. Mix the solution. (The type of solution used will determine how long you can reuse it before making a new batch.)
3. Boil the necessary amount of water for sterile rinsing.
4. Wash your hands with soap and water, then dry them and put on your gloves. (In a pinch you can manage without gloves, but you will find the solu-

tion irritating to your skin, especially if you have any scratches or wounds on your hands.)

5. Take apart each piece of equipment to be washed and pour any remaining medication into the sink.

6. Wash everything first in hot, soapy water if your doctor recommends it. Be sure not to use soap that contains much fat, for the fat particles can leave a film on the equipment.

7. Place parts into the cleaning solution, making sure each is completely submerged with no trapped air. Let the parts swim for 30–60 minutes. Do not just dump the parts in the solution and forget them for a few hours: the rubber and plastic parts may start stretching, disintegrating, or showing other signs of adverse reaction to the chemical. (If on a given day you do not have time to soak the parts, a quick cleaning of the machine is still *far* superior to not cleaning the machine at all.)

8. If the solution you use requires rinsing, take each part out of the solution, give it a shake, and drop it into the sterile rinse water. Swirl the water around to make sure everything is well rinsed. Your child can inhale the unrinsed solution, which can cause irritation.

9. Take the parts out one by one, give them a shake, and place them into the colander. (You can hook hoses to your respiratory machine and blow out most of the water, but do not use a hair dryer.) Then hang hoses over your line to drip dry. Do not dry any parts with a towel, for unless your towel is sterile you simply ·recontaminate the parts.

10. Let everything dry thoroughly (overnight or 24 hours) in a clean place before using again. It is handy to have double sets of everything as well as a few extras of parts that are apt to break, stretch, or get lost so you have one set to use while the other is drying. You may want to cover the colander with a clean paper towel while the parts are drying.

11. Fill the bottle of an ultrasonic nebulizer with the chemical solution from your pot and let it sit for a while or overnight (if you have two bottles) before emptying, cleaning, and letting the bottle air dry.

12. Rinse any cleaning brushes or funnels in the remaining sterile water and put out to dry in the colander.

13. Rinse your gloves in water and hang them to dry; rinse the pot with tap water and dry. Both the gloves and the pot will deteriorate if exposed to saline for extended periods of time.

14. Put the equipment together again when everything is dry.

OBTAINING THE EQUIPMENT AND INFORMATION YOU NEED

Your child will probably not need all the equipment we have mentioned at once; rather, as your child's condition changes over time you may add or subtract components as you develop an individualized respiratory therapy program. Your doctor will help you as much as possible, but unless he or she specializes in lung diseases a respiratory therapist, a respiratory nurse, or a physical therapist may be able to help you more with information on home respiratory care. Many visiting nurses associations have nurses or therapists specializing in helping clients with home respiratory therapy programs.

If your child is hospitalized and is having respiratory therapy, learn as much as you can from the therapist there so you can carry on at home. If your child is not hospitalized and there is no respiratory therapist providing home care in your community, you can phone the local hospital and ask the respiratory therapist specific questions. Be polite, explain your needs, and ask when he or she will have time to talk with you. Many things can be explained over the phone.

If there is more than one supplier of respiratory equipment in your community, try to find the one that has the most qualified person working in respiratory therapy for children. Your hospital's head respiratory therapist or local Lung Association may be a good source of information, for most suppliers try to keep in contact with these people. Ask such professionals which services the various firms in town provide.

Some medical suppliers hire respiratory therapists to work with their clients in the home. These visits are usually nominally free but may be reflected in the higher costs of the items the company sells and rents. If your needs are very simple and routine, the additional cost of such a respiratory therapist may not be worth it. But if your child has complicated, ongoing needs, you may find such professional services well worth the additional cost.

Whomever you consult on your child's home program should also be able to advise you on equipment. Usually a month's rental can be deducted from the purchase price of the machines, so it's wise to try before you buy. Before you buy any machine, discuss the comparative virtues of the available equipment with the supplier and inquire as to which machines have the best performance record, whether spare parts are readily available, and whether the company will give you a loaner should your machine need cleaning or repair. If your child needs to use a machine daily, a reliable firm, even if it charges a little more, is well worth the cost. Some suppliers will also assist you in submitting your insurance or Medicaid claims, for they have learned what wording and support information is necessary.

EVALUATING YOUR HOME RESPIRATORY THERAPY PROGRAM

You should know how your doctor decides whether your child's therapy program is effective because respiratory problems aren't always visible. Also, it is frequently difficult to see the results of any treatment. Changes are often gradual, and because many respiratory conditions can't be cured treatment may simply help your child continue to function at the present level.

There are certain factors which can help your doctor and you assess changes in your child's condition:

- Does your child look different? (Gray or bluish lips, tongue, ear lobes, and finger nails are indications of severe oxygen deprivation in most children. However, an anemic child's oxygen can get very low without any color change.)
- Does your child act differently? (Insufficient oxygen may cause a child to be sluggish, tired, depressed, forgetful, or to lose appetite.)
- Is your child breathing differently? (Any changes— shallower, deeper, noisier, quieter—can be significant.)
- Does your child's breathing sound different through a stethoscope? (Your doctor may have recommended that you use a stethoscope so you can hear less obvious problems. It takes time to learn what different sounds mean, but if you use a stethoscope regularly you will learn what your child sounds like and will know if changes occur.)

- Are there any changes in your child's sputum? (Color change, increased or decreased amount, increased difficulty in raising sputum, thicker sputum, mucus plugs, or change in odor should all be noted.)
- Does your child say it hurts when he or she breathes?
- Is your child coughing more or less?
- Does your child have a fever?
- Does your child tell you he or she feels different? (Sometimes this will be only a vague statement, like "I feel tight," which he or she can't further elaborate but which indicates that something is wrong.)

If your child has asthma, your doctor may recommend that you purchase a "peak-flow meter," with which you can monitor your child's airway obstruction. Your respiratory therapist can teach you how to use one at home.

Sometimes it is easier to pick up illness in a child than in an adult, for your child may not be as active, may act sluggish or irritable, or have a poor appetite. Whenever you get any clues, it is important to discuss them with your doctor immediately, for if your child gets medical attention at the first signs of an infection, while this may not prevent illness, it can often lessen its severity.

When you report changes to your doctor, he or she may wish to do some or all of the following:

- See your child.
- Run a sputum culture.
- Take an X ray to see what the lungs look like if he or she suspects significant problems.
- Measure pulmonary function.

On the basis of all this information your doctor may then suggest:

- Continuing the present program.
- Checking that your child is receiving treatments correctly.
- Changing or adding treatments.
- Changing or adding medication.
- Modifying your child's diet or increasing your child's fluid intake (both of these can help liquify secretions).
- Checking how you are cleaning your equipment (inadequately cleaned equipment can be the source of recurring infections.)

While some problems are common to many individuals, each child has unique needs. So you may have to be inventive and try out different ways of doing things. But you will find out what works best with your child. And if he or she follows the respiratory therapy program regularly, you will find it can make an incredible difference in your child's life.

PART 2

MEETING YOUR CHILD'S DAILY PHYSICAL NEEDS

7

Positioning Your Child: Beds, Wheelchairs, and Other Orthopedic Equipment

It is important to learn how to help your child get positioned lying, sitting, and standing so he or she is not only comfortable but can use and further develop existing muscle strength. The greater the controlled motor movement, the more independent your child will be in moving about and caring for himself or herself, learning and playing, and interacting with other people. Moreover, correct positioning and maximum movement aid normal body functions such as circulation, respiration, and elimination while reducing physical deformities and pressure sores.

Rehabilitation doctors and orthopedists, as well as pediatric physical and occupational therapists, can be of great assistance to you. These health-care professionals are skilled in determining not only how but also in what a child can best be positioned. With some children you can simply use standard equipment such as beds, high chairs, strollers, and so on. But you may have to either adapt such equipment or purchase special equipment for the disabled child. A pediatric therapist should have a good idea of what special equipment is available, as well as what standard children's items can either be used as they are or adapted to meet special needs.

Equipment for positioning and mobility is expensive; and it is useless if it does not meet your child's particular needs. Therefore, try out any equipment before you buy it. Ideally, your local vendor will carry samples of what is available so you can actually see the equipment and have your child try it in the store. Alternatively, your therapist may know children using the same or similar equipment in your area and may be able to coordinate your therapy appointment with that of another family, allowing you to try out the item in the clinic.

A longer trial period with a piece of equipment is, of course, ideal. Sometimes your vendor can arrange this, perhaps allowing the monthly rental charge to be deducted from the final purchase price.

If you live in a rural area, and resources for trying out equipment are limited, try to find a large distributor of medical supplies and equipment located in a city who is willing to send a salesperson (and the equipment you are interested in) to your home. Try to coordinate this with a home visit by the therapist. If your child receives therapy at a clinic, perhaps the meeting can be held there. You have to apply any basic principles your doctors and therapists teach you to the specific needs of your child. It is through providing insights into the particular needs of your child that you can work most effectively with health-care professionals.

Don't despair if there are no therapists in your area. Work with your orthopedist and rehabilitation doctor, look through equipment catalogs and magazines for the disabled (see Appendix 3, "Suggested Reading"), and phone companies to speak with their salespeople to discuss their products and perhaps even arrange for them to come and show you their wares. You can then make an intelligent purchase based on the information you have gathered. While this isn't ideal, you can manage, although you will have to do a lot more of the thinking and legwork yourself.

In determining how best to position your

79

child, consider also where to position your child so he or she can be as actively involved in family life as possible. Don't be trapped by what you consider to be normal functions of rooms in your home or routine methods of procedure. If, for example, your child has to spend some time lying down immobile, as with a body cast, and consequently will have to spend almost the whole day in bed, put the bed, or even a hospital bed, close to the action in the living room or dining room. If your child is permanently immobile and has to spend much time lying, arrange for your child to lie on the floor, couch, or table, using padding or bedding as necessary.

Remember, no one position by itself is adequate. Rather, you must establish a repertoire of positions and change them frequently. If your child cannot reposition himself or herself, you will have to help him or her do so at least every two hours. Pressure sores, one of the greatest hazards of the disabled person, can result from remaining in one position too long. So it is not only important to reposition your child frequently but also to watch for early signs of pressure sores, more fully described in Chapter 10. Bodily functions are also greatly helped by changes in position.

LYING

When we lie down, we are prone (on our stomachs), supine (on our backs), or on our sides. Do the following exercises to see how your child might feel in these positions.

First lie flat on your back on the floor. You'll have a fine view of the ceiling or anything right above you but a limited view of the rest of the room. Lying with a wedge-shaped pillow under your head increases your range of vision forward and to the sides as long as you are able to move your head. The longer you lie on your back—level, head-up, or head-down—the more you will feel the difference in each position.

Now if you roll over and lie on your stomach you either turn your head to one side or mash your nose into the floor. Again vision is limited, especially if you cannot turn your head to the other side. When lifting your head, you can look

about yourself very nicely, but if you use your arms to support yourself, they not only get tired but their movement is restricted. If you use a rolled-up pillow or blanket as a bolster placed under your chest at a level just below the armpits, it is easier to move the shoulders, use the hands, and move the head.

Now lie on your side with your body completely relaxed and limp. If you hold this position long enough, the arm on the floor will get sore and fall asleep. Your legs will get stiff unless bent somewhat, and the bony parts of your legs (ankles and knees) will hurt unless there is some padding between them and between your legs and the floor. If you can make your body go really limp you may begin to roll onto your back. However, if you position yourself properly you will probably find lying on your side most comfortable, and this is why many of us sleep this way. This is a safe position for those children having trouble with vomiting or swallowing secretions.

Now lie in the various positions in different parts of different rooms and try to imagine not only how your child feels but also where he or she can be most stimulated and involved in the environment. You may discover that your child will be much more involved with you when lying in one part of a room than another. For example, looking out a window is more interesting than looking at a blank wall or a bare ceiling. And being in a room with people is more interesting than being shut off in a bedroom.

If your child must spend a great deal of time in a bed set against the wall, alternate the end on which the pillow is placed so your child does not always lie on the same side to face the center of the room. If your child tends to keep his or her head turned toward one side, position your child so he or she will have to turn it toward the opposite side to see the interesting objects or activities in the room. This is not only good for the muscles of the whole body but can also help to prevent asymmetry of the skull or bald spots on the side of the head that is always against the pillow.

Discuss with your doctor or therapist the advantages of lying prone, supine, or on the side.

Pediatric physical and occupational therapists can be especially helpful with positioning.

The supine position (on the back) provides a limited range of vision. Your child can see more if you prop his or her head up, and you can improve postural drainage, should your child have respiratory problems, by tilting the head down. (Any home respiratory therapy program involving postural drainage should be set up in consultation with your child's health-care team.) You can tilt your child by placing him or her on a wedge-shaped cushion or by placing blocks of wood under the feet of the bed. You can make the space above your child more interesting by stringing toys or mobiles overhead. Hammocks can make supine lying very relaxing.

There are several disadvantages to the supine position. It is dangerous if a child vomits, for he or she may aspirate and this can be fatal. Also, the supine position puts a strain on the lower back. Though this can be reduced by placing a pillow under the knees, such positioning makes it impossible to straighten the legs fully and can therefore cause contractures due to shortening of the muscles, particularly with cerebral-palsied children. Finally, mobility is very limited.

The prone position (lying on the stomach) can be a good position for sleeping. There is much less danger of aspiration, and contractures of the hip and knee can be prevented, since the muscles that flex the hips and the knees, which are always bent during sitting, get stretched out. However, prone positioning is often contraindicated for children who have trouble breathing or who have severe cardiac problems.

The prone position is good for playing and taking in the sights, particularly if your child can hold his or her head up (fig. 7-1). However, your child may have the strength to hold up his or her head for only limited periods. If your child lies on a bolster placed at the level just below the armpits, the arms are more free for play and the head for movement. You can make such a bolster by rolling up a towel or blanket (your linen closet can be a valuable resource in positioning).

However, if your child will need to use a bolster regularly, either buy or make a permanent one. The prone position also helps develop the weight-bearing capacities of the upper extremities. But the prone position may not be recommended for the child whose pelvis or legs are twisted or who already has severe contractures. Moving about is possible for the child who can hold his or her head up in the prone position and has some use of arms or legs.

A *prone crawler* is a platform with wheels (fig. 7-2). This supports the child's trunk while the child moves with his or her hands and legs. A prone crawler can offer a helpful intermediate step between lying and crawling for small children. If your young child is temporarily restricted to a lying position because of surgery or a body cast, you can use a wooden platform and add four casters. Always use very good casters, or your child may become frustrated in attempting to move, especially on carpets. Another alternative is simply to use a little red wagon. Your child can learn to use it as a prone crawler; if you are going longer distances, you can just pull your child. Pad the wagon as necessary.

A disadvantage of this mode of movement is that the child is close to the ground and therefore you have to continually bend over to care for him or her. Also, the child gets a good look at table legs but not at anything much higher than your knees.

A *gurney* will get your child up higher, where the action is, for this nonfolding padded five-to-six-foot stretcher on wheels usually has an adjustable height of 24–30 inches (fig. 7-3). It has eight-inch rear casters and 24-inch front wheels, which a child as young as five can learn to propel. You may be able to borrow a gurney from an organization like the Visiting Nurses or rent one from a hospital-supply house. It is a great aid for any child who is restricted to lying down, even if only for a few weeks. The amount of room needed to maneuver a gurney is significant and should be considered. A danger in making a child in a cast mobile on a prone crawler or gurney is that the cast makes the child much heavier while impeding coordination and sense of balance. If a child falls off any vehicle, such as a prone crawler or a gur-

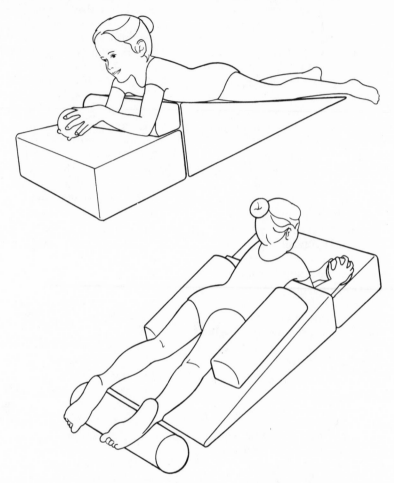

Figure 7-1   Child playing on wedge-shaped pillow. Foam shapes may be added for positioning as necessary.

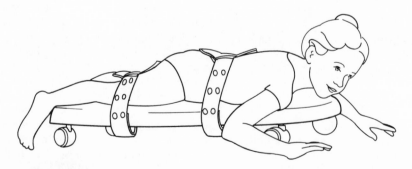

Figure 7-2   Prone crawler.

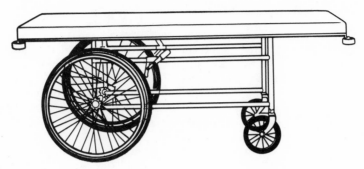

Figure 7-3   Gurney.

ney, he or she can damage not only the cast but himself or herself as well. Therefore you may need to add adequate restraints such as seat belts or railings to keep your child from falling off the vehicle.

The side-lying position can be very beneficial for palsied children, since it helps achieve relaxation of tight muscles, helps decrease uncontrolled flailing movements, and helps the child bring his or her hands together so they can be used for bilateral manipulative activities (fig. 7-4). This position is best when the head is supported slightly and the lower arm is pulled forward from under the body so the hands can be used for play. The hips and knees can be slightly flexed, and pillows can be placed between the legs for better positioning and the prevention of pressure sores.

Beds

Beds, as we all know, can enhance or interfere with sleep. If the bed is too hard, too soft, or too lumpy, we do not sleep well. Think of how much harder it must be for a child to get to sleep and stay asleep if he or she can't shift position or adjust the covers or has difficulty breathing. Try to analyze your child's needs in order to help your child (and you) get a good night's sleep.

A standard bed may be appropriate for your child, especially if you make some modifications. You may find it easier to care for your child if you raise the bed by placing wooden blocks under the legs. If your child needs to sleep head-up or head-down, just put blocks under one end. While increasing the height may hinder your child's ability to get into it and out of it

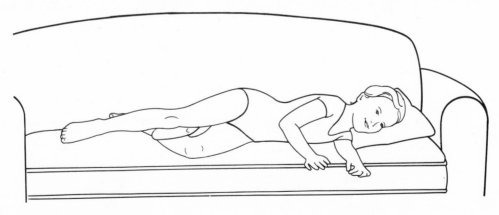

Figure 7-4   Side-lying position.

alone, it may make it possible to use a mechanical lift.

A hospital bed can be rented for short-term use or purchased if you think your child will need one for a long time. The advantages of such a bed are:

- The bed is on casters, so it can be moved about.
- The height of the bed can be adjusted, which can facilitate transfer and help save your back, since you don't have to bend over so much.
- The angle of the head and foot can be adjusted to allow for a variety of positions.

However, don't let these advantages tempt you to leave your child in bed too long.

Water beds help relieve pressure and consequently help prevent pressure sores on people who cannot move. The movement of the water can also make for comfort. Your child may even be able to use the water movement to roll over. (But many people find it easier to roll over on a firm surface.)

Water beds have disadvantages too. Because they rest on platforms, it is difficult to use a lift with one. And since water beds must remain level, they may not be effective if your child has respiratory problems and needs to sleep tilted head-up or -down. Finally, water beds are heavy and can cause a minor flood in the bedroom if they spring a leak. Water pads, which can be placed on a regular bed, can be useful alternatives, but they can't be heated and therefore need insulating covers of foam or some other material.

Rolling beds are the only mechanical answer for the child who cannot roll over alone at night (fig. 7-5). Such beds are very expensive. If you decide your child might need one, be sure the equipment is carefully evaluated by a professional working with your child before you purchase it. If you cannot find an appropriate bed, a last resort is to try enlisting the help of engineers, such as those in a university or business, to custom-build a bed. You can have a bed built that rolls from side to side and from head to toe. You may have to experiment to discover the best timing and frequency at which your child should be rolled.

Bedding will vary according to your child's needs and preferences. Experiment with regular sheets, flannel sheets, blankets (wool, synthetic, electric), and comforters. A foot-cradle device that holds the bedding off the feet at the end of the bed is helpful if the weight of the blankets causes discomfort or makes it difficult for your child to roll over. You can also make a cradle to hold the covers off the body, which might be necessary if your child is recovering from a pressure sore and needs to lie with no weight on the affected part of the body. If covers make it hard for your child to roll, try to find an extra-warm sleeper so he or she needs fewer, if any, covers.

The sleeping surface can influence how frequently a child must change position during the night and whether he or she can do so without assistance. It is also important in the prevention of pressure sores, a real danger for any child with loss of mobility. Therefore when choosing your child's sleeping surface, consider how well he or she could roll over and transfer and whether the surface would help prevent pressure sores.

Consider the following:

Sheets must be fitted and wrinklefree.

A sheepskin can be placed on top of the sheet to provide for some air circulation and cushioning. While real sheepskins are somewhat more effective, synthetic ones are cheaper and can be easily laundered at home in your washing machine. Remember, as your child grows a longer sheepskin will be needed so the heels are still padded.

A foam insert can be placed under the sheet. These are often used in hospitals and can be obtained from medical-supply and rental stores. Consult a rehabilitation specialist for the best kind.

An "air bladder" mattress provides optimal protection but is also very expensive.

A water bed, discussed earlier, distributes weight and therefore prevents pressure buildup under vulnerable bony parts, making it possible for some people to sleep longer in one position. Some find it easy to roll over on a water bed, others do not.

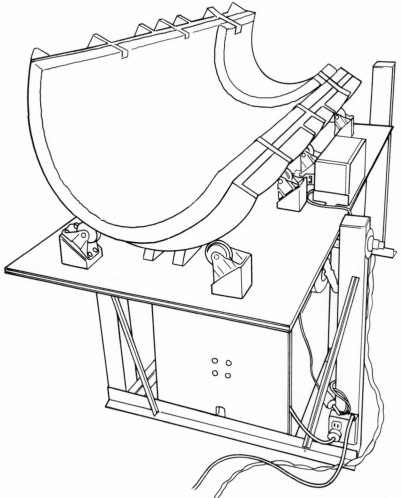

Figure 7-5 Custom-made moving bed: half cylinder rotates from side to side; platform tilts from head to toe.

If your child uses any respiratory equipment at night, read Chapter 6 for advice on keeping him or her comfortable while sleeping.

SITTING

Sitting upright or at least in a semireclined position is good for almost all children, since it is easier to see and interact with the surroundings when sitting than when lying down. The follow-

ing exercise will demonstrate the need for the correct chair(s) in which your child can sit. First, get a pebble or similar hard object. Place it under your bottom while you sit on the edge of a table with your legs dangling over the edge. Now sit this way for at least a few minutes, preferably half an hour, while you read this book or do something else. Your dangling feet are stretched beyond their normal 90-degree angle and may begin to hurt; your thighs will feel pressure where the table ends; your back would appreciate some support; and that pebble gives you some idea how uncomfortable wrinkles and folds beneath the immobile sitting child can be.

Obviously you would be more comfortable if your back were supported and if you could rest your feet on the floor. The same is true for your child. Chairs with maximal weight distribution and adequate support are, of course, more comfortable for extended sitting. Armrests and supportive surfaces of an appropriate height need to be considered. A headrest may or may not be indicated, depending on what your child is doing, such as sitting in one place, eating, moving about in a wheelchair or car. If your child cannot get in and out of chairs alone or lacks sensation from the waist down, any chair he or she sits in should be padded for comfort, support, and the prevention of pressure sores.

Padding should be soft enough for comfort yet firm enough to prevent any further deformity or asymmetry, especially in children with spinal curvatures. Many types of foam are now available, varying in density (which influences firmness), durability, ease of care, and price. While you may need padding made by a medical-equipment company, it may be more practical and inexpensive to buy foam from an upholsterer and maybe even have it covered.

Remember that, whereas you know through experience that some chairs are more comfortable than others, some children cannot communicate their discomfort to you. Even those who can talk sometimes think that discomfort is a part of life and can't see by themselves how their position could be changed to bring greater comfort.

Have a variety of chairs in which your child can sit. Not only will he or she sit differently in each one, but if you have a variety of places to seat your child you will be more apt to move him or her to change positions and less apt to leave your child in one chair for more than an hour or two.

Seats for Infants

A car seat may have been the first seat your child ever sat in, if you brought your child home from the hospital after birth in a car seat.

Some car seats are designed only for infants

(birth to 17–20 lbs.). Some are only for toddlers and preschoolers (17–20 to 50 lbs.). And some are called "convertible" because they can be converted from the infant mode to the toddler mode according to manufacturer's instructions when your child reaches 17–20 lbs. Any car seat you buy should be marked "dynamically tested," which means it has passed federal safety standards. Car beds and flimsy plastic feeding chairs are *not* safe for car travel.

No one car seat is best. You must choose which seat best suits your needs by considering the following factors:

- Does your child sit well in the seat? If your child has a poor sense of balance or cannot sit unsupported, try to find a seat that offers as much support as possible. When you have chosen the best available chair, you can, if necessary, fill long tube socks with foam and wedge these in on either side of your child between his or her body and the seat.
- Does the seat fit well in the car? Since the shapes of the seats of different models of cars differ, you will have to try out which seat fits best in your own car(s).
- Is the seat easily attached to the car? Particularly if you want to use the seat in more than one car (and maybe also in the house), you'll want a seat that can easily be moved, for the seat does any good only if your child is actually in it every time you go for a ride in the car.
- Are your seat belts long enough to hold the car seat in place?
- Does the car seat need a top harness or tether strap to prevent the top of the seat (and the child's head) from falling forward? Such tether straps must be permanently installed in each car your child will ride in. If you think a tether strap is too much of a hassle to install and use, try to find a seat that doesn't require a tether strap.
- Do the harness straps fit comfortably around your child and can you put them on easily?
- Is the seat wide enough for your child, especially if he or she is wearing bulky clothing or orthopedic appliances?
- Is the backrest high enough to protect your child's head? If your child needs head support on the side, are the side "wings" long enough?
- Is the seat of proper height? There should be at least three inches between the top of the seat and the roof of the car for safety.
- Can you still see well out of the rear mirror when your child is seated?

Carefully consider these factors when buying a car seat for your child. If your child is over four and needs support while sitting, try to get a car seat designed for the larger disabled child. After buying your child a car seat, use it so every ride is a safe ride.

A cloth baby-carrier, with which you strap your baby to the front of your body, can, after the car seat, provide the first sitting experience for an infant. Full body support is provided, and the baby profits from the closeness to you, although the child's vision may be limited. The advantage of baby-carriers is that most babies are happy being held by you and moved about. If you "wear" your child, you have your hands free to get on with the tasks of the day. This can be important, for it can be very frustrating if your baby starts to cry when you put him or her down and want to get to work. The baby-carrier also gives you more mobility outside the home if, for example, you want to do errands or go for walks.

A frame baby-carrier that fits on your back is better for older infants and toddlers. Their trunks will be fully supported (and you can make them sit more securely by stuffing foam pieces or a small blanket between their body and the frame). In case your child has limited head support, some deluxe carriers have detachable headrest extensions. Further support can be provided by using a headband to attach the head to the headrest, as with American Indian papoose packboards. If you can't devise something like this yourself, call on your local orthotist or prosthetist, who may be very innovative and helpful. A padded backpack waistband comes with some deluxe models and can be attached to most other baby-carriers. This distributes some of the weight from your shoulders to your waist, making it possible to carry a much heavier child with ease. As with cloth carriers, frame carriers are great if you need your hands free or if you want to walk over terrain too rough for the average baby stroller.

A sling can be used to carry a light, young child who lacks sufficient trunk and head support to sit in a frame baby-carrier. The sling goes under your child and then up and across your opposite shoulder. You support the back and head with your arm. Slings are a good alternative for short distances if you don't have a stroller with you or want to walk short distances over rough terrain.

Plastic infant seats provide the first sitting support for most infants. If your child has uncontrolled movements or wears orthopedic appliances, be sure to try your child out in the seat before you buy it, so you can check that he or she sits comfortably and won't capsize the chair. If you can't find a suitable plastic infant seat, using the more stable car seat or a reclined bath seat in the house may be a solution.

High chairs are excellent for the child who outgrows an infant seat and can sit with some support. If you are buying a high chair and you think your child will spend more time in it than most children, explore the latest innovations and see if any would be helpful. For example, an oversized tray provides additional play area. If the tray swings down and stores at the side of the chair, it is easier to support your child while getting the tray positioned than if the tray has to be completely removed.

Some high chairs come with casters, but you can take the rubber guards off the bottom of any high chair and attach wheels, purchased at a hardware store. As with most things, the more expensive the wheel, the better it will probably work. If your child is too heavy to carry in the chair, consider attaching good casters. And if you know before you buy a chair that your child will be spending a lot of time in it, the additional cost to give your son or daughter a better chair is well justified.

If you find a standard chair in which your child sits comfortably and well, with the help of your orthotist you can modify it through the years as necessary, perhaps adding a chest strap to stabilize your child's trunk, a backrest to support the head, a head strap to keep the head from falling forward, chest and neck supports to align the trunk, a wheelchair seat cushion, larger and lower footrests as your child grows, a mobile arm support, and bigger and better casters (fig. 7-6). Although you might consider this the "Band-Aid" approach to making a good chair, adding to

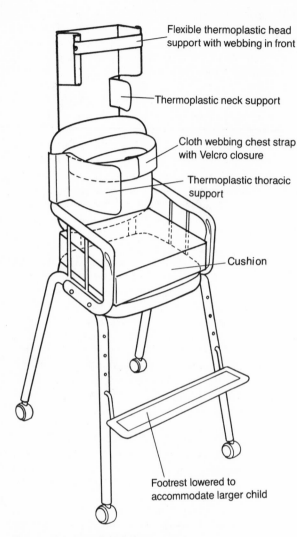

Flexible thermoplastic head support with webbing in front

Thermoplastic neck support

Cloth webbing chest strap with Velcro closure

Thermoplastic thoracic support

Cushion

Footrest lowered to accommodate larger child

Figure 7-6　Modified high chair.

the original chair as needed can give your child what he or she needs. The adjustments may be costly, but they will probably be much less than the cost of a commercial chair designed for the disabled; besides, your child's chair will be "custom-made."

A play table is an alternative to a high chair. It looks (and folds up) like a card table and has a seat that folds open in the middle of the table. The child has a greater play area than with a high chair. The child also sits lower, which can be nice if he or she wants to be closer to other children, but the child may be able to see less of what is going on in the room since he or she is lower than in a high chair.

Strollers and Pushchairs

A standard stroller may be the best way to get about with your child if he or she can sit reasonably well unassisted. Seated almost upright, your child will be able to look around, and he or she will have a small tray for toys. If your child has poor balance, make a chest strap of cotton webbing and Velcro or buy a commercial harness or support vest.

Modified strollers, which provide more positioning aids, such as hip abductors and chest and head supports, are expensive. You may want to consider doing your own modifications with some professional advice from your pediatric physical therapist or occupational therapist. For example, if your child is in a body cast, you can position him or her in a semireclining position by readjusting the seat with padding or by sewing a new canvas seat. For the child who would rather stand than sit or lie, you can take the seat out and make a platform on which to stand. Strollers are designed for stability and with the correct center of gravity for a young seated child of average weight. If your child is heavier than normal due to a cast, or is positioned differently than usual due to condition or age, be sure to check whether the stroller is stable. If not, you may need to weight one end or make other modifications.

Collapsible umbrella strollers are so named because the folded stroller vaguely resembles a folded umbrella. The lightweight models offer little support for a child with spasticity or extreme muscle weakness. However, large-size and extrasturdy umbrellastyle strollers are available for children with disabilities. Special features include trunk harnesses, seat inserts, footrests, and heavy-duty castered wheels.

Even with these modifications, an umbrella stroller may not offer the same kind of support as a modified stroller. However, the umbrella stroller is much lighter and more portable. Some children sit better in these, since the cloth material of the seating molds to their bodies, thus providing support.

Push and travel chairs position the child to be somewhat reclined (fig. 7-7). Accessories to position the head, trunk, and hips are available. The advantage of a travel chair is that the rear wheels retract, turning it into a car seat. This is a big advantage if your child has outgrown standard car seats yet needs support while sitting in the car or cannot transfer unassisted. You may find a travel chair that converts into a car seat far superior to a standard pushchair, which necessitates transferring and repositioning the child whenever you go out by car, bus, train, or plane.

An ultralightweight wheelchair with push handles may be appropriate for a very young child who can usually propel himself or herself but needs help over longer distances or up inclines (see fig. 7-10).

WHEELCHAIRS

A wheelchair (often simply called a chair) can give a disabled child some greatly needed independence and mobility—two things many able-bodied people take for granted. A child may be able to walk short distances, but if this requires great effort he or she will not be as mobile as other children and may spend more time than necessary inactive, alone, or sitting or lying in improper positions. (Of course, a wheelchair should not be used as an excuse for not teaching a child to walk or not helping a child develop the muscles and coordination he or she has.)

Almost every nonambulatory child should have a wheelchair in which he or she can sit reasonably upright (even if only for short periods) and can wheel or be wheeled from place to place and take in the activities of the day.

Even if a chair offers your child independent mobility or the ability to sit in the correct posture, he or she should still have periods out of the chair during the day to get a fuller range of motion than just sitting would provide. Time spent out of the wheelchair might include walking, playing, or just lying on the floor or couch, sitting

in other chairs, or having a midday nap.

Not only is the traditional chair, with big wheels in the back and small wheels in the front, available with a variety of options, but there is also available a range of motorized wheelchairs that might be more appropriate for a child unable to operate a manual wheelchair. No one chair is best for all children. With the help of health-care professionals you will have to consider in which type of chair your child can be correctly and comfortably positioned and whether he or she can safely maneuver such a chair to achieve maximum independence.

The Manual Wheelchair—Driving Parts and Their Accessories

Following is important information on different types of wheelchairs and their components. With this information you should be able to decide on the best type of chair for your child.

The framework is made of metal tubing (fig. 7-8). While the type of tubing used will affect the cost and durability of a chair, the more important factor to consider is the weight of the chair, for this can greatly influence how your child can maneuver in it.

The large wheels in the rear are used for propelling and are available in different sizes, from 20 to 24 inches. Pneumatic tires with inflatable inner tubes are the most shock absorbent. Some manufacturers now offer "thorn-proof" inner tubes, which are somewhat more durable. A solid-rubber tire is the most durable but also the least shock absorbent. A compromise is a polyurethane tire with a hollow or internal foam core; this provides some cushioning yet requires no maintenance.

The handrim or pushrim, which a person grips and pushes to propel himself or herself, is slightly smaller than the large wheel and attached to the rim of it.

For the child having only one arm with which to push a chair, one-arm wheelchairs are available.

If your child has limited range of motion or strength, you can make the handrim easier to

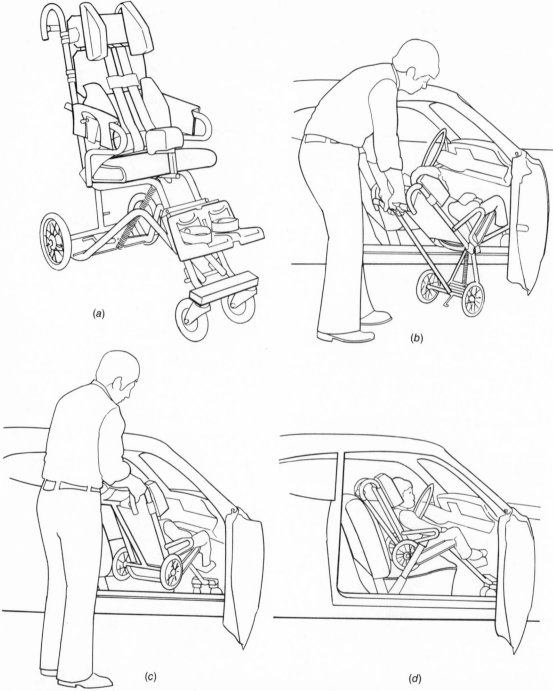

Figure 7-7   Travel chair converts into car seat: *(a)* the chair; *(b)* raise front wheels, pivot chair, and place front wheels on car floor; *(c)* press hand trigger to retract rear wheels; *(d)* position chair on car seat and fasten safety belt around child in chair.

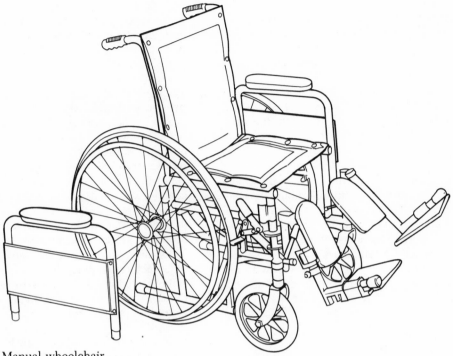

Figure 7-8   Manual wheelchair.

push by adding plastic coated vertical or oblique projections, known by those who use them as quad pegs. If your child would have difficulty gripping the handrim, many manufacturers will now add a friction coating. As the stickiness of this surface varies among companies, be sure you and your child examine a sample of the coating before ordering it. You can wrap the rim yourself with foam, friction tape, or IV tubing. Your child might also want to consider wearing a wheelchair glove or cuff, which not only provides friction but protects the hand.

Levers can be attached to the wheels for children who lack the hand control needed to propel the rims but who can perform the forward-backward motion a lever requires. These are hard to find and usually need to be ordered with the chair; the most common ones are European.

The small front wheels, often called casters, swivel. The larger the caster, the easier it is to push the chair over rough, soft, or irregular terrain, like dirt, sand, lawn, rugs, and doorsills. While an eight-inch caster will provide more maneuverability, it will make the chair a bit less stable than a five-inch caster. Small front casters are traditionally made of solid rubber. As with the large tires, the biggest innovation in casters has come through the use of polyurethane. Since these casters are narrower, they often roll and turn better than conventional solid-rubber casters.

Spring-loaded caster forks absorb some of the shock into the forks when going over an obstacle, such as a rock or a doorsill. Thus less resistance goes into the frame, making it easier to move the caster wheel over the obstacle.

Brakes (also called wheel locks) are crucial for stopping and parking. They should be located within easy reach. Sometimes a single lever operates the brakes on both large wheels; sometimes each big wheel has a separate brake. Brakes are commonly applied by pushing the lever forward and released by pulling. However, if you think your child could operate a pull brake better than a push brake, see if you can get that option. Extensions can be attached to brake handles for persons with restricted reach, but since they can get in the way when transferring (getting out of the chair) sideways, it is best if the extensions can be removed. Look into the various types of brakes available to see which would be best for your child.

Wheelchair narrowers are devices with which you can decrease the width of a nonmotorized standard wheelchair up to four inches. Such a device is marvelous if your child has trouble getting through narrow doorways or maneuvering in small spaces. A temporary narrower can be made out of a belt or rope; this is handy to remember if you are ever away from home and find a doorway just a bit too narrow for your child's chair.

The Manual Wheelchair—Supporting Parts and Their Accessories

The seat is one of the most important parts of the chair, because it supports most of the weight and can therefore help cause or prevent pressure sores. The standard collapsible-wheelchair seat is made of an easily folding material, such as Naugahyde or nylon. Such a sling seat and back of a folding wheelchair may not be appropriate if your child has weakness, paralysis, or spasticity, for they can contribute to deformities such as spinal curvatures and pelvic obliquity. For such children a padded solid seat and back inserts, which you can remove to collapse the chair, may be recommended. A sling seat or padded insert may be sufficient for children sitting in chairs for short periods of time. But if your child is going to spend much time in the chair, you will have to consider getting an appropriate cushion.

Wheelchair cushions come in all shapes, sizes, and costs. They are designed to help distribute pressures, especially over bony prominences, thus preventing the problems associated with prolonged sitting, the greatest of which are skin breakdown and pressure sores. An expensive cushion is far cheaper than the cost of healing a pressure sore. Obviously, the lighter a child, the less pressure he or she exerts while sitting and the smaller the problem with tissue breakdown. Therefore a lightweight or young child may not need as sophisticated a cushion as an older or heavier child. But any child lacking sensation below the waist needs to have the buttocks and other pressure-sensitive areas checked daily for redness and other signs of skin problems.

Rehabilitation centers are equipped to do complete evaluations of your child's sitting needs. If you have such a center nearby, utilize its services. You may need a referral from your doctor to get an appointment. Investigate the wide variety of cushions available, considering such factors as durability (especially if your child is incontinent or likes to poke holes in things), weight (which will influence how well your child propels himself or herself), and ease of care.

No one cushion is consistently better than another. It depends upon your child's needs. A simple foam cushion may be sufficient in the beginning for a small child, but remember that it is cheaper and easier in the long run to seat your child properly. At some time *before* pressure sores develop, a professional evaluation may be in order. It is best if your child can try out different cushions to see how he or she actually sits on them.

Cushions are expensive and prices can vary greatly from distributor to distributor, even for the same model. So once you find out what your child needs, shop around. Wheelchair cushions should be covered by funding sources mentioned in Chapter 17, if the claim is correctly submitted.

The back of the chair is usually made of the same material as the seat—Naugahyde or nylon. The back height is determined by the child's upper-body stability. An active, strong child wants a lower back, because the back interferes with the ability to propel the chair. (In fact, some wheelchair athletes have back heights so low that the back's only function is to keep the athlete from sliding out the rear of the chair.) On the other hand, a child with great trunk instability may need a very high back, possibly even restraint belts and abductor pads to assure proper positioning.

Solid backs or back supports, flat or contoured, are commercially available for those needing more rigid back support.

Back cushions can be added to help with a variety of problems. For example, they can aid in contouring the seat to fit, have cut-outs for pressure relief along the spine, help position the child farther forward in a chair he or she is going to grow into, or help with ventilation in hot weather.

Thoracic supports can be added to some chairs to support the chest so the child sits straight and does not develop a spinal curvature. Often such pads have to be custom-made and attached. If it is difficult to align your child, you may need neck supports too.

Opening backs have a zipper down one side of the fabric so the child can transfer to or from the wheelchair, bed, or toilet by sliding through the open back.

Reclining backrests are manual or power-driven. A reclining backrest may not be necessary for a small child whom you can move about from place to place. But if you have a heavy teenager who needs to alternate positions or cannot sit upright, consider reclining backrests. A power recliner does, of course, add a lot of weight to a chair, but if you need a power recliner your child is probably already in a power chair, which is so heavy that the additional weight is irrelevant.

Headrests are necessary if your child needs to be reclined or has weak neck muscles. A weak child who can support his or her head most of the time may sometimes lose his or her balance so the head falls backward or may sometimes intentionally throw the head backward. For such a child, consider getting a headrest, for when the head snaps backward your child could sustain a spinal-cord injury.

Many chairs now have headrest extensions as an available option: ask the manufacturer if it makes one, for this may be cheaper than having one made by your orthotist.

Armrests should be chosen according to your child's needs.

A fixed full-length arm provides arm support in the front of the chair. However, any fixed armrest makes transferring difficult.

Detachable desk arms allow a child to get up close to desks and tables. When the arms are removed, the child can transfer laterally.

Adjustable-height desk arms may be important to facilitate standing, encourage correct posture, or do increasingly difficult wheelchair push-ups.

Wrap-around armrests can decrease the overall width of the chair.

Armlocks should be added to all removable arms to secure them when positioned.

Legrests and footrests must also be chosen with care. Unless your child is propelling the chair by moving his or her feet along the ground, the chair will need to have foot- and legrests of some kind. Get adjustable footrests to allow for growth. Removable (swing-away) or low-profile footrests enable your child to get close to the object to which he or she is transferring. If your child has leg spasms or is extremely active, you may have to get extra foot or leg accessories such as heel loops, ankle straps, toe loops, or a fabric legrest. An elevating legrest is useful if you want to vary the position of your child's legs or if your child needs the leg elevated and supported while wearing a long leg cast. However, these increase the overall length and the turning radius of the chair.

Electrically elevated footrests should be considered if you order a power recliner. Unfortunately, powered footrests don't generally swing away unless they are custom-made.

Chairs with adjustable support structures provide postural control for children with impaired neuromuscular systems. As you can see from figure 7-9, such a chair can be used with legrests, hip abductors, thoracic supports, armrests, shoulder stabilizers, and neck and head supports. That may look like a lot of extra equipment, but it can enable some children to sit very well. It does take time initially to adapt such a chair to fit your child since it is fully adjustable, but you can keep modifying the dimensions of the chair as your child grows. Some chairs can also be purchased with power units. Such a chair can be excellent indoors but poor outdoors since the whole frame may jiggle too much on rougher surfaces. Sometimes the seat can be separated from the base so it can be used as a car seat. However, since it is very difficult to lift the child in the seat into the car, it may be better to bring your child to the car in the chair and then transfer him or her into a car seat or use a travel chair that can be wheeled to the car and then pivoted onto the seat (see page 89).

If such an extensively adapted chair does not seem necessary, but your child needs careful positioning, consider simply buying a modular postural-control adaptation system (the medical term for a positioning system) that can be inserted into the chair your child is presently using.

Wheelchair Safety Accessories

The following are important safety accessories you may want to consider:

- Antitip devices are helpful if your child's chair is unsteady when he or she transfers or makes other movements.
- Antifold devices attach to the cross members of the chair to prevent it from accidentally folding while your child is getting in or out.
- Spoke covers are flat sheets of plastic that cover the spokes, protecting them and preventing objects (including hands of other children) from getting caught in the spokes.

Wheelchair Convenience Accessories

There are many convenience accessories available for wheelchair users. Following are some useful accessories:

- Trays provide a play and work area for your child when in the chair. They come in various models. You can make your own tray, but you will probably find that a good tray that can be easily positioned is well worth the cost, even though commercial trays run between $50 and $150.

- Pouches can be attached to the armrest and are handy for carrying small objects.
- Wheelchair backpacks, attached to the rear of the chair, are great for carrying larger items such as schoolbooks, lunch, or jackets.
- Transfer boards have smooth surfaces for easy sliding while transferring in and out of the chair.
- Crutch- and cane-holders consist of a metal cup mounted on the bottom of the frame and a snap lock at the top.
- A horn or bell on the chair enables a child to gain the attention of another, particularly if the child is nonverbal or can't speak loudly.
- Lights and reflectors are necessary if the chair will ever be used outside after dark.
- Reaching tongs enable your child to pick up anything dropped or beyond reach. (If your teenager is too weak for tongs, you might consider a canine companion, a dog trained to help an older adolescent or adult do what he or she can't do alone.) In spite of such aids, some children will need people to help them.
- Handcrank unicycle attachments are easily attachable to the front of standard wheelchairs. A child with good trunk balance can use such a device to go farther and faster without getting tired.

Special Manual Wheelchairs

The ultralightweight chair and the sports chair were first marketed by Jeff Minnerbraker, an athletic youth injured in an automobile accident at the age of 18 who wanted to continue to participate in sports but was frustrated by the weight and lack of maneuverability of the standard manual wheelchair. With the help of George Linder, an importer of racing bicycles, Minnerbraker designed a sports chair. The new chair was so radical that when he appeared with it at an international wheelchair sports competition in Germany in 1980 the officials conferred before allowing it on the court. The interest of other athletes inspired Jeff and George to manufacture the Quadra sports chair.

When athletes found they'd rather use such a chair all day long, it became apparent that there was not only a market for a sports chair but a need among the whole disabled population for an ultralightweight chair that had the maneuverability of a sports chair plus such standard wheelchair options as a folding frame, higher

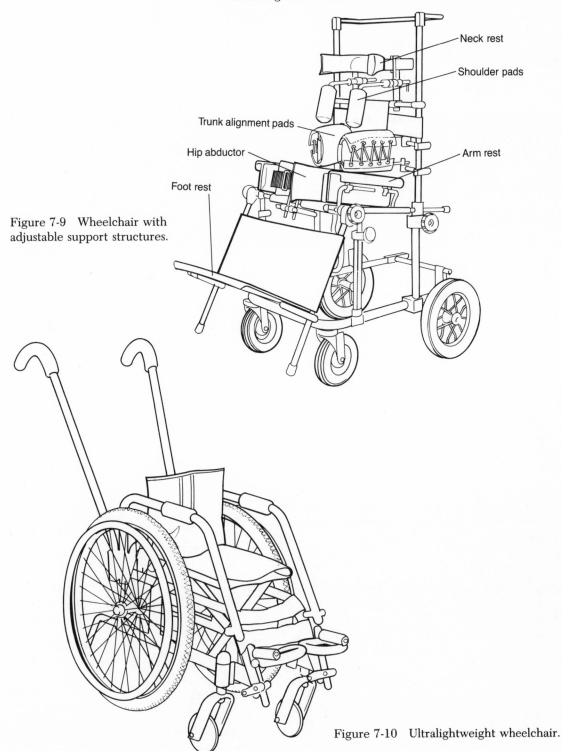

Neck rest

Shoulder pads

Trunk alignment pads

Hip abductor

Arm rest

Foot rest

Figure 7-9 Wheelchair with adjustable support structures.

Figure 7-10 Ultralightweight wheelchair.

backrest, armrests, caster-pin locks, clothing guards, chest straps, body harnesses, modular seating devices, and push handles for those needing assistance over longer distances or up inclines (fig. 7-10). The child's chair provided mobility for children as young as three years old.

The ultralightweight chairs are favored by so many people that new companies as well as established wheelchair manufacturers are now marketing them.

An ultralightweight chair may increase the mobility of a child in a standard manual chair or may eliminate the need for a power chair with some more disabled children. If your therapy or rehabilitation center has not placed many children in such chairs, contact ultralightweight chair manufacturers directly to discuss their products and, if appropriate, to arrange to have your child actually try out such a chair.

Although these chairs are often simply called "sports chairs," insurance companies will pay only for lightweight chairs, not sports chairs, since the latter are deemed recreational vehicles. Therefore, when filing an insurance claim, be sure to designate the chair as "lightweight"

only, not as "sports" or even "lightweight sports."

Medical justification for such a chair might include a statement to the effect that, due to the upper-extremity weakness of a child, such a chair increases the child's endurance, ability to maneuver, and independence in the activities of daily living.

Commode chairs are discussed fully in Chapter 10, but it should be noted here that if transferring to the toilet during the day is a major problem, as with a retarded child who can neither transfer alone nor propel the chair, a commode chair may be a good alternative. Such chairs are discreet in appearance.

Motorized Wheelchairs—Special Features to Consider

Motorized chairs can give mobility to many people who can't push their own chairs (fig. 7-11). However, before you decide to buy a motorized chair, remember that propelling one's own chair develops arm and shoulder muscles, which are

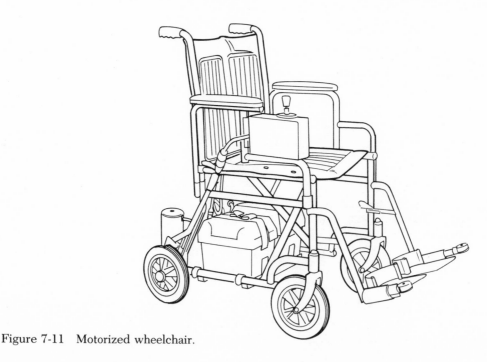

Figure 7-11   Motorized wheelchair.

helpful for general mobility, especially transferring. There are adults who insist on propelling their own chairs because they know they will lose strength if they don't get daily exercise. But while a motorized chair can be inappropriate for a child who can propel independently with ease, it can be marvelous for a child who cannot get around alone or only with great difficulty. For general information about motorized-wheelchair features, read the section on manual wheelchairs (pages 89–94), for much of this information applies to any type of wheelchair you buy. Specific features you will have to consider when purchasing a motorized wheelchair include the following.

The frame of a motorized chair contains many of the same features as a standard wheelchair, although the rear wheels may be smaller than those used on a manual chair. The overall construction must be sturdier due to the weight of the motor unit and the batteries. Many power chairs do not fold easily, making it necessary to have a van in order to transport them.

The power unit on most chairs consists of two motors between one-quarter and one horsepower in strength. You can get a chair with a direct-drive system, in which the axle rotates as on a tricycle; a belt-drive system, which incorporates a pulley system such as on a bicycle (although wheelchairs use belts rather than chains); or a combination system, which incorporates advantages of both belt drive and direct drive.

Protection circuits are similar in function to the circuit breakers in your fuse box at home. In case of mechanical malfunction, they limit the damage to one part of the total electronic circuitry. This is an important feature, since electronic repairs can be very expensive.

Automatic correction circuitry monitors wheel speeds so if in uneven terrain one wheel slows down extra power will be sent to the slower wheel.

The control unit determines the responsiveness of the chair to signals sent by the operator, who pushes a joystick in the direction he or she wants to move. The joystick can be placed wherever your child can most easily reach and maneuver it, including near the shoulder, chin, or any other part of the body if your child lacks hand control or strength. Control units vary greatly in power, range of motion, and convenience and safety devices. As innovations continue to be made, you should investigate what is available.

Consult with your rehabilitation or special-education professionals about what would be best for your child. Ask them for the names of the distributors who work with them so you can contact them directly if necessary to discuss the latest technological innovations and arrange for your child to try out a variety of devices to see what works best. While it may be appropriate to postpone the purchase of a specific item because it will become commercially available in a few months, don't put off buying something your child needs now because you think something better will be produced later. It probably will be, but your child may need the device now.

Batteries need care and attention and may be your biggest expense in keeping a chair running. Most chairs do not come with batteries, since they are expensive to ship and there is a danger of acid leakage. When you buy a chair, check your manufacturer's recommendations, for the battery needs to be the right size, shape, voltage, and amperage. A car battery will work, but it will not last as long or be as efficient as a deep-cycle battery. You should buy a battery made specifically for wheelchairs.

Batteries contain either wet cells (sulfuric acid and water) or gel. Wet cells are preferable for daily use, since they last longer and are cheaper, but many airlines will accept only gel cells in a spillproof container, even if the wet-cell batteries have spillproof caps or are in spillproof containers.

Most chairs come with battery chargers, but you need to know when the battery needs recharging. Some batteries come with built-in remaining-charge indicators. Otherwise you can manually measure the charge with a hydrometer; or you can purchase a range indicator, which tells you how much charge is left. It is important to recharge the battery completely each time, for if a battery is frequently given an incomplete recharging it will soon not take a total recharging.

The driving time (or how long an electric chair can be driven between chargings) depends on the weight of the person, the terrain, the efficiency of the motor, and the size and charge of the battery.

The maneuverability depends on the size of the wheelbase, the efficiency of the motor, the sophistication of the control unit, and your child's ability to control the chair.

Types of Motorized Chairs

A standard motorized chair can be adapted by the addition of various accessories. Generally a more expensive chair will also have a more responsive control system and a smoother ride. However, such chairs are heavy and bulky, and sometimes difficult to maneuver in tight spaces in the home. And they require a van for transport.

A portable motorized wheelchair is reasonably light and can be transported in a car by removing the batteries and then folding the frame. However, lightweight chairs usually have less power than a standard motorized chair, so while it may be very appropriate for indoor use and for short drives on sidewalks it would not have the driving time and maneuverability over rough terrain of a standard motorized chair.

Portable power units can be attached to your child's manual wheelchair either by replacing the rear wheels with a direct-drive system or by using a spline drive that exerts force on the existing large rear tires, causing them to rotate.

Generally a motorized chair is more effective than a manual chair with a portable power unit, since a manual chair is not designed to take the stress and weight of a power unit. Therefore, if your child needs to move from a manual to a power chair, you may want to purchase a motorized chair and keep the manual as a backup. However, if your child will need a motorized

chair for only a short period of time or occasional use, a portable power unit is a less expensive option. Before buying a portable unit be sure that it will provide your child with the needed mobility and that it will fit on the present chair as well as on other chairs he or she may need in the future.

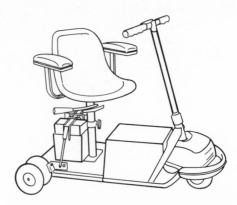

Figure 7-12   Three-wheeled motorized wheelchair.

Three-wheeled electric wheelchairs are like electric scooters with a seat on them (fig. 7-12). While such a chair can be handy for a child who can walk some and wants to drive some, the seats do not give extensive support, and the small wheels make it difficult to maneuver on rough terrain.

Custom chairs are a last resort if you cannot find an appropriate chair on the market. A custom-designed and -built chair is an expensive alternative to a commercially available chair. If you cannot find the appropriate chair for your child commercially, discuss having a custom chair designed and built with your doctor and therapist. Some insurance companies will pay for a custom chair if you submit the claim correctly.

How to Choose the Right Wheelchair for Your Child

Unfortunately there is no one chair that is best for all children, and there is not always one chair that is best for your child under all the conditions he or she may encounter. Before you buy a chair, you should, with professional advice if possible, carefully assess your child's needs, considering the following factors:

- *Correct comfortable positioning:* Do the basic structural design and materials make it possible for your child to be positioned correctly and comfortably when the chair is both stationary and moving?
- *Transferring:* Can your child get in and out of the chair alone? If he or she needs help, how easily can you assist?
- *Maneuverability:* Can your child go where he or she wants to go and as fast (within safety considerations) as he or she likes? Can your child move about the house, through doorways, over doorsills, over pile carpets, turn into different rooms and even within given rooms (such as the bathroom) so he or she has access to your whole house? Outside, can your child maneuver curbs, wet grass, bumps, the sidewalk, and other uneven terrain? Maneuverability is determined by the basic construction of the chair, its overall size and weight, its turning radius, and the construction of the wheels (size, pressure, and tread). If it is a manual chair, will your child be strong and coordinated enough to maneuver it? If it is a motorized chair, will your child be coordinated enough to drive it? Will the overall construction, including the efficiency of the motor and control unit, the size and weight, and the driving time, make it possible for your child to go where he or she wants to go? Is there enough driving time in the battery system to get there and home before the batteries need recharging?
- *Safety:* Can your child sit in and maneuver the chair safely without capsizing, running into objects, or having some other accident?
- *Portability:* How does the basic construction and weight of the chair influence how easily you can take it with you in a car, a van, or on public transportation?
- *Maintenance:* What needs to be done to keep the chair in good running order? What routine maintenance can you do at home to prolong the life of the chair? What is the warranty? What repairs might be necessary? Where and how quickly can it be repaired?
- *Cost:* How much does it cost to buy the chair and to keep it running? How long can your child use the chair before outgrowing it? As with cars, comfort and maneuverability are often related to cost. Since your child will spend many hours a day in the chair, it is wise to select the chair that best meets your child's needs, searching for outside financial assistance if necessary.

In trying to choose the best chair for your child, you may find that you have to compromise on some of these factors. Have your child try as many chairs as possible. Talk with professionals (rehabilitation doctors, therapists, coordinators of state medical services, etc.), the medical director of a hospital-supply store, parents of other disabled children, and disabled adults in chairs. Information from someone with a similar disability and similar interests is most helpful; for example, a college student interested in wheelchair sports might give better tips than an elderly housewife as to the best chair to mobilize your ten-year-old son. Phone organizations assisting the disabled, such as the local health department, Easter Seal, the Muscular Dystrophy Association, or the disabled students' coordinator at the local college, to get names of people who may be able to offer advice.

Representatives of medical-supply stores should be able to tell you about what they sell and how their chairs compare with others. Do not expect them to recommend chairs their competitors sell, but they should be able to advise which chair would be best for your child. Even then, they may not be fully informed about recent innovations or their company's ability to make a chair to your specifications.

The fastest way to do comparison shopping is to go to an exposition of rehabilitation equipment (if there is ever one near your home) so you can actually look at the equipment, try it out, and discuss your needs. As you move from booth to booth and talk to the salespeople, you may well become aware of factors you never considered before. It is perfectly reasonable to ask someone how his or her chair compares with other chairs and why he or she thinks it is best. However, listen with a critical ear, particularly to the factors he or she criticizes in another company's product.

If you can't get to an exposition, write or phone manufacturers. The advantage of phone calls is that you get the information faster and you also often get more candid information than a person would want to put in writing. Many businesses have tollfree numbers. (Call 800-555-

1212 to see if the company has such a number.) Some will accept collect calls from prospective customers. If you have specific questions, ask them. Otherwise, ask why they think their chair is best. If you are considering another chair, ask why their chair is better. Through such discussion, points to consider may arise you hadn't thought of before. Request written information so you can review what they have said later and also compare products. Many companies will send a sales representative to your home to demonstrate their product, and that way you can talk to them in person.

No one manufacturer, even if it sells the largest number of a particular type of chair, makes the best chair for all people. It is worthwhile to investigate small companies that are making interesting innovations.

This research is a lot of work, but a wheelchair costs a lot of money, and with insufficient research you may buy the wrong one.

How to Measure Your Child for a Chair

Wheelchairs, like shoes, have to fit. But since most wheelchairs are custom-made to a child's measurements, they cannot be returned if they do not fit. Therefore, it is best if your child can actually try sitting in a number of different chairs before you make your final choice. If your community does not have a well-stocked durable medical equipment store, it may be possible for the area distributor of the chair(s) you are seriously considering to meet you at your therapist's or in your home.

Measurements should be made by a qualified person experienced in measuring children for that particular type of chair, because different companies have different ways of taking measurements. Only as a last resort should you measure your child yourself, and if you do so, make sure you know exactly which measurements are needed and how they should be made. To do the measuring yourself, seat your child, wearing shoes and any braces, in a firm-bottomed chair. If wheelchair cushion(s) will be used, make sure you add information about the height of the cushion(s), or your measurements will be wrong.

You will probably be asked to give the following physical measurements:

1. *Seat width:* Measure distance across the hips or thighs, whichever is wider.
2. *Seat depth:* Measure from the back of the buttocks to behind the calf. In some chairs you can add a back cushion and then remove it as your child grows. If this is possible, you will have to order a longer chair depth.
3. *Seat height:* Measure from the bottom of the thigh at the knee joint to the bottom of the shoes while your child is sitting. Be sure to measure your child with the type of shoes he or she usually wears, since the height of the shoe heel will influence this measurement. Some chairs come with standard seat heights measured from the floor, but there must be a minimum two-inch clearance between the footrest and the floor.
4. *Arm height:* Measure from the outer bend of the elbow to the bottom of the buttocks.
5. *Back height:* Measure from extended arm to bottom of buttocks. Again, if a cushion is to be used, include its thickness in your measurement.

These numbers will help when you read literature and specifications for different chairs. A manufacturer may be able to make some changes. If your child is growing fast, consider whether the chair frame is adjustable or whether you could use cushions when first purchasing the chair and then remove them as your child grows.

Certain pointers can help you evaluate whether your child fits in the chair. As your child grows, you will periodically have to check the fit. The table on page 102 may be helpful.

Wheelchair Care

Wheelchair maintenance and repairs are crucial: if your child depends on a chair, when the chair is out of commission so is your child. Most manufacturers give you a maintenance-information booklet when you purchase a chair. If they don't, ask for one. There are wheelchair-repair businesses in some larger communities. In other localities a wheelchair distributor or a bicycle shop may do wheelchair repairs. Still, you should learn to do as much as possible yourself. Then if you periodically check the chair, you are more apt to know if something is about to go wrong and can make repairs (or have them made) if necessary.

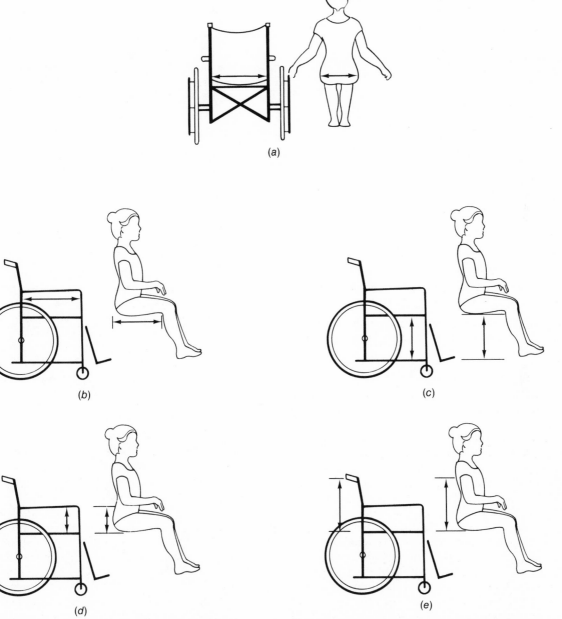

Figure 7-13   Measuring child for wheelchair: *(a)* seat width—measure across hips or thighs (whichever is wider); *(b)* seat depth—measure from back of buttocks to back of calf; *(c)* seat height—measure from bottom of thigh at knee joint to bottom of shoe and add two inches; *(d)* arm height—measure from bottom of buttocks to outer bend of elbow; *(e)* back height—measure from bottom of buttocks to armpit.

Footrests too high:

Knees forced up, weight not evenly distributed on thighs, putting too much pressure on sacrum or tail bone (which can cause pressure sores).

Seat too shallow:

Weight poorly distributed and excessive pressure on the ischium. Balance lessened. Legs and feet not correctly positioned in respect to footrest.

Arms too high:

Shoulders forced up as child tries to use armrests for support; unnatural position restricts range of motion necessary to propel chair.

Seat too wide:

Child tends to lean to one side, promoting scoliosis.

Back too high:

Restricted arm and shoulder movement when child propels chair. Head may be pushed forward.

Footrests too low:

Foot not firmly supported at a 90° angle to the leg. When foot drops downward, plantar flexion or "foot drop" can develop.

Seat too deep:

Legs extended or child slides forward in chair. Back cushion can be used to create correct seat depth and then thickness reduced as child grows. Child should not be positioned so far forward that he or she has difficulty reaching handrims.

Arms too low:

Child tends to lean to one side or forward for support, which can cause scoliosis.

Seat too narrow:

Restricted ability to move and change position. Difficult to transfer and wear warm winter clothing.

Back too low:

Insufficient support. If child leans back, he or she may catch shoulder blade (scapula) over the top of the back or lose balance.

STANDING

Our bodies were made to spend some time upright. Bones become brittle and do not grow and develop properly if they do not bear weight. And the muscles in the lower extremities weaken if we do not spend time upright. Therefore your child should spend some time tilted in as upright a position as possible.

Tilt tables or prone boards allow you to position your child on the back or stomach at an angle as close to upright as possible (fig. 7-14). This helps bodily functions, helps prevent contractures in the hips and legs by lining your child up straight, and lets your child have a look at the world from another position.

Body-suspension systems or jumpers are excellent if your child needs less support than a tilt table provides, yet is not strong enough to walk. Body-suspension systems are similar to baby

jumpers. The child is placed into a cloth body jacket with rings around the top and is then hung in this vest from a walker frame designed for full body suspension. Or you can use a ceiling-mounted suspension system.

Walkers are appropriate for children who can support some of their body weight yet still need assistance in maintaining the standing position and balance. A more disabled child may need a walker that has positioning controls for the chest and hips, as well as a padded seat. A more mobile child may only need a more traditional walker, as illustrated in figure 7-5. Other walking aids for children needing even less assistance include canes and crutches (see pages 117–118).

Transferring

Transferring, moving your child from one place to another, can place great strain on your back. As back problems can become chronic, you must be extremely careful when you transfer your

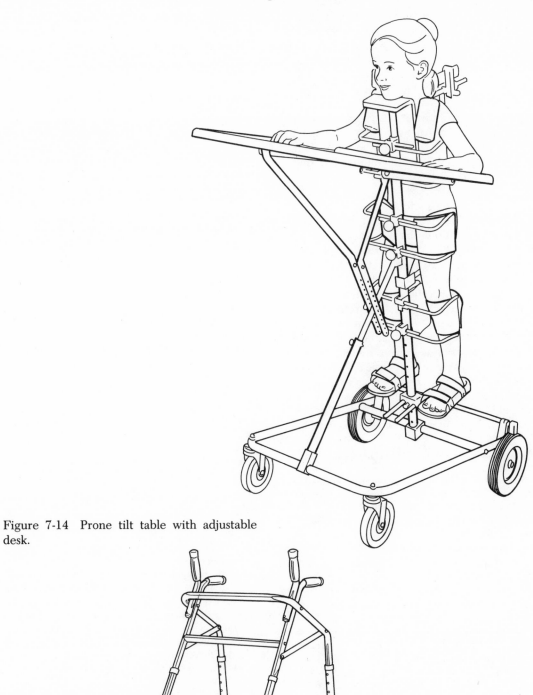

Figure 7-14 Prone tilt table with adjustable desk.

Figure 7-15 Walker.

child. Always bend from the knees, keeping your back as straight as possible. Ask your therapist or an orthopedist how best to transfer your child. These professionals can also show you exercises to help strengthen your back muscles as well as those in the abdomen, which are used when you lift.

Should your back hurt, don't wait for it to get better. Get professional help from a qualified orthopedist, therapist, or chiropractor. As your child gets larger and heavier, you may find that you need to use a lift.

What is the best way to lift your child? Not only is there no "best way" to lift all children, but as your child's condition changes and as he or she grows, you may modify your lifting technique. Therefore discuss with your doctor or physical therapist the best way to lift your child. (As physical therapists are specifically trained to teach transferring, henceforth we shall refer to the health-care professional helping you with transferring as a physical therapist, although you may actually be receiving help from someone else.)

It is most valuable if the physical therapist is willing to come to your house for an evaluation; in your home, he or she can better assess what your daily transferring needs actually are. The therapist will consider the following factors:

- Where and when does your child need to be transferred?
- Can your child learn to transfer independently? (Remember, the more independent your child can become, the better it is for everyone.)
- Can your child be taught to assist in the transfer if unable to transfer alone?
- Is there any way to adapt your child's chair(s), wheelchair, or bed so you can transfer between places of equal height?
- Do you need any mechanical devices such as lifts to facilitate transferring?

Once your therapist has considered these factors, he or she is ready to teach you how to transfer. This process has two major components: preparation and the actual transfer itself.

Preparation. While you may not need to consciously consider each of these steps every time you move your child, do keep them in mind:

- Evaluate your child's size, weight, and where he or she is going to transfer. If you think your child is too heavy for you to lift, get a mechanical lift or call for help. Don't risk back injury trying to play Superman.
- Make sure the floor around you and along the route you will travel is hazardfree. The surface should be as skidproof as possible. Waxed floors, throw rugs, and wet, slippery surfaces are dangerous. Check the route for obstacles such as toys or other clutter that you may not see while carrying your child but upon which you could trip.
- Check that where your child is now and where he or she is to be placed are both stable. This means making sure wheelchair brakes are on, chairs are sitting squarely on all four legs, and so on.
- Decide how best to transfer your child. The technique will vary depending upon whether the surfaces are of equal height and upon the distance you will have to travel.
- Check the appropriate features of any lift or adaptive equipment you are using to assist in the transfer.
- Be barefoot if possible, or wear flat shoes with skidproof soles. When you carry your child, he or she will usually be in front of you. Consequently, you will be heavier in the front and any heels will throw your body weight even farther forward, making you unstable.

The transfer. The following factors are important every time you move your child, for poor position and movement over time, or even just one false move, can cause back problems. While exactly how you transfer your child may vary, try to do all of the following during each transfer:

1. Talk to your child about what you are doing together. It is easy to feel that since your child cannot get about unassisted, you should just get on with the job of lifting and transferring. However, being moved by another person can be a bewildering experience. If you explain your actions to your child, you not only prepare him or her mentally for what you are about to do but you also provide the opportunity for your child to learn the process and to cooperate as fully as possible. Anything your child can do so you do not have to lift his or her whole weight will be good for both of you.
2. Face your child squarely with your feet 10–12 inches apart. This gives greater stability and lifting power.
3. Bend your legs, get a good grip, then lift your child

by straightening your legs. Remember that your arms and legs are levers; your back is not. So use your limbs and the strong muscles in them, not your back, to carry the weight.

4. Keep your back straight, though not necessarily vertical.
5. Lift slowly and evenly without quick or jerky motions. It is not true that the faster you can move your child, the better. You are much more apt to move your child safely if you use slow, deliberate movements.
6. Keep your child as close to your own body as possible throughout the entire lifting procedure. The farther your child is from your body, the more difficult it will be to lift him or her safely.
7. Change direction only by turning your feet and legs. Never twist your back. Twisting during a lift is one of the most common causes of back injury.
8. Try to keep one hand free to hold onto the bannister if you have to carry your child up and down stairs.

If you and your physical therapist devise methods of transferring taking the factors above into account, you should be able to transfer your child well. As your child grows or his or her condition changes, you may have to modify your transferring techniques.

Lifts. As soon as it starts to become difficult to lift or transfer your child, you need to get a lift (fig. 7-16). Get a lift *before* you injure your back. Since a variety of lifts is available, discuss with your physical therapist which type(s) best suit your child's needs. For example, you may need

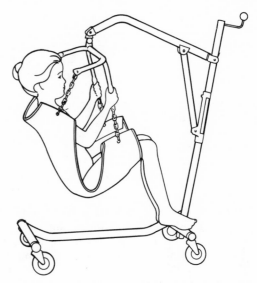

Figure 7-16 Patient lift can be used to lift child from supine to sitting position and for transfer to wheelchair, commode, bath, and car.

one in the house to get your child from the bed to the chair, toilet, or bathtub. You may need another to get your child in and out of the car. A lift is an expensive investment, so if possible try out the type you think would be best before purchasing it. Get advice from professionals familiar with the lifts that might be appropriate for your child. It takes time to learn how to use a lift.

8
Exercises and
Orthopedic Appliances

You may have consciously to help your ill or disabled child to develop the optimal use of whatever physical capabilities he or she may have. Since your child is growing, deformities and other problems can develop very quickly. Therefore appropriate physical therapy to exercise the body and keep it properly aligned, coupled with any necessary orthopedic appliances, is vital. This is not for the sake of future beauty contests but rather for the child's health, comfort, and maximum independent mobility.

When you and a health-care professional recognize that your child has an orthopedic need, a number of persons may work with you to help your child. Your pediatrician, who monitors your child's overall care, may have you consult an orthopedist, who specializes in the correction or prevention of skeletal deformities. Often these doctors will work with therapists. A physical therapist will help your child with exercise and training to prevent deformities and maintain maximum use of all remaining functions. An occupational therapist will aid with the development of skills needed in the activities of daily life, such as dressing, eating, and so on. An orthotist will construct any braces your child may need.

Periodic consultations with such health-care professionals is a good idea for any physically disabled child and for some who are terminally ill. These professionals will offer recommendations as to how the child can maximize capacities for movement and deter problems.

In most large communities "team consultation" is available at clinics set up to help children with specific diseases and disabilities, such as muscular dystrophy, cerebral palsy, spina bifida, cystic fibrosis, and amputations. When a whole clinic team works with your child, his or her needs are viewed in a more holistic way.

EXERCISES

In order to understand why most children with orthopedic problems need an individualized exercise program, let's look briefly at the mechanisms behind simple bodily movement. The human skeleton consists of 206 bones joined together by ligaments. Muscles, extending from one bone to another, are attached to the bones by tendons. To control every joint, there are sets of muscles that oppose each other. For example, when you bend your elbow, your bicep muscles contract and shorten while the opposing triceps on the back of the arm simultaneously relax and lengthen. Sometimes there is a stronger muscle in the set that constantly outpulls the weaker one, so a limb is constantly bent or straight, or the spine is constantly pulled over to one side. Or, as a result of paralysis of one muscle group, the opposing muscle group wants to shorten because it finds little or no resistance to its pull. This can rapidly result in contractures and fixed deformities. It is important to understand that even when you are totally relaxed, as when asleep, there is still some pull on your muscles. It is not apparent, because the two opposing groups balance each other. This pull is called "muscle tone." Whenever muscles do not operate normally, there is a chance of deformity developing.

When you consider that, in addition to the above, movement depends on messages from the brain traveling down the spinal cord out to the muscles, you can see that problems of movement and even simple body alignment can be very complex. The results of exercises and therapy can never be guaranteed, and what works with one child may not work with another.

You can play an active part in determining your child's needs and developing an exercise program to meet them. Since you are with your child all day, you can give your doctor and therapists valuable insights into your child's capacities, weaknesses, and needs. Keeping written notes can help because, as changes often occur slowly, you may have trouble remembering exactly what your child could do two months ago and how that compares with today. Or you may want to keep a record of physical ability by making home movies. However, even if you are a good record-keeper, it may be very difficult to analyze how your child's body and ability to move are changing, because as children grow the relationships between nerves, muscles, and bones and the ability to move can be constantly changing as well.

Ideally, your child should be able to do more today than six months ago. If this isn't so, it could be that the muscles haven't become weaker but that your child's body has become heavier. Also, although most physical deterioration and improvement are gradual, it doesn't always seem that way. Rather than seeing your child go "uphill" or "downhill," you may believe the condition has leveled out, and then suddenly your child's capacity goes up or drops down a step. In fact, your child was probably gaining or losing skills slowly, but the change has suddenly become outwardly apparent. Therefore it is sometimes difficult to evaluate exactly how your child's condition is changing. If you do keep mental (and, it is hoped, written) notes, you can report any changes you observe to your doctor.

Setting Goals

An alternative to keeping continual notes on your child's progress is to work with the therapist to set goals for the exercise program, documenting what your child is able to do at that time, and then reevaluating after a given time his or her ability relative to the goal. For example, Sally's goal might be to sit unsupported during "Sesame Street" without getting tired.

- *September 1:* After 10 minutes Sally tires and needs support to continue sitting.
- *December 1:* Sally can now sit unsupported for 15 minutes at a time.

The goals of your child's exercise program may include the following:

Maintain or improve muscle strength and endurance. After illness, children sometimes have to exercise to regain strength. A disabled person may have to exercise certain muscles in order to become strong enough to live independently. A child may also have to learn to use different muscles than previously if a set of muscles is weakened by an accident or illness.

Maintain or improve joint range of motion. If your child cannot move independently or can move only with difficulty, exercise must be done to maintain maximum range of motion or limberness.

Even paralyzed or otherwise severely physically disabled children need to be limber. First of all, a limber child can move more easily and achieve more independence. Second, the child will be more comfortable if his or her body is not stiff. Third, the ability to move helps prevent medical problems such as pressure sores. Fourth, a limber child is much easier to provide with daily nurturing care, such as dressing and bathing. And last, deformities such as scoliosis, which of themselves can be severe, disabling, and life-shortening, may be prevented.

Maintain or improve mobility. For some children walking unassisted is not a realistic goal. But even if your child can't walk unassisted, he or she may be able to learn to crawl, walk with crutches, or propel a wheelchair.

Attain the maximum level of independence. The more your child can learn to do independently, the better it will be for both of you. Areas to consider are daily living skills such as eating, dressing, bathing, and so on.

Your child should understand whenever possible the purpose of the goals. As your child gets older, he or she can even help choose goals to work toward, such as being able to open a door or to shower alone. This will lead to a more realistic understanding of his or her abilities and limitations.

For some children, goals may be only to maintain present levels of function. If your child has a progressive disorder and is losing independent function, goals may include finding or inventing a piece of equipment that will enable your child to continue doing what he or she has previously done with a few adaptations. At any rate, the goals of an exercise program should be achieveable; achieving the goals will help your child gain a positive self-image.

Doing the Exercises

There are four kinds of exercises, which may be classified as follows:

Passive exercises are exercises someone else will do for your child, such as moving your child's arms and legs to keep them limber and prevent contractures. Passive exercises are done most easily if the body is warm and relaxed. You may find it effective to do stretching exercises while bathing with a young child.

Active-assistive exercises are employed if your child has some strength but is too weak to go through the total range of motion. Someone or something helps your child move a part of the body. For example, you can either help your child exercise an arm by assisting as he or she moves it backward and forward, or you can strap the arm to a skateboardlike device and your child can roll the arm back and forth.

Active exercises are exercises that your child can do independently to stretch or strengthen specific muscle groups as well as to increase general endurance.

Resistive exercises, if a child can move with ease, enable him or her to increase strength by applying resistance to the muscle. For example, to strengthen arm muscles, your child can lift weights, which applies resistance to the muscles and thus strengthens them.

Ask your doctor and other professionals as many questions as you need to. The questions you want to ask may include:

- *What is the purpose of the exercise?* Although exercise in general is done to achieve or maintain the highest possible level of functional independence and efficiency, you should understand why each specific exercise needs to be done.
- *Which body parts are to be affected?* With exercises to strengthen specific muscles, it is helpful to know where they are attached and how they function. If you are trying to increase the range of motion of a joint, it is important to know how it is constructed. If you are exercising a part of your child's body that he or she cannot move independently, remember that bones that are not used to bearing weight are very fragile (in a paralyzed child, all the bones are at risk) so you must be sure to do the exercise properly.
- *What is the correct way to do the exercise?* If your child does an exercise incorrectly, it will not help and may actually do harm. Before beginning stretching or strengthening exercises with your child, get instructions on how they should be done from your doctor or therapist. It is advisable also to have your doctor or therapist watch you do them with your child.
- *What problems might occur?* You need not only to know what positive results you may see but also to be able to recognize indications that things are going wrong. Some exercises produce discomfort. But if your child finds something truly painful, be sure to check with the doctor. You may be doing the exercise incorrectly, your child may be unable to tolerate the exercise as prescribed, or the pain may indicate a medical problem such as a sprain, fracture, internal bleeding, etc. While the latter is highly unlikely, if your child experiences pain with the exercise, and if you think there is a problem, don't wait; call the doctor at once.
- *How frequently should the exercise be done?* It is important to know this, and to do each exercise as often as prescribed.

Maintaining the Program

Once you and your doctor or therapist have developed an exercise program, you must stick to it. This can be difficult with an exercise program since you don't get instant rewards for your efforts, and sometimes you never see a spectacular result. However, perseverance pays off, for even if you don't see any improvement you may have minimized other complications. And you don't see the result of not doing the exercises until the damage is done.

Your efforts may also influence your relationship with your orthopedist or rehabilitation doctor. Carrying through on a prescribed exercise program is an excellent way to convince a professional that you and your child do care, that you are willing and determined to work with the doctor or therapist and to have him or her work with you.

Most exercises are not inherently interesting. Teach your child why they are necessary and make exercise time as interesting as possible: sing songs, tell stories, make up games—do anything to keep interest up. You should also set up special exercise times. Choose times that fit into your routine and are not times when your child would definitely rather be doing something else: perhaps before dressing in the morning, after a nap, and then before bed.

While most of us err on the side of being too lax about exercises, you may sometimes see elements of the drill-sergeant mentality in yourself. Try to keep things in perspective and don't be so rigid that you lose sight of your child's emotional needs in your concern for the physical ones.

Any exercise program should be monitored periodically by a doctor or physical therapist since your child's needs may change due to growth or alteration in his or her physical condition. Many children can and should come to assume responsibility for doing their own exercises. It should be considered a daily routine, like brushing teeth. Especially as a child gets older, attitude and motivation become vital. A teenager may resist your enforcement of the exercise program. By the time he or she is a young adult, self-motivation will have to take over.

Massage

While massage is no substitute for a regular exercise program, it can help increase circulation (thus decreasing the risk of pressure sores), relieve soreness, relax muscles, and sometimes lessen muscle spasms. While massage may not significantly alter your child's physical condition, it may make him or her more comfortable.

Your doctor or therapist can tell you whether massage would be helpful for your child. Get verbal instructions and watch the therapist massage your child. Note whether the therapist uses lotions, mineral oil, or powder to keep the hand moving with less friction. Then have the therapist watch you give your child a massage and ask for constructive criticism. If you want to read about massage, ask your therapist for recommendations. While some people seem to be born with the knack of giving good massages, the rest of us need to learn how.

Whirlpool baths are helpful for some conditions. Not only are they relaxing, but they sometimes help reduce muscle spasms. For some children a warm whirlpool bath in the evening may help alleviate spasms during the night. Vibrating the chest in the warm whirlpool bath may help some children with respiratory problems.

You can either buy a portable unit or have one built into your tub if you happen to be remodeling your bathroom. Units vary greatly in effectiveness, so be sure you not only get advice from your health-care professional but also talk with distributors and users of various units before making any purchase. Whirlpool units may be covered by insurance if you have sufficient support information.

ORTHOPEDIC APPLIANCES

Even with a good exercise program, your child may need braces to support body parts that lack sufficient muscle power to function without assistance. Or bracing may be required to achieve good joint alignment or to minimize deformities caused by structural abnormalities or muscle imbalances.

You should not brace anything a child can support independently because that will compromise the use of the muscles your child does have. Sometimes a brace can support one of a set of muscles that work together. Or the constant adjustment that a brace provides can equalize uneven pull in a set of muscles. When paralysis is extensive, braces can either stretch out contracting muscles or support that which lacks muscle support of its own.

Unless your child has a simple and common problem, it may take a certain amount of thinking to figure out what should be done and how. Again, since you live with your child and know what he or she can and can't do, your insights into your child's strengths and weaknesses are valuable. You should understand what your doctor thinks needs to be done and then be willing (and allowed) to make suggestions.

If your child has a physical therapist, the therapist should also be involved in this process. You will have to discuss:

- The nature of your child's specific problem.
- How an orthotic device will help.
- How the device will be made.

The Orthotist

An orthotist is the professional who makes your child's orthopedic device. Some large rehabilitation clinics have orthotic units, but in most communities you will use an independent orthotics shop. If there is more than one shop, get suggestions from your doctor, therapist, and maybe even other parents as to the best place. For guidelines on how to pick a good orthotist, review the advice on finding a doctor in Chapter 2, for the same considerations apply. Generally, it pays to have someone nearby, as numerous fittings are often necessary. But if you hear that people continually have problems using the local shop, it may be worth driving a longer distance and making fewer visits. You may want to check with knowledgeable people before your first visit to see if there is one particular person in a shop who might work best with your child. If you know who you want to see, tell your doctor, since he or she (and sometimes also the physical therapist) usually discusses the order with the orthotist and wants that person to make the appliance.

The appointment should be made for a time of day when you, your child, and your orthotist are all at your best. Although orthotists, like everyone else, try to run on time, this isn't always possible. (See Chapter 2 for suggestions on scheduling and making your office visit as pleasant as possible.) Be sure to bring any equipment your child has been wearing or using, since the orthotist will want to check it and may want to use it as a guide when filling a new prescription.

The procedure can differ from case to case. Try to understand what will be made, and how, before your visit. If your doctor's information to you was sketchy, when you make your appointment with the orthotist by phone you can ask him or her to discuss the general procedure with you. Then when you have your first appointment, which will probably be just for measuring or casting, discuss the alternatives in the basic shape of what is being made, what materials are to be used, and what closures or fastening devices are available. Sometimes your orthotist will ask you for suggestions. At other times it may be important for you to offer suggestions about your child and his or her life style. If you know another child who has a similar appliance, try to talk with one of the child's parents *before* your appointment.

Measurements and castings are the first step. Sometimes the orthotist can modify commercially available equipment, but most appliances are custom-made. In that case the orthotist may make a plaster cast of the body part, then use that cast to make a mold so the appliance can be made to fit exactly to the contours of your child's body.

To make a cast of an arm, for example, the orthotist makes a plaster cast similar to that for a broken arm. First the arm is covered with a jersey-knit material so the plaster won't stick to the hair on the arm. Then rolls of plaster bandages are dipped into water and unrolled around the arm.

Chest castings are done in the same way. (Ask your orthotist if your child should eat before the appointment for a chest casting.)

If your child's trunk is being wrapped in plaster, make sure he or she breathes deeply, for otherwise your child may have difficulty breathing when the plaster starts to harden.

If your child is very weak and his or her body tends to sag together under the force of gravity, consider carefully how to position your child while the casting is being done. Always try to keep the body as aligned as possible. This may entail manually supporting parts of your child's body while the plaster is being applied and while it dries. Discuss positioning with your orthotist.

Orthotists generally favor cutting casts off

with power cast-cutters. But a power cutter can make what many children consider to be a loud and frightening noise, and they feel helpless when this saw comes at them. Cutting the cast off with scissors, before it is fully hardened, is more difficult. However, it is well worth the extra trouble if it makes your child happy. After all, you have to come to view castings as outings, and if they are frightening they are no longer fun.

Once the casting is done, you go home. The orthotist fills the cast with plaster to have an exact model of your child's body, then makes the brace to fit the plaster mold. Often you will be asked to come in for fittings as the orthotist works. Finally, the appliance will be complete and your child can wear it.

Even though the appliance has been fitted carefully, you may find places that rub or hurt. If your child complains, take the appliance off and check the body for red spots. If a red spot does not disappear in 15 minutes, too much pressure is being exerted in that area and the appliance will have to be adjusted. But even if you don't find a red spot, take your child's word and get the appliance checked.

Although it takes time to get used to a new appliance, your child has to understand that wearing it regularly as prescribed is very important.

Types of Orthopedic Appliances and Adaptive Devices

Trunk supports range from lightweight vests that look like Victorian corsets with whalebone stays all the way to molded plastic body jackets that vaguely resemble armadillo shells (fig. 8-1). A trunk support can support the trunk of a very weak child in correct alignment, help straighten the trunk of a child with a spinal curvature, or both support and correct. Since spinal curvatures are easier to prevent than to cure, and since they tend to get worse and more rigid as a child grows, getting a child fitted and then having him or her wear the trunk support regularly is vital.

The trunk support designed simply to support a weak child generally provides only as much support as needed so the child continues to use any muscle strength he or she has. Such a trunk

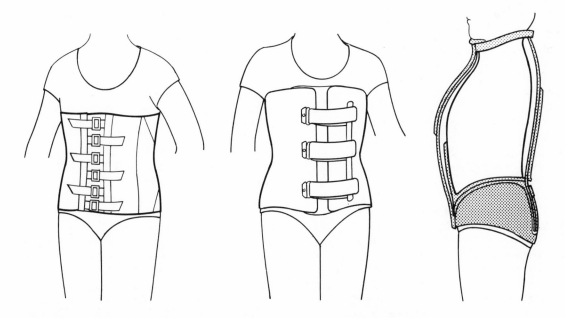

Figure 8-1   Cloth corset (Hoke corset); molded body jacket; Milwaukee brace.

support may simply be a lightweight cloth corset with stays. If a child gets weaker or larger, the back may need a firm support panel so spinal curvatures do not develop or are at least controlled as much as possible. The type offering the most support is a molded body jacket. Due to its rigidity it actually holds the spine in one position, either holding a weak spine straight or providing constant pressure to push a spine straight through what is called passive correction. Some such trunk supports, such as the Milwaukee brace, have neck supports to align the spine all the way up to the head. Your doctor or therapist may want your child to do spinal exercises while wearing the support. A well-made Milwaukee brace is much more effective if the child actively pulls away from the support pads on and off over the course of the day than if he or she just accepts the passive correction by the brace. Since not every child wants or remembers to do this regularly, your doctor or orthotist may recommend building in a tactile feedback device. This is an electronic unit that pokes the child until he or she does the exercise and then stops until it is time to do it again about 40 minutes later.

Neuromuscular stimulators, which provide passive stimulation for the muscle, are also sometimes incorporated into trunk supports or other orthopedic appliances. Stimulation causes muscle contraction, and a neuromuscular stimulator is designed to cause a specific muscle to contract. Unfortunately, muscles cannot always be isolated, so the usefulness of a neuromuscular stimulator is limited.

Your child must wear an undershirt beneath all trunk supports to prevent rubbing and to absorb perspiration. All-cotton undershirts are best. Cut off the sleeves for summer wear, leaving a flap of sleeve under the arm to protect the skin from rubbing.

"Air-conditioning" trunk supports is a problem, for the more substantial the support, the hotter it is to wear. Also, some children may not tolerate heat well due to temperature-regulatory-system problems. The simplest way to make a molded jacket cooler is to have your orthotist drill quarter-inch holes throughout the support. Since this will definitely weaken the jacket, it may not be possible if a child's condition causes much stress to be placed upon it. However, with some children you can have the orthotist drill holes and then glue leather patches over any cracks that occur. Such patching is unsightly by the time the support is outgrown, but it will be much cooler. Comfort is more important than looks. If your child has a problem with heat, ask your orthotist or another qualified and interested person to help you.

Neck and head braces call for ingenuity. The easiest way to hold the neck rigid is to use a foam cervical collar. A foam cervical collar might stabilize the neck enough so your child can do some things that would otherwise cause too much jiggling, like riding in the supermarket cart or riding the elephant at the circus. However, unless your child needs that type of support all day, consider using a variety of modes. Some wheelchair manufacturers make headrest extensions. Your orthotist can help make extensions for other chairs by extending a piece of molded plastic up the back of the chair to the top of your child's head. The plastic can have flaps to support your child's head on the sides. Then a piece of cotton webbing can be attached to the side flaps so your child's head won't fall forward. Such a headrest can be constructed to have some give and some space for movement, so your child can move his or her head from side to side and also bend down to look at things (see fig. 7-9).

Arm supports help the weak child utilize the strength he or she has by supporting the weight of the arm in a trough so the muscles can concentrate on movement.

Suspension slings simply aid the arm movement by supporting the weight of the arm. They are relatively easy to adjust.

Mobile arm supports not only support weight but, through a complex and carefully balanced set of ball-bearing joints can greatly aid a child in moving the arm back and forth and up and down (fig. 8-2). Mobile arm supports are difficult to fit and to learn to use, but if your child is strong enough to use one it can greatly increase arm mobility and independence. It may enable a child to feed himself or herself and perform other actions involving arm movement.

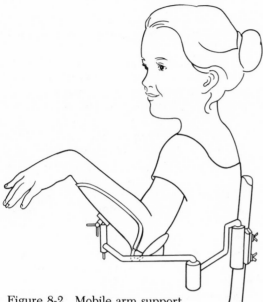

Figure 8-2   Mobile arm support.

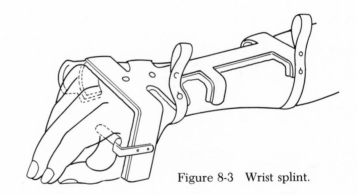

Figure 8-3   Wrist splint.

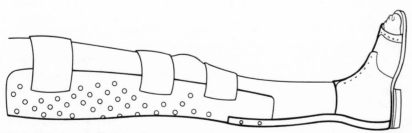

Figure 8-4   Night leg splint.

Wrist and hand splints are designed to increase hand function, which may be limited because of a loss or imbalance of muscular power, a loss of flexibility, or skeletal malalignment (fig. 8-3). The relationship of these factors will determine how to choose the best splint for your child. Although a variety of ready-made splints that can be adjusted to the individual's hand are available for adults, splints for children often have to be custom-made and experimentation may be necessary.

Precise fitting is important for optimal use. The effort to develop workable hand splints will definitely pay for itself in your child's increased hand mobility and consequent independence.

Night leg splints are leg braces meant for sleeping only and are worn in bed to prevent contractures or fractures (fig. 8-4). Since they do not have to bear weight, they are usually made of lightweight material. If your child is weak and doesn't have strong muscle spasms, you can "air-condition" plastic night splints with holes. Instead of drilling little holes, your rehabilitation doctor, orthopedist, or orthotist can cut out whole shapes of plastic for cooler wear.

It is best to use attachable shoes rather than make the splint out of a continuous piece of plastic that includes the foot. Then, as your child grows, you can lengthen the piece of metal that connects the splint with the shoe. But you must periodically check that the splint does not become too snug around the leg, particularly at the knee.

If you have to put shoes on your child, you may find it difficult to get the foot into the shoe. It is better to cut the toes out of the shoes, or even cut the shoe open all the way to the toe, rather than to cram your child's feet into them, since if the toes cannot lie flat in the shoes the feet can become permanently deformed or damaged.

If the shoes do not have Velcro closures, your orthotist can replace laces with Velcro, making it easier to put on and take off the shoes.

If you have to get your child out of bed, ask your orthopedist whether you should remove the night splint first. This is very important, for if you lift your child with night splints on, there may be so much stress on the femur (the big

bone connecting the knee with the hip) that it will fracture.

Leg braces support the leg so it can bear weight (fig. 8-5). Your child may need to have the ankle, the knee, or even the hip supported, depending on the condition or problem. Your doctor will probably give the orthotist a prescription for a standard type of brace. However, if you feel that your child's mobility is limited by the weight of the brace, tell your doctor or orthotist so you can try a different design or material.

The length of a brace depends on how much of the leg needs support for maximum function. If the brace is to aid with body control as high as the hip, you cannot compromise on length and need long leg braces that attach to a low back support system. A long leg brace extending above the knee (also known as a knee-ankle-foot orthosis, or KAFO) provides more support than a short leg brace extending to below the knee (also known as an ankle-foot orthosis, or AFO). But since the closer a short leg brace extends up to the knee the more support it provides, skillfully fitted and designed high short leg braces may eliminate the need for long leg braces.

The brace *must* fit well and be the correct length. As your child grows, the brace must be adjusted regularly.

A metal stirrup on the bottom of the shoe traditionally attaches the brace to the leg. The thinner the metal used in the stirrup, the easier it is to find suitable shoes for attachment. However, whether or not a lightweight or heavy-duty stirrup is to be used depends upon the child's needs for support, and there may be no room for compromise.

Ankle-foot orthoses, which go under the foot, around the back of the ankle, and up the leg, are sometimes used instead of metal stirrups. They are much lighter and enable your child to wear a variety of shoes, including soft soled shoes. Your child's condition will determine if plastic inserts are feasible.

The type of shoe, as we already mentioned, will in part be determined by whether the brace has a stirrup or an insert. Consult your doctor before adding any padding to the shoe, especially under the heel, for this could alter the alignment of the entire foot. Leather shoes are dangerous when new because their soles are

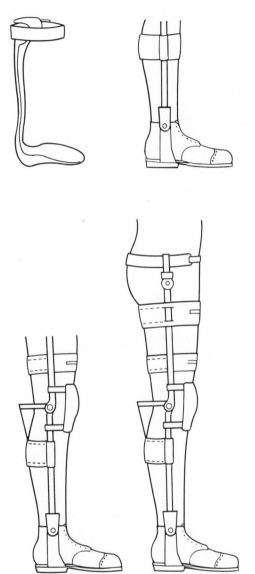

ches and swings the legs through, the toe of the shoe can stop the foot suddenly as it hits the ground, preventing it from sliding on through and perhaps capsizing your child in the process.

If the front ends of your child's shoes wear down very quickly, see page 155 for suggestions.

It is important to check the heels regularly for wear, for if the heel is worn down even as little as a quarter inch, your child will have a much different feeling of mobility. If one heel wears down faster than the other, it can throw the sense of balance off and affect your child's range of motion. These are subtleties that a child may not be able to articulate, but they are nevertheless important details.

Cuffs attach the brace to the leg along the calf and along the thigh in long braces. Most closures are made of Velcro, which is adjustable and lightweight.

Since the area where the cuff itself meets the upright is under a lot of stress, check it for tears.

Knee locks keep the leg rigid when bearing weight. They can be released so the child can sit. Drop locks are most commonly prescribed, since they are the easiest to use and the most reliable.

The material of which the brace is made can vary. A brace made of plastic with lightweight metal-alloy parts is obviously much lighter than a brace made of metal. The lighter the splint, the more possible it is for the child to walk distances with ease. However, lighter-weight plastic braces, especially when riveted to metal joints, wear out much faster than conventional metal braces.

Maintenance and repair of orthotic devices is extremely important. Active children are very hard on braces. Rather than get annoyed when repairs are necessary, check the devices and make minor repairs regularly to avoid more costly major repairs, which can also immobilize your child if he or she has only one pair of braces.

Nuts and bolts throughout the brace need periodic tightening, since they can work themselves loose quickly.

Joints need regular maintenance, for if they get dirty inside they do not move as easily. Many people simply give joints an occasional squirt of WD 40 or oil, but as the brace is used these

Figure 8-5 *(Top)* Plastic ankle-foot orthosis (AFO); metal ankle-foot orthosis; *(bottom)* knee-ankle-foot orthosis (KAFO); hip-knee-ankle-foot orthosis (HKAFO).

very slick, especially when wet. Roughen all smooth soles with a rasp before your child wears the shoes. Crepe soles can also be dangerous, for as your child supports his or her weight on crut-

liquids leak out, staining whatever they touch. It is preferable to learn to disassemble the joints and lubricate them with a special grease your orthotist can provide. If a joint is not properly maintained, it will stiffen and make it much harder for your child to move. Keep extra springs on hand, since the springs in the ankle joint can break.

The size of the brace must be checked regularly. This is crucial, especially in times of rapid growth. If the brace does not fit properly, your child will begin to walk incorrectly. Such a brace can also cause medical problems, including skin breakdown due to rubbing or pressure sores. (Extra-long cotton tube socks can help protect the skin, especially under plastic braces.)

Prostheses, as with braces, help the body function; but whereas braces support what is there, prostheses replace what isn't. In some minds, the word "prosthesis" may conjure up images of peg legs and hooks. But prostheses have come a long way.

A prosthesis is made to order for your child, on the basis of your doctor's prescription, by a prosthetist. Some prothetists are also orthotists. Read the guidelines in Chapter 2 on choosing a doctor, for similar considerations apply here.

The age at which a child should get a prosthesis depends on whether the child is a congenital or surgical amputee, on the age of the child who needs the device, and on the limb the device is replacing. By and large, the earlier a child is fitted with a prosthesis, the sooner he or she will learn to use it and the more consistently he or she will wear it. A child who learns to compensate for the missing limb by using the body in a different way is more likely to reject the prosthesis. Babies with congenital leg amputations are usually fitted with legs when they start to attempt standing. Upper-extremity prostheses are more complicated and require more mechanical coordination. Nonfunctional (no hand function) below-elbow prostheses are fitted as early as 10–12 months. Above-elbow types are fitted between three and four years.

Congenital amputees usually have a fleshy area surrounding the end of the limb and can be fitted for prostheses fairly easily. By contrast, the end of the limb of a surgical amputee is often slow to heal, does not have much fleshy covering, and consequently is much more difficult to fit with a comfortable prosthesis. Nevertheless, an initial temporary prosthesis can be applied at the time of surgery in the form of a rigid cast dressing with a pylon attached. A permanent prosthesis may be made as early as four weeks following amputation.

There is not only a physical difference between surgical and congenital amputees. The two groups also tend to view their bodies differently. Surgical amputees are often more desirous of replacing the missing limbs, whereas congenital amputees are sometimes more apt to accept their bodies as they are.

To make a prosthesis, a cast is made of the remaining part of the limb, or the "stump." Fitting arms and legs are often different specialties, and a prosthetist may specialize in one or the other. Ask your doctor or therapist where you should have the prosthesis made.

The construction of any joint will influence how closely that joint can simulate normal body movements. Since many innovative joints are available, give careful consideration to which type would be best for your child.

Lower-extremity prostheses are made of wood or plastic, with metal joints at the knee and sometimes at the ankle. Prostheses below the knee are usually held in place by a suspension cuff, which can be tightened snugly around the leg above the knee, often with Velcro. An above-the-knee prosthesis can be held in place with shoulder or waist straps, or it can be kept in place with a suction device, which eliminates the need for straps. Usually, the shorter the part of the body replaced by the prosthesis, the easier it is to use the prosthesis. As it is difficult to learn to walk with an artificial knee joint, it may take your child some time to gain mobility if the prosthesis leg is that long.

The weight of prosthetic legs can also greatly influence your child's ability to walk. Ultralight plastic legs might allow your child to walk much more easily than he or she ever could with a standard plastic or wooden one. So look into and keep informed about which materials can be used.

Upper-extremity prostheses are made in much

the same way as the lower-extremity types, but since they do not have to bear weight they can be made of much lighter materials. The stump usually fits into a shell, and the whole arm is then attached to the body with a harness. Since the hand is activated by arm and shoulder movement, your child has to learn how much movement is necessary for the desired hand movement. A myoelectric arm, first used in 1968, amplifies currents produced by muscle contractions in the stump and uses these to activate the arm. Some people can gain much more precise movement using myoelectric-type arms.

Missing hands are usually replaced by hooks, the most efficient replacement. If your child uses one, you will both come to view a hook as a hand and be delighted with what it can do.

Stump care is crucial, especially with legs, for much pressure is exerted on the stump when a person stands and walks. Ask your prosthetist which type of stump sock is best for your child. The stump size of new amputees may vary, so over time it may be necessary to increase the thickness of the sock used. When the diameter of the stump stabilizes (usually within the first year), it may be appropriate to replace the stump socket with a better-fitting one.

Stump stocks *must* be dry. Skin softens when wet and consequently is more apt to break down. On a hot day the stump sock may need to be replaced one or more times. The sock must also be clean, for clean cloth is not only more comfortable and absorbent but, should skin breakdown occur, infection is much less likely.

Stumps must be carefully washed and dried every night. At that time check the skin carefully for any red pressure spots. If these do not disappear within 10–15 minutes after removing the prosthesis, your prosthetist should check it. Since children grow, a prosthesis that fits well today may not fit in six months. Fit is particularly important with legs, for an ill-fitting prosthetic leg not only puts a lot of pressure on the stump but can also cause your child to walk with an uneven gait. Some shops build in some telescoping capability so the artificial leg can grow with the child. However, your child may need many legs before he or she grows up.

Learning to use a prosthesis takes time. Usually members of your medical team—your doc-

tor, physical therapist, occupational therapist, and prosthetist—will help you and your child learn how to use the prosthesis most effectively. It is your responsibility to understand what is necessary, to ask questions if you don't understand, and then to carry through with the prescribed program. Progress may be slow, and everyone involved may sometimes get frustrated. However, the effort will be worth it. In general, children acquire functional use of a prosthesis much faster than grown-ups. (For information on learning to walk with crutches, see pages 117–118.)

Must your child wear the prosthesis? Lower-extremity amputees are usually surgical and not congenital. Such children, many of whom have walked previously, tend to persevere in learning to use the prosthesis, since it gives them the ability to move about without a wheelchair.

By contrast, upper-extremity amputees, particularly those with congenital amputations below the elbow, can function quite well without a prosthesis, for they come to use the elbow like a hand without fingers. A person who is proficient with the use of one hand and a stump may find that even when wearing a prosthesis he or she tends not to use the artificial hand. It can also happen that congenital amputees, who have accepted their prostheses and have used them for a few years, suddenly just don't want to wear them anymore. This is particularly true of children with one congenital amputation below the elbow.

However, research has shown that below-elbow amputees are the most successful users of prosthetic hands and are most apt to use them if the prosthetics are introduced early enough.

If your child has and rejects a prosthesis, discuss with your medical team the pros and cons of insisting that he or she wear it. If the child can function well without the prosthesis, there is no clear-cut answer to the problem.

Crutches are needed by many children with leg braces and prostheses. Although the word crutch still conjures up the wooden underarm model (axillary crutch) in most people's minds, such a crutch is no longer used very often, since if used improperly it puts a great deal of pressure on the armpit and can pinch the nerves that lie just under the skin. Therefore, people using crutches regularly often use Canadian or forearm crutches (fig. 8-6).

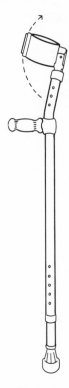

Figure 8-6   Canadian crutch.

Your child can walk most efficiently with crutches when he or she has a relatively long and effortless "swing through." This is influenced by total body weight, the strength of the arms, the weight of the braces or prosthesis, and the material out of which the soles of your child's shoes are made. There are two-, three-, and four-point gaits in which one uses combinations of moving the crutches alternately or together. Whatever method is used, crutches must be of the correct length. If your child is still growing in height, periodically check that the crutches are long enough.

Your physical therapist will work with your child to teach him or her how to walk, for this is a very individual matter influenced by your child's capabilities. But you can also consult adults on crutches, who may have helpful tips to pass along. The crutches should be as lightweight as possible.

The handgrip must be comfortable, for your child's hands bear some portion of his or her body weight. You can pad the grips with plastic bicycle handgrips. If your child needs more padding, have the orthotist pad the handgrip with foam rubber and then cover this with soft cowhide.

The crutch tips get a lot of wear. Cheap crutch tips may wear out in two weeks, whereas good ones may last for six months. You can extend the life of the tip by rotating it 90 degrees every week. The slug in the middle of the crutch tip tends to work itself loose, so reset the slug with a screwdriver when rotating the tip. Narrow crutch tips are lighter but provide less traction and may wear through faster. Wide crutch tips provide more traction on slippery surfaces but can get caught on objects when your child "swings through." If your child has to move about a lot in snow and ice, you can attach spikes or screw-in cleats, which have to be removed when your child is indoors. Experiment with different tips until you find which works best for your child. Then keep an extra pair on hand for repairs.

Learning to walk with braces or prostheses, with or without crutches, takes time, effort, and patience. Some braces and prostheses need little adjustment and are immediately effective, giving your child the desired mobility. But in most cases a child will have to learn how to use them to gain proficiency and to derive maximum benefit. This will be achieved only if the child really uses them.

Some children are in their braces or prostheses all day. In families of such children, these appliances are treated like clothes, something to put on in the morning and take off at night. Such children usually learn to use them well. But other children put on braces or prostheses only for certain exercise periods. When this is the case, it takes much longer for the child to accept them and learn to use them well. If your child is learning to use lower-extremity braces or prostheses, consider getting a set of parallel bars. (This can be easily made using pipes from your local plumber.) It is extremely helpful to have a mirror or punching bag at one end to encourage movement. Place these bars wherever the action is—in the living room, family room, or kitchen.

Many severely disabled people, as teenagers or young adults, decide to use only a wheelchair. While it is good for most children's bodies to spend some time upright, walking is not for everyone, and upright positioning and parallel-bar activity are sometimes contraindicated physically or from the standpoint of nurturing false hopes in families and their children. Walking can be laborious and can damage muscles and nerves of the hands and arms if they have to bear much weight, as with an older, heavier child. It requires much less energy to propel oneself in a wheelchair. A child can cover longer distances with speed in a chair and can carry things about in his or her lap. When you consider how much more active children are than adults, you can appreciate how a child might value the increased mobility a chair can provide. However, if your doctor feels it is appropriate to work with your child on walking, follow this advice. A child who can stand even briefly can transfer more easily. If he or she can walk short distances, a child can go places on crutches that are not wheelchair accessible, such as up steps and through narrow doorways. When your child is a teenager, he or she can choose whether to retain the ability to walk, but at least there will be a choice.

It is obvious that for a child to walk with braces or prostheses he or she has to be able to move his or her body weight. Hence the lighter and stronger a child is, the easier it is to walk. Plan your child's diet with care to prevent excess weight. Exercise programs to build up the arms and shoulders, such as lifting weights, are also helpful.

Combining a wheelchair with a walking program can give a child the best of both worlds. Therefore, when a child has the potential to walk, many rehabilitation programs now combine using a wheelchair with braces and learning to walk.

9

Vision, Hearing, and Communication Problems

It may be difficult to tell that your child needs glasses or a hearing aid unless the impairment is severe, and even then it may take some time, especially with a baby, to discover exactly what the problem is. Even an older child may not tell you about a problem, for he or she may not know what "normal" vision or hearing is. You will, of course, know if your child can't communicate verbally, but precisely for that reason it may be difficult to determine how best to help.

VISION PROBLEMS AND CORRECTIVE DEVICES

A full discussion of vision problems that cannot be corrected with glasses or contact lenses is beyond the scope of this book. If your child does have severe vision problems, contact the various organizations that serve the blind (see "eye and vision disorders" in Appendix 4, "Helpful Organizations"), for they offer much helpful information and support. However, if your child's eyesight can be improved through the use of glasses or contact lenses, it is helpful to have a fundamental knowledge of how the eye works and how best to buy and use glasses or contact lenses.

How Does the Eye Work?

The eye functions very much like a camera (fig. 9-1). When we look at something, the iris opens or closes to allow just the right amount of light

to enter the eye so we can see clearly. The lens focuses the image. If the light rays focus on the retina, a clean image is produced. But if the eye is the wrong shape, the rays will focus in front of or behind the retina, causing the image to be blurred.

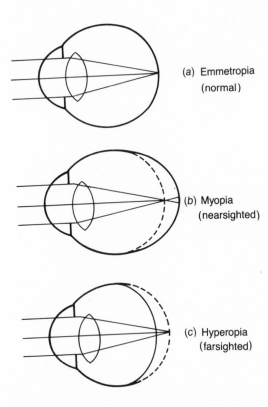

Figure 9-1 The eye: (a) normal vision, (b) nearsightedness, (c) farsightedness.

Nearsightedness (myopia) results when the eyeball is too long and the focus falls in front of the retina. Nearsighted people see objects that are up close clearly, but objects farther away, such as the writing on a blackboard and faces at the playground, get blurred. Since nearsighted children may do well at desk work, it can be difficult to detect a problem.

Farsightedness (hyperopia) occurs when the eyeball is too short and the focus falls behind the retina. Farsighted people can see distant objects clearly but have difficulty with small objects right in front of them, like the letters on this page. Such children often have difficulty with reading or written work; the correction of their problem can make a tremendous difference in their schoolwork.

Astigmatism results from abnormalities in the shape of the cornea or lens: some of the light rays are focused on the retina, but other rays fall in front or in back, causing eyestrain and blurring of both nearby and distant objects. Some children have only astigmatism; others may have astigmatism combined with near- or farsightedness.

Strabismus occurs when the eyes do not work in unison. Then the person sees two superimposed images, which is so distracting that often one eye simply ceases to function, letting the other take over the job of seeing. The major disadvantage of this is that if the eye is not used, it never develops the ability to see. Therefore, if you notice that your child's eyes cross or do not move together, have an eye specialist check your child.

Visual acuity is a measurement of the fineness of detail a person can see. The normal measurement is 20/20. The person with 20/200 vision, for example, must stand at a distance of only 20 feet to see what a person with normal vision can see from 200 feet. Anyone with vision that cannot be corrected to be better than 20/200 is considered legally blind, but many such partially sighted people function very well and can do almost everything necessary to live independently.

What Professionals Can Help You?

Ophthalmologists are physicians who have had the training of a general practitioner as well as additional training in the diagnosis and treatment of eye problems. They are qualified to do eye surgery. If your child has medical problems, an ophthalmologist is most qualified to treat the eye, taking into account how it relates to the rest of the body.

Optometrists are professionals carefully trained to give eye examinations. They are not medical doctors trained to diagnose and treat diseases of the eye. Most optometrists also dispense glasses; occasionally one may be more likely to encourage the buying of glasses than an ophthalmologist would be, since an ophthalmologist doesn't dispense glasses and, therefore, has less vested interest in people buying them.

It is best to consult with your child's regular doctor as to whether your child should go to an ophthalmologist or an optometrist. Although either can give a prescription for a simple problem such as nearsightedness, an ophthalmologist is probably a better choice if your child has a complicated vision problem or other medical problems. In either case, follow the pointers given in Chapter 2 to help find a qualified person who likes to work with children. Your child should see the ophthalmologist or optometrist at regular intervals, usually either every six months or once a year.

The dispensing optician fills the prescription for glasses and may well be the professional you interact with most, for you may have to go to the optician frequently if your child bends his or her frames out of shape, breaks the frames or lenses, needs frequent new prescriptions, or loses the glasses altogether.

The optician should like to work with children, have a good selection of children's frames, and be willing to take the time necessary not only to select the glasses but also to keep them in good working order. Ask for recommendations from your ophthalmologist and talk to other medical professionals, friends who wear glasses, and parents of children who wear glasses. If your ophthalmologist has a dispensing optician in his or her complex, do not feel compelled to use that optician.

An optician with a finishing lab will give you much better and faster service than one who sends work out to be done, because the former will work as quickly as possible for a customer in great need—such as a little girl who has just broken the lenses in her only pair of glasses. In addition, such an optician will probably stock a variety of replacement parts, so if your child breaks something, the chances are good that the optician can fix you up with something so your child can use the glasses until the broken part can be ordered and replaced. (When a child is initially fitted for glasses, it is usually sufficient to order only one pair. If the glasses need repairing, your child can usually manage without them. Then when the lenses or frame need replacing, you may consider getting an entirely new pair, and the old glasses can serve as a backup pair.)

What Kind of Glasses Should Your Child Have?

When you and your child go to get a prescription filled, your optician will give you a number of choices of frames and lenses. Look for frames with a warranty on the parts that your child is likely to break. You will probably have to buy an expensive frame, but buying an expensive frame and the occasional new temples is more cost-effective than buying a cheap frame with no warranty or replacement parts. Before coming to a decision about which frame to buy, consider the following.

The components of the frame are very simple.
The front is the part into which the lenses are set. The bigger the lens size, the heavier the glasses will be, so if your child needs thick lenses, remember that the smaller the size of the lenses, the lighter the glasses will be.

Large-diameter frames do *not* give a wider field of vision, and they exaggerate distortions near the edge of the lenses.

The bridge is the piece that fits across the nose; it must fit correctly if the glasses are to fit well. A properly fitting fixed bridge requires the least maintenance. If your child has a difficult nose to fit, you might think (or be told) that adjustable pads are just the thing. They might be best for a day or two, but they will be the first thing to go out of whack on the frame, causing the glasses to fit incorrectly. If an adjustable bridge breaks, repair involves a major solder job.

The temples are the side pieces that go around the ear. These come in different lengths and must be ordered to fit your child. A variety of temples are available, so discuss with your optician which seem most appropriate for your child.

- *Skull temples* are the type you see on most glasses. With most children, if these are correctly adjusted to the shape of the head, they hold the glasses securely in place.
- *Spring temples* contain a spring in the hinge. If these springs function properly, they keep the glasses adjusted correctly longer than skull temples. But be sure you only buy hinges that have a lifetime (or at least a one- or two-year) guarantee, because poor springs tend to loosen—usually at different rates; a frame with loose or uneven temple springs never fits correctly.
- *Cable temples* are made of flexible wire and fit around the ear. These keep the glasses in place better than skull or spring temples, but the glasses are more difficult to take on and off. As cable temples are more expensive than other temples and need to be replaced if not used correctly, they are usually not recommended unless it is known that a child has trouble keeping glasses on.
- A *pediatric harness* consists of half temples attached to an elastic harness that goes around the back of the head. This is often recommended for young children under three years of age or for an older child with impaired motor skills.

Since your child may well break the temples, make sure before ordering any frame that your optician can order replacement temples. Often frames on sale are closeouts of discontinued styles, and replacement temples are no longer available. It is also helpful if your optician carries some temples in stock which he or she can attach temporarily in place of the broken temple until the correct replacement arrives.

The composition of the frame is of primary importance. Frames are made of plastic or metal.

Plastic frames are cheaper than metal frames and require less adjusting, as they have some elasticity. However, they generally have a shorter lifetime than those made of metal because plastic is more apt to break. Even if plastic is taken care of properly, it will become brittle with age.

Metal frames cost more and are stronger. However, metal bends out of shape more easily and requires more adjusting than plastic. As metal frames are much narrower than plastic, your child may find them less distracting when looking above, below, or out to the side of the frames.

The composition of the lens also makes a difference in the feel and practicality of glasses. Lenses can be made of glass, plastic, or polycarbonate. Most prescriptions can be filled in any of these, yet there are factors to consider before making your choice.

The weight of the lenses should be considered, especially if your child has very poor vision, because the thicker the lens, the heavier the glasses. Glass is much heavier than plastic or polycarbonate.

The "breakability" of the lens is always a factor to consider with active children. Plastic and polycarbonate are highly impact-resistant but are not unbreakable. Glass lenses are treated to be shatter-resistant, but they will still break if you drop them just the right (or wrong) way. Once glass lenses are badly scratched, they are no longer shatter-resistant and should be replaced, especially if you think your child's glasses might get hit by a ball, a rock, or another child's fist.

The "scratchability" of the lens is the greatest problem with children's glasses. Glass may be heavy and may break, but it is much more resistant to scratches than plastic. Plastic may work for a very quiet child, but not for an active one.

The latest invention in lenses is the polycarbonate lens. Polycarbonate is the hardest type of plastic—almost as hard as glass. These lenses cost more than glass or plastic, but they may be worth the extra money if your child needs thick (and consequently heavy) glasses and is active (so the lenses may break) but is not so hard on glasses that the lenses would become quickly scratched.

Tinted glass is available but is usually not necessary for children.

The appearance of the glasses is very important, because a child who doesn't like the looks of his or her glasses may not want to wear them. You may rightly think that you have to look at your child, whereas he or she doesn't see the glasses once they are on. But your child has to wear them and should find them attractive. Once you have decided how much you can afford, let your child take an active part in choosing the frames.

Your child may need time to adjust to glasses, particularly if this is the first pair or if the new lenses are very different from the previous ones. A complaint about the fit of the frame and redness on the nose or behind the ears may be due to incorrect adjustment or rubbing of the frame. Even if you cannot see any redness, it is worth having your optician check the fit.

If after your child has been wearing glasses for about two weeks he or she still complains about vision or about related symptoms such as sore eyes or headaches, first take the glasses back to the optician to check the prescription. Mixups are rare, but they can occur. If the lenses are correct, call your ophthalmologist and have your child reevaluated, for a change in prescription may be necessary. If you have ever had your own eyes examined, and been asked, "Which is better, lens number one or lens number two?" you know there is a subjective element in lens prescriptions. This is why your ophthalmologist may have to try another prescription. However, as such problems are rare, it is best to assume that your child's prescription is correct unless he or she actually complains.

How Can You Best Care for Glasses?

Taking glasses on and off requires two hands. Grasp each temple right behind the hinge that mounts it to the front. Adjustments will last twice as long if you and your child learn to use two hands (even though, admittedly, most adults use only one hand).

Adjustment of the frames may frequently be necessary. If your child's glasses look crooked on his or her face, if the temples bend out rather than going straight back, if your child says the glasses hurt, or if your child cannot jump up and down looking at the floor without the glasses coming loose, they need adjustment. If your child can get to the optician alone, you may want to make him or her responsible for taking the glasses in for adjustment.

Athletic straps are extremely helpful if your child plays active sports where glasses are apt to come off. However, wearing glasses with a strap in place is apt to bend the frame out of shape. If the frame is well adjusted, it should be tight enough for most activities.

Cleaning glasses is a daily chore with most children—and a more frequent one with some. You can wash all lenses in the sink by running hot tap water on them, squirting on some liquid dishwashing detergent, rubbing them clean with your fingers, and drying them with a towel. You can blow on slightly dirty glass lenses to fog them up and then rub them dry. But don't try this with plastic or polycarbonate, as they are apt to scratch.

How Can You Tell if Your Child Needs New Glasses?

If your child cannot communicate well with you and tell you when things are fuzzy, rely on your ophthalmologist's recommendation as to how frequently your child needs to be examined. If your child can communicate, you can do some periodic checking yourself, for your child may need a change in prescription at least yearly until both head and eyeballs stop growing, in the teens or early twenties. If your child is nearsighted, practice reading freeway signs and the like. If your child can no longer read as well as when he or she first got glasses, an eye examination is in order. If your child is farsighted, periodically read books or look at pictures together.

If your child has an astigmatism, you can also make a general vision check using the methods suggested above. (As a rule, however, astigmatism is constant, while nearsightedness increases as the child matures. Farsightedness usually stays the same until adulthood.)

Remember, though, that none of this takes the place of the checkups your doctor recommends. Rather, it provides you with a means of periodically giving your child a superficial eye check that will indicate problems needing prompt attention.

Contact Lenses

Contact lenses are small plastic eyeglasses worn directly on the eye, floating on a thin layer of tears on the surface of the cornea.

Hard lenses are about the consistency of your finger nail.

Soft lenses are rather like a thin piece of cooked noodle. Some people find soft lenses to be more comfortable. This is not only because they are soft but also because they allow some oxygen to pass through them to nourish the eye. Also, since a soft lens is larger and doesn't move so freely on the cornea, dirt is less apt to get under it. The disadvantages of soft lenses are that they cannot correct astigmatism, they must be sterilized, and they usually must be replaced within two years, if not sooner.

Extended-wear lenses are made of an even more porous material and can be worn continuously for a couple of weeks at a time.

Contact lenses correct most vision problems and sometimes give better correction than glasses, particularly for people who have had cataracts removed. They are in fact the obvious choice for very young children, even infants, who have had cataracts. As these children need contact lenses in order to see, they rapidly get used to wearing them, but the parents must assume responsibility for care of the lenses.

Children with other vision problems are usually not fitted for contact lenses until reaching their teens, when they become responsible and motivated enough to care for them. Yet while contact lenses are usually not the solution for an active elementary-school child, as your child gets older you may nevertheless want to consider how well he or she could see and function in normal daily activities with contact lenses. If a child is very active and needs strong, expensive frames and many repairs, contact lenses may not be that much more expensive than glasses, and they do eliminate the need for repairs and the danger of having the glasses break while being worn, which might injure the child. And there are some children who just don't like the looks of glasses and therefore want contact lenses. Today children as young as 11 years of age have demonstrated the ability and willingness to assume responsibility for taking their contact lenses out and cleaning them, particularly if they are fitted with extended-wear lenses.

Not all people can comfortably wear contact lenses—at any age. If the cornea is not exposed to air, it can become oxygen-deficient, causing blurred vision and discomfort. This may be so slight that it either doesn't matter or is easily overcome, but for some people this causes major problems. Therefore, before purchasing any contact lenses for your child, check on your optician's guarantee period. Some opticians will let your child try them for one day free of charge. Others will charge for the fitting but give a 50% refund on the lenses and case within a 45-day trial period. If your child experiences pain during or after the trial period, seek prompt medical attention.

HEARING IMPAIRMENT AND DEAFNESS

If you think something is wrong with your child's hearing, have your doctor check your child right away. Hearing impairment can greatly affect your child's learning ability, and the sooner you take steps to help, the better. Even if nothing is evident on physical examination, your doctor should refer your child for further testing, probably by both an otorhinolaryngologist and an audiologist.

There are two major types of hearing disorders—*conductive* and *sensorineural*. A conductive disorder is a disorder in the functioning of the middle ear; a sensorineural disorder is a disorder of the inner ear. Some individuals have both.

Both types of hearing disorders can be caused by birth defects or disease. Whereas sensorineural disorders cannot be treated medically because the damage to the inner ear is permanent, conductive hearing loss can often be treated with medication or surgery.

Who Can Test Your Child's Hearing?

Otorhinolaryngologists are commonly known as ear, nose, and throat specialists. Such a doctor will determine the medical nature of the problem and whether anything can be done medically to improve hearing.

Audiologists are trained to detect and assist in the diagnosis of the acoustical nature of the hearing problem—how great the hearing loss is.

After the nature and amount of hearing loss have been determined, your child may be given a recommendation by the otorhinolaryngologist for a hearing aid. In other cases medical or surgical treatment may be preferable.

What Is a Hearing Aid?

A hearing aid works on the same principle as a telephone. It converts sound into electric energy, amplifies the energy, and then changes the energy back into sound. To understand what one hears with a hearing aid, think of a radio. If you turn up the radio's volume, what you are hearing gets louder. If the reception is good, it remains good; if you are hearing static, you hear louder static. An expensive radio may give you better, clearer tone and reception than a cheap one. A hearing aid has the same limitations as a radio. But it can selectively amplify different frequencies, like an expensive stereo that can be set to increase the volume of tones in specific registers.

Hearing aids come in a variety of forms. The most common type is worn behind the ear and connected to the ear by a piece of plastic tubing (fig. 9-2). For people with profound hearing loss who require more powerful aids, a body-type instrument is usually recommended. This is worn around the neck or in a pocket, and the

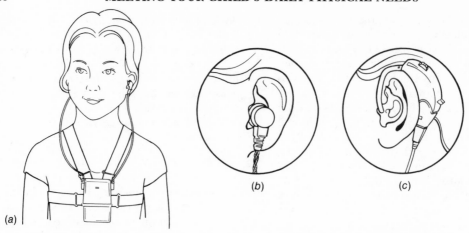

Figure 9-2   Hearing aids: *(a)* body aid; *(b)* earphone for body aid; *(c)* behind-the-ear hearing aid.

receiver (loudspeaker) is held in the ear by an earmold.

The disadvantage to either of such hearing aids is, of course, that they they amplify all sounds, not just those a person wishes to hear. Therefore, for children with profound hearing loss, FM auditory training systems are sometimes recommended. With such a system, a person can speak into a small microphone, the words are transmitted by FM waves, and the deaf child receives the information through the receiver of the body-type instrument with less amplification of the environmental noise. Such FM auditory training systems can be used in the home and are particularly useful in educational settings. The final basic type of hearing aid is the all-in-the-ear type, but its small size limits its power.

A hearing aid can successfully help a child with a conductive disorder. It may, however, have only limited value in a case of sensorineural impairment.

While a hearing aid may help your child hear, it cannot restore normal hearing. Nevertheless, it is crucial that your child be fitted with the hearing aid that can help best.

From Whom Should You Buy the Hearing Aid?

The recommendation for your child's hearing aid can be filled by a dispensing audiologist or a hearing-aid center. Use someone who carries a variety of reputable brands so you can pick the one that will best suit your child's hearing needs. You need a qualified person who works well with children and who is willing and able to give your child the follow-up care that may be needed. A dispensing audiologist is trained and licensed to do this, and if there is one in your community or nearby he or she might be preferable to a hearing-aid center. After being fitted with a hearing aid, your child should probably be seen twice during the first week, once a week for the next three weeks, once a month for the next five months, and then again before the end of the first-year warranty period.

All hearing aids come with a 30-day trial period. Although the audiologist's information can give the dispenser an indication as to which hearing aid would be best, dispensing hearing aids is an art as well as a science, and your child may have to try different aids to determine which helps most. Your dispenser should be willing to take back a hearing aid and let you try others should the first prove unsatisfactory.

Before deciding from whom to buy the hearing aid, get recommendations from your otorhinolaryngologist, audiologist, parents of other hearing-impaired children, and from hearing-impaired adults. You may also want to call local dispensing audiologists and hearing-aid centers to see what kinds of follow-up care they provide. Beware of anyone who tells you that he or she does such a superlative job that no one ever has to come in for a follow-up visit. And beware of anyone offering hearing aids at very low or very high prices, for the prices of hearing aids are usually standardized in a community among those selling reputable brands and offering the necessary follow-up care.

What Are Potential Problems Involved in Wearing a Hearing Aid?

The joy of wearing a hearing aid is that your child will be able to hear better than without it. But problems will occur.

Getting used to wearing a hearing aid may take time, and your child will need your encouragement as well as friendly, firm insistence that he or she wear it. Your child may take the earmolds out in the beginning until he or she gets used to them.

Improperly fitting earmolds can cause discomfort or pain, and your child will undoubtedly try to take them out. Since you will be seeing your dispenser at least every week in the beginning, discuss your success at keeping in the earmolds. If the molds fall out by themselves, they probably do not fit properly. It is sometimes difficult to get a good mold on a very young child who has small ears and may have wriggled during the fitting. However, your dispenser should be willing to make new molds if the first pair really doesn't fit. In rare cases sedation may be needed to keep a very wriggly infant still enough to get a good impression, but your dispenser probably won't suggest this until the first one or two impressions have not been successful. You may also find some dispensers are able to make better-fitting earmolds than others.

Ear infections can occur when a child wears the earmolds all day, so ear care is important. Your doctor will recommend how often and in what way your child's ears and the earmolds should be cleaned. Be sure the ears and earmolds are completely dry before inserting the earmolds. If your child starts taking out earmolds that he or she was previously willing to wear, an ear infection may be developing. Ask your doctor whether you should buy an otoscope (which your doctor uses to check ears) so you can detect early signs of inflammation or infection.

A malfunctioning hearing aid that produces distorted sounds can be detrimental. Before you even take a hearing aid home, be sure you understand how it works and how to check that it is functioning correctly. Ask your dispenser for a written checklist of how you can determine the nature (and, it is hoped, the cure) of minor hearing-aid problems. Then if you have a problem you can try to solve it yourself. If you can't, take the hearing aid to your dispenser and have it tested. If your dispenser thinks the hearing aid is functioning properly but you still have your doubts, try to explain this and work with him or her to solve the problem. Often small distortions can make a great difference to your child. On rare occasions a person will get a hearing aid that malfunctions more often than it should. If you are convinced you have a "lemon," discuss this with the dispenser, who should be willing to ask the manufacturer to replace a defective aid.

Lost or broken parts are something you will have to learn to take in stride. If your young child frequently loses earmolds, it may be worthwhile to ask your dispenser to get the earmold impressions back from the lab so you can get replacements made without needing new impressions, or even have a spare pair of earmolds made. But remember that a growing child may outgrow earmolds every few months. If your child uses a body-worn hearing aid, keep an extra cord.

Worn-out batteries are a frequent problem. Experiment with different brands to see which works best. Ask your dispenser which type of battery-testing device works best, for you should check the batteries daily, preferably in the evening after they have been used all day. Store spare batteries in the refrigerator, where they will last longer.

The hearing-aid setting must be checked daily to be sure it has been set at the proper amplifying level. A hearing aid can only amplify the sounds your child can hear, so while turning it *too low* prevents him or her from getting the full benefit of the aid, turning it *too high* will not improve hearing.

How Should Your Child Communicate?

The disagreement among different schools of thought on how best to teach the hearing-impaired or deaf to communicate has raged long and hard. Should a child be taught to communicate orally (by learning to speak and lipread), by manual communication (using sign language), or by Total Communication (a combination of the two)?

The vast majority of hearing-impaired children do not have profound losses, so the oral method is preferred for them. The controversy really centers on those children who are profoundly hearing-impaired and whose impairment was present at birth or before they learned to speak.

The oral method is often favored by hearing parents, who feel that, since most people in the world communicate by speaking, the only way for deaf people to participate fully in society is by doing likewise. They fear that if their children cannot speak and lipread, they will segregate themselves. However, studies have indicated that, whereas an average speaking child has a vocabulary of about 5,000 words by age five, an oral deaf child may know fewer than 50. The oral deaf child may therefore feel great frustration at not being able to communicate with family or friends. The deafer the child, the harder it will be to learn to speak, since the child cannot hear the sounds he or she or others make. While some profoundly deaf children can learn to speak intelligibly, most cannot.

A complication with lipreading is that more than half of the sounds in English look like other sounds. It is difficult even for experienced lipreaders always to understand what is being said.

The manual method is taught by deaf parents to their children. Manualists contend that a signing child can build a vocabulary about as fast as a hearing child and can thus communicate well from an early age. But the signing child is limited to communicating with others who can sign.

Total Communication is a new approach that began to be accepted in the mid-1960s. It encourages deaf children to integrate speech, lipreading, hearing aids, and sign language.

Whereas many now favor Total Communication, there are still staunch oralists and manualists. You will have to make the difficult decision as to which method of communication you want your child to learn. It may be helpful to speak not only with educators and parents of other deaf children but also with deaf adults who have grown up with this disability and can give you their perspective. Write for information from the different national organizations for the deaf listed under "ear and hearing disorders" in Appendix 4, "Helpful Organizations."

The Silent Garden: Understanding the Hearing Impaired Child (see Appendix 3, "Suggested Reading") presents an impartial discussion of the advantages and disadvantages of these various approaches, illustrated with descriptions of the lives of people who have lived with deafness. The authors, one of whom has been profoundly deaf since birth, also address other dilemmas faced by parents of deaf children.

NONVERBAL AND NONVOCAL COMMUNICATION

If your child is unable to acquire intelligible speech or legible writing skills, you should make every effort to provide alternative modes of communication such as nonverbal (without words) or nonvocal (without voice) ones. Nonverbal communication includes any way of conveying a message without using words, from eye blinks to sophisticated electronic devices. Nonvocal communication is used by an individual who cannot speak. Such a person may be able to communicate nonverbally, or verbally through the use of a device that employs words. Although you may think you can intuit what your child wants, the more communication skills your child can develop the greater will be his or her ability to communicate with anyone he or she wants. You have to work with a speech therapist to determine exactly what modes and methods are best for your child.

The Use of "Yes," "No," and "I Don't Know"

If your child can learn to respond to questions that can be answered in one of those three ways, a conversation can flourish to the extent that you can ask meaningful questions, intuiting the direction of the conversation and the next question to ask. In order for a child to use a yes-no response, he or she must be able to make at least one movement that is distinctive from all other movements to signify "Yes." The absence of the movement can then mean "No." If the child can make two movements, then one can signify "Yes," the other "No." The third response option of "I don't know" requires another reliable movement. A child may learn to move his or her head or even just the eyes as responses. If a child cannot do any of these he or she may be able to activate with some part of the body a switch connected to a buzzer or light. Then one buzz could mean "Yes" and two buzzes could mean "No."

Once a reliable system for indicating "Yes," "No," and "I don't know" has been established, everyone who interacts with your child should know about it. You might want to make an attractive sign that reads something like this:

Hello!
My name is Mary.
I cannot talk because of motor problems.
I can think and I like to visit.
I say "Yes" by looking up.
I say "No" by looking down.

If the rules for communication and interaction are clearly stated, most people will adjust to them in a few minutes. But if they are not known, communication is frustrating for both parties. An older child may have a much more explicit sign:

Hello!
My name is Ben.
Please give me time to express myself.
Don't interrupt me.
Don't guess at what I'm trying to say.
Look me in the eye.
Take turns so we can have a conversation.
You get three chances!

Whatever sign you decide to make, make sure your child has it when he or she goes out. It could be attached to a wheelchair or worn around the neck or wrist.

The Use of Other Nonverbal Signs

Gestures are valuable if your child has controlled bodily movements. But many children learn to express a whole range of emotions with their eyes by varying the direction, duration, and intensity of their gaze. Your child may also learn to look in a particular spot to indicate one or more things. For example, looking up could mean "Yes" as well as other things your child frequently wants to say, such as "Please reposition me." Looking at your forehead could indicate "Think some more" or into your eyes could mean "Please read my mind."

General Rules for Nonverbal Communication

You can make it easier for your child to communicate if you do the following:

- Teach your child to make signals as clearly as possible.
- Ask one question at a time, wait, and give your child a chance to think of an appropriate reply and to indicate his or her response. Delays in response may indicate either that your child didn't understand the question or that he or she is thinking about the most appropriate way to indicate a response.
- Ask yes-no questions to help your child communicate. If it is obvious that your child is trying to tell or ask you something, it helps if you narrow the options by finding the classification or category: "Is it about home? School? Someplace else?" "Are you thinking of telling me something? Asking me something?" "Do you want to talk about someone? Some place? Some thing? A feeling?" "Is it about the past? The present? The future?" Whereas it is easiest to ask factual questions like these, remember that your child also has feelings that she or he may wish to communicate with you, so you may want to ask, "Are you angry? Frustrated? Bored?"
- Continue the conversation until the messages are clear. The range of what your child can communicate often depends on how well you can reflect upon what yes or no might mean, for your child

depends upon you to think about, guess, interpret, or restate what he or she would like to say. Repeating and clarifying what you think your child is saying can help prevent distorting the message.

• Recognize deadlocks. Sometimes you may really just not understand what your child is trying to communicate. At that point you can say, "I really don't understand. Do you want me to go on trying?" Often deadlocks are reached because the questioner reached premature conclusions without clarifying what was "heard." The best method to check for erroneous assumptions is to recheck information phrase by phrase. For example, "Are we talking about your class at school? Is it about your teacher?" and so on.

Sometimes you may ask questions that your child doesn't want to answer, relating perhaps to feelings or personal concerns. But a nonvocal child has no way of saying, "I don't want to talk about it." Or your child may want to talk about a topic that makes you uncomfortable. But if open communication is your goal, try to overcome such barriers if they arise.

Communication Devices

Since there is a severe limitation to the range of thoughts and ideas that can be expressed by answering questions with "Yes," "No," or "I don't know," additional communication methods can be most helpful. You must be resourceful and innovative in providing ways for your child to communicate. Finding or developing the right communication aids may depend upon collaboration with speech therapists, occupational therapists, physical therapists, and rehabilitation-engineering specialists. It may take patience, effort, and cooperation on the part of many individuals, but this will certainly be worth it if ways are found to help your child communicate more effectively.

Communication boards (or conversation boards) are charts of pictures, symbols, phrases, words, letters of the alphabet or numbers, and, of course, "Yes," "No," and "I don't know" (fig. 9-3). Your child might have such a basic information chart, placed in a protective plastic cover, to take along as he or she moves about during the day. If your child uses a wheelchair, you might attach basic information to the chair or tray. When planning the size and shape of the board, be sure to space the items so that even with uncoordinated movements your child can convey one response and one response only. A child can point with one finger, use a hand-held pointer, a pointer held in the mouth, or one attached to the forehead. Direct-focus headlights, as used by dentists and doctors, may also be effective. If your child does have fine motor coordination, a pocket-sized notebook with words and phrases may be very helpful.

You will have to make new charts for your child as his or her interests and ability to communicate change. Early charts may contain only pictures, but if your child can read and spell, words and the alphabet can be most helpful. Since spelling each word is a laborious way to communicate, if you know the word being spelled, say it so your child can converse more rapidly.

COMPUTER TECHNOLOGY FOR THE DISABLED

Recent technological advances in microcomputer technology can be utilized by children with a wide range of disabilities, such as mobility, motor, language, hearing, visual, or vocal impairment, as well as educable mental retardation, psychological and social disorders, autism, learning disabilities, severe multiple handicaps, and long-term illness.

If you do not know a lot about computers and/ or how they can be helpful to your child, the *Microcomputer Resource Book for Special Education* (see Appendix 3, "Suggested Reading") can provide basic information. It is written specifically for parents and special education professionals in nontechnical terms about how microcomputers can be used to help disabled children (and adults), and it includes an extensive appendix containing specific information on products and available resources. *Closing the Gap* (see Appendix 3, "Suggested Reading"), a newsletter on computer technology for the handicapped, can help keep you informed on new products. Regional conferences and university extension courses for adults often provide

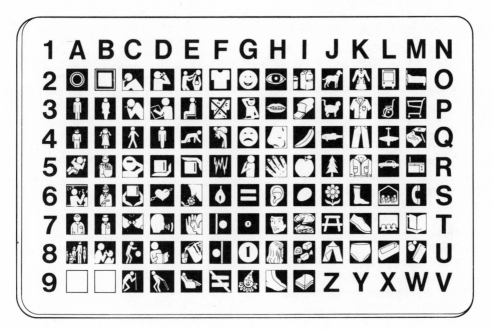

Figure 9-3 Picture communication board.

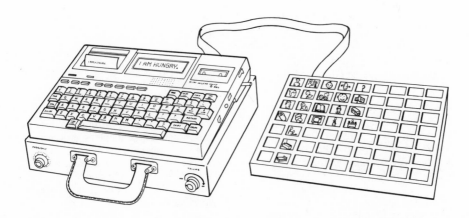

Figure 9-4 Computerized communication system allows for keyboard and/or expanded keyboard input and provides for vocal, printed, and/or visual output.

not only basic information but also the latest in innovations in this rapidly changing field. Unless someone working with your child is well-informed and enthusiastic about computer technology, you may have to learn what is necessary to find the appropriate computer technology for your child.

Available equipment can range all the way from small, relatively inexpensive hand-held devices to complete computer work stations. Since equipment is constantly becoming more sophisticated and new devices are being invented, choosing the right equipment for your child may be a difficult task. While you could become dazzled by all the equipment you could buy, you shouldn't become deluded into thinking that the most complicated and/or expensive system is best. If you think your child might be aided by some equipment, his or her current skills and potential abilities should be reviewed by professionals involved in his or her care. Such a review team might include a physical therapist, occupational therapist, speech pathologist, teacher(s), rehabilitation engineer, expert in communication technology, yourself, and your child. The team might consider basic questions such as:

- What is the nature of your child's disability?
- What can't your child do now that you would like him or her to be able to do?
- What kind of a system using microcomputer technology could be of assistance now?
- What are your child's projected needs in the future?

These areas might then be considered in light of the following basic factors:

- *Input systems:* While most of us think of typing onto the keyboard of a computer, expanded keyboards with pressure sensitive plates that can be used for alphabet letters or symbols are also available. If a child has limited motor control but does have at least one controlled movement, he or she can utilize a switch to run the system. There are even voice-controlled systems. (The first with high recognition accuracy is Computer Aided System for the Handicapped [CASH] by Cascade Graphics Development—1000 South Grand Avenue, Santa Ana, CA 92705).
- *Speed of communication:* When you consider that

normal conversation can approach speeds of 200 words per minute, anyone with limited motor control will be greatly aided if the number of input actions needed to produce output can be reduced. So if sentences, phrases, and/or words can be stored and called up by typing in an abbreviated form, this can significantly increase the speed of communication. Ultimate speed will be influenced to some extent by the speed of the computer and its peripheral devices, but much more by the speed of the software and the acceleration methods it provides to reduce input actions.

- *Output systems:* It is possible to have dynamic visual display (such as one sees on a computer terminal screen or a calculator), a static visual display (such as a light appearing behind one of the images on a display board), hard copy (printed paper or Braille), or vocal output (speech synthesizer). Just as a normal child learns to speak and to write down information, a disabled child is aided in his or her development if given a range of modes of expression.
- *Flexibility and growth:* It is very important to consider not only what your child needs now but also what he or she will need in the future. For example, a five-year-old who can't read and who has limited understandable speech could use a computer with an expanded keyboard with symbols, which could be continually reprogrammed by the family to assist the child in expressing himself or herself. As most of the child's friends probably can't read either, voice output via a speech synthesizer would be important now. When he or she gets a bit older and can spell and read, the keyboard and hard copy would be important. Types of available software (programs) should also be considered. In computer jargon, what you want is an "upward expandable system," or one than can be modified to meet your child's changing needs in terms of input and output modes (hardware) as well as programming (software).
- *Environmental controls:* A physically disabled child might gain greater independence by having an environmental control capability, which would enable him or her to telephone (dial, answer, hang-up) and control lights (on/off), page turners, electric bed, television, radio, and nearly any electrical device. If your child needs these now or might need them in the future, it is important to consider how they could interface with the computer system.
- *Telecommunications devices:* Hearing- and/or speech-impaired children should be able to communicate by telephone. While telecommunication devices (known as TDDs and TTYs) have tradition-

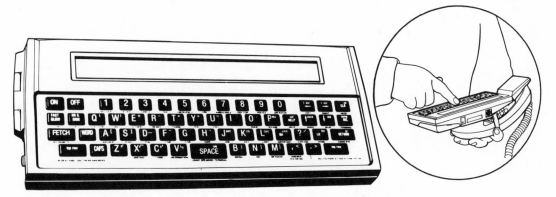

Figure 9-5   Pocket-size personal communicator.

ally been used, these typewriterlike devices can be used only to send typed messages over telephone lines to another person with a compatible system (unless one pays a special message center to convey the information). Computers with modems are now frequently used, and any two persons with home computers need only each get a modem in order to communicate by telephone. The first small, pocket-size personal communications device is made by Audiobionics (9913 Valley View Road, Eden Prairie, MI 55344, Voice + TDD 612-941-5464). This multifunction minicomputer can be used to send typed messages or text, which can be created and stored in advance, to home computers or TDDs. To communicate with people who have no computers or TDDs, such a personal communicator can use speech produced by its built-in voice synthesizer, thus making it possible for disabled individuals to use any telephone. Its other functions, such as telephone number listing, autodialing, autoanswering, and phone-line monitoring, will help make telephoning much easier. Noncommunicational functions important to hearing-impaired individuals, such as alarms and alarm couplers, are also included.

- *Reliability, maintenance, and repair:* Obviously any system is only of use when it works. Therefore, check for warranties and guarantees, as well as by whom, where, when, and for how much the system can be repaired. Unless you live in a metropolitan area that has a dealer who will provide same-day service or offer you a loaner while your unit is being repaired, this can be a major consideration.

- *Convenience and portability:* Consider the size and weight of the system (although this is less important for wheelchair-mounted systems). You also need to know if the system can be run on battery power and, if so, for how long between rechargings.
- *Trial period:* Once you have determined which device(s) might be appropriate, try to arrange for a trial period so that you can see whether your child can actually learn to use the device or whether something else might be more appropriate.
- *Cost:* Communication systems are expensive, in part because most of them are produced in relatively small quantities. (The most innovative approach to providing reasonably priced systems was started by Words +, Inc.—1125 Stewart Court, Suite D, Sunnyvale, CA 94086—which decided to use mass-produced hardware and to customize only the switch interfaces and software.) However, your initial aim is to identify which system would be best for your child now and in the near future. While it may seem best to postpone the purchase of a specific item because it will become commercially available in a few months, don't put off buying something your child needs now because you think something better will be produced in the future. In the rapidly changing field of computer technology it probably will be, but your child needs to be able to communicate as effectively as possible *now.* Such equipment is often covered by insurance if you can provide *medical* (not psychosocial or educational) need. Local service organizations will also sometimes be of assistance. (See Chapter 17 for information on funding.)

10
Bathing, Toileting, and Personal Hygiene

BATHING AND PERSONAL HYGIENE

Little children should be allowed to play and get dirty. After all, children are washable, and they can be cleaned and made tidy when appropriate. Since cleanliness can be very important for physical well-being, you have to devise methods to clean and bathe your child.

Soap can make your child slippery and difficult to hold. It can also irritate the skin if not properly rinsed off, and it can dry the skin. Therefore, use a mild soap in a convenient form, perhaps a pump dispenser or a soap bar on string that can be hung within reach or placed around your child's neck if he or she is doing the washing. Add bath oils to the water if dry skin is a problem.

Baths

Baths are the easiest way to clean the whole child if he or she can be immersed in water. If your child can safely sit alone and wash himself or herself you have no problem. But water is very dangerous, especially for children with limited mobility. *Never leave such a child unattended in the bath.*

Bathing with your young child makes very good sense. You both get clean, you don't strain yourself kneeling and leaning over the tub to clean your child, and you can make it into a playtime, with toys and storytelling in the tub. You can also help your child exercise in the tub, since he or she will probably be more limber

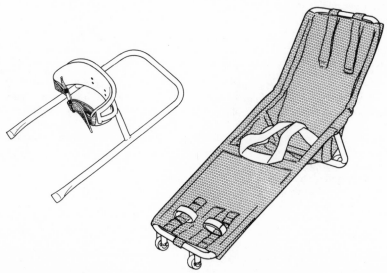

Figure 10-1   Children's bath seats.

there (see pages 106–109). If you have another young child who needs supervision, he or she can get in with you, should the tub be large enough.

If your child cannot get in and out of the tub unassisted, it is safest to get into the tub first yourself, kneel, and then reach out to lift your child off the floor and into the tub. When it is time to get out, simply kneel and lift your child onto the floor. It is not safe to step in and out of the tub while holding your child.

Children's bath seats offer not only support but also the security of being strapped in (fig. 10-1). Such seats can be made of molded plastic, tubular metal with fabric seats, and even foam. These can be helpful if your child cannot sit safely alone and you do not want to or cannot bathe with your child. However, even with such a chair you should never leave your child in the bathroom alone.

Safety stripping can be installed to make the bottom of the tub less slippery. This rough-surfaced plastic tape with strong adhesive backing is available in most hospital-supply and many home-improvement and hardware stores. The tape can easily be cut with scissors in appropriate-length strips, which should be placed about two inches apart on the bottom of the tub.

Plastic safety mats with suction cups on the bottom are somewhat less satisfactory. Initially you have to put about half an inch of water in the tub and then press the mat down hard at several points to make it stick. The mat must then be removed at least weekly for cleaning to prevent an accumulation of soap and dirt underneath that could cause it to smell and slip.

Permanent safety guard or grab rails can be screwed into the wall vertically, horizontally, or diagonally. Be sure you screw these into the wall studs. If they are screwed into plaster or wallboard they can easily pull loose when someone relies on them for support. Bathtub safety rails can also be mounted onto the side of the tub.

Bath mats can be made out of foam Ensolite pads used for backpacking. These high-density pads are skidproof, waterproof, and insulating, which is particularly useful if your child lies on the floor while being dried and dressed.

Bathtub thermometers are crucial if anyone in your family lacks sensation in any part of the body. Such a person can use the thermometer to test water temperature and avoid scalding.

Showers

Many disabled or ill children cannot take showers unassisted. However, with the following modifications, you may find showers to be better than baths.

A hand-held portable shower head that connects into your regular bathtub faucet or shower head can be used to direct the spray so the water doesn't stream down on your child from above. With such a shower head the various parts of your child's body can be washed with ease. Massage force is available on some of the more expensive models. (However, a whirlpool bath is far superior if massage is necessary.) Of course, these shower heads also make cleaning the tub easier.

Bath seats or bath-seat-and-commode combinations are usually made of tubular metal with plastic seats (fig. 10-2). If you will want to roll your child in and out of a shower, make sure the chair has casters and locks to facilitate safe transfers. The chair you choose should be safe and stable for sitting as well as for transferring. When choosing a bath seat to be positioned inside the tub, consider a park-bench-type transfer bath seat, which facilitates transferring and is stable.

A wooden ramp can be built up to a shower stall (fig. 10-3). A platform made of parallel slats of wood can then be placed in the shower, level with the lip. Then a bath chair on wheels as mentioned above can be rolled right into the shower. Flooding is prevented because the water runs between the slats. If you buy or build such a platform, carefully consider in which direction to run the slats so the wheels of the bath chair won't get stuck between them. You can also drill holes into wider boards or a piece of plywood, but since the holes weaken the wood a slat construction is more durable.

lem, examine different models and get some professional advice as to which model would best meet your needs. Some lifts can be used for bathing as well as for transfers at other times.

Bed Baths

Bed baths may be necessary for several reasons: your child may be too ill to move, may have a large cast or bandage, or may have uncontrollable movements that preclude baths or showers. Soap the entire body only two or three times a week. Only the genitals and armpits of an older child need soaping daily. The following basic routine can be modified to meet your child's individual needs:

1. Get your supplies ready:
    a. A washbasin or dishpan
    b. Soap
    c. A washcloth or mitt
    d. A large bath or beach towel to cover your child
    e. A towel to place under the section being washed
    f. A towel with which to dry your child
    g. Warm water
2. Remove the bedspread, blankets, and top sheet.
3. Cover your child with the large towel, uncovering only the part you are washing in order to prevent chilling.
4. Fill the basin with warm water.
5. Put the towel under each part as you wash it, using a new one should it become damp.
6. Use only as much soap as is necessary, since soap residues can irritate the skin. Rinse the skin well.

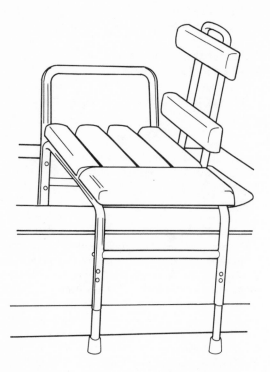

Figure 10-2   Park-bench transfer bath seat.

Bath lifts are expensive and take up much tub and bathroom space. This can be a disadvantage if your bathroom is small and the tub is used by persons other than the disabled. But if a lift seems like the best solution to a bathing prob-

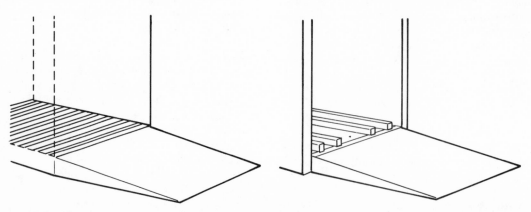

Figure 10-3   Shower stall with wooden ramp and platform or with tracks for shower-chair legs.

Change the water often to keep it clear and warm.

7. Dry each part of the body after it has been washed and rinsed before continuing, being especially careful to dry any areas with skin folds, such as the genitals.

8. Bathe in the following order so you use the cleanest water on the areas where it is most desirable. If you always follow the same order, it aids you in remembering what you have yet to wash:
   a. Eyes
   b. Face
   c. Neck and ears
   d. Chest and abdomen
   e. Far arm
   f. Near arm
   g. Hands
   h. Far leg
   i. Near leg
   j. Feet (You can even put a foot or hand right in the dishpan.)

9. Get clean water and then wash:
   a. Back
   b. Buttocks
   c. Genitals (You can place your child on a bedpan and pour water over the genitals to moisten the area. When washing, remove the accumulated secretions [smegma] from behind the foreskin of an uncircumcised boy and from behind the hood of the clitoris of a girl. Then rinse again. Wash girls from front to back to prevent infections of the bladder and vagina from germs from the anal area.)

Inflatable bed-bath tubs are an alternative if it is difficult for your child to use a conventional

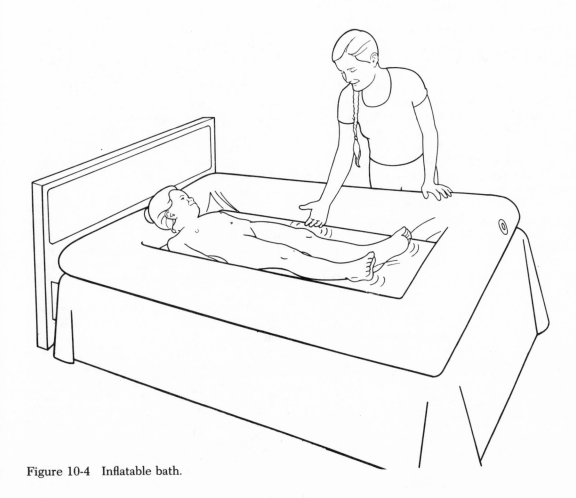

Figure 10-4   Inflatable bath.

bathtub or shower, for sponge baths are often unsatisfactory over an extended period of time (fig. 10-4). An inflatable bath must be well designed and made of a strong leakproof material (such as urethane-coated nylon) and engineered so it can be inflated, filled, emptied, and deflated quickly. The size and weight of the whole unit will also influence how easily it can be stored or taken along when traveling. Before you buy one, talk not only with the manufacturer but also with families and therapists experienced in using that specific product. You will then have to decide whether using an inflatable bath or making any necessary bathroom adaptations and buying equipment would be more appropriate for your child.

Hair

Keep your child's hair clean and tidy.

Length is important when a person spends considerable time lying down or having his or her position radically and rapidly changed. Long hair can become hopelessly tangled and untidy. The most convenient styles for girls are very short hair or hair that is long enough to braid. Braided hair becomes less tangled, looks neater, and probably stays cleaner longer than other styles. A quick braiding twice a day will keep your child's hair neat. If you cut shoulder-length hair (which could be braided) somewhat shorter before surgery, you may find that after the surgery it is too short to braid but still long enough to become tangled.

Shampooing is disliked by many children. Those who cannot move themselves come to fear or hate situations over which they have no control. This is probably why so many ill or disabled children dislike having their hair washed. It is your responsibility as an adult to make shampooing as pleasant as possible. If your child can be bathed in a tub or shower, wash the hair there. You can also wash it in the sink. A small child may lie on the kitchen counter while you wash his or her hair, supporting the head with an object such as an inverted dishpan. For a bedridden child, you can buy a special shampooing tray.

How frequently hair should be washed cannot be determined by a set rule. If it looks dirty or your child's scalp itches, it's time. But if your child is really ill or dislikes having his or her hair washed, you can procrastinate.

A very mild shampoo, such as baby shampoo, is less irritating if it gets into the eyes.

A good conditioner (as sold by beauty-supply stores) used after shampooing helps prevent tangles. The conditioner is most effective when actually combed through the hair with a "rake comb." A regular comb will just comb the conditioner out of the hair. After conditioning, a final rinse is needed. If the hair still tangles when drying or between shampooings, try a spray-on conditioner.

Skin

Skin is a most important covering of the body, protecting it against disease. Any breaks in it can lead to the entry of bacteria. Skin care is particularly important for the child who has limited mobility or uses orthopedic equipment. Pressure, friction, rubbing, and moisture can all lead to a breakdown of skin tissues.

Pressure sores (decubitus ulcers), which result from a lack of blood supply and consequent lack of nourishment to the skin and underlying tissues, can be serious. They most commonly occur over bony prominences, such as heels, knees, lower back, sacrum, and buttocks—wherever the blood supply is restricted and the padding poor (fig. 10-5). Pressure sores are often caused by unrelieved pressure, such as occurs when one sits or lies in one position for an extended period of time.

A child with limited mobility often endures the discomfort of being in one position for too long because he or she can't move. A child lacking sensation in a part of the body doesn't even feel the discomfort that is the signal to shift positions and therefore is much more at risk. Pressure sores can also be caused by friction under braces, moisture from perspiration, and in an incontinent child by the moisture and chemical content of bodily discharges (stool and urine).

In the early stage, a pressure sore appears as a warm, tender red spot that turns white when

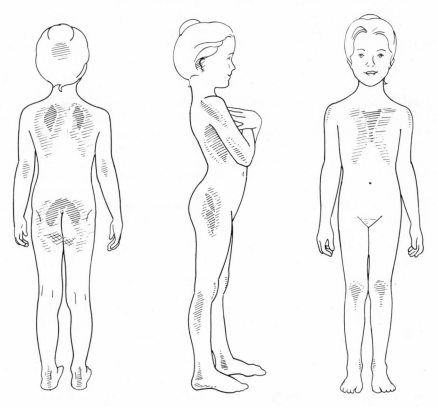

Figure 10-5   Areas susceptible to pressure sores.

you push it with your finger but that becomes red when you release pressure. Any area that stays red for over 15 minutes is a potential problem area. In later stages, the skin becomes blue or purplish-red and is often mottled. It is no longer warm and does not pale when pressed with your finger. Now an open sore is almost inevitable because impaired nourishment has caused the tissue to die.

Pressure sores are deceptive in that we see only the skin dying on the surface, but layers of undernourished tissue can die all the way to the bone, causing wounds that heal only very slowly and that sometimes require surgery. Prevention is the key.

A daily skin check can aid in the early detection of pressure sores. Check your child for any pressure spots first thing in the morning and also when taking your child out of the wheelchair or when taking off any orthopedic appliances at the end of the day. As soon as your child is old enough, involve him or her in these daily skin checks. First you can do it together, making verbal or written notes of any skin problems. You will have to use mirrors so he or she can see his or her back, but the effort is well worth it. Pressure sores are one of the biggest health hazards of disabled people, particularly if they lack sensation. If your child is going to grow up and be independent, this is certainly one health-care area in which he or she must learn to assume responsibility.

Ensuring good circulation is the best prevention of decubiti. Circulation is assisted by massage. It is important to take pressure off any vulnerable area by changing positions. During sleep, this means devising a means to change your child's position if he or she cannot do so alone. During the day, it means preventing your child from staying in any one position too long. If your child is in a wheelchair but has arm mobility and is strong enough, discuss with your doctor or therapist whether wheelchair push-ups done periodically throughout the day will prevent pressure sores caused by sitting. (Wheelchair push-ups are done by grasping the armrests with the hands and pushing the trunk up off the seat of the wheelchair.) If your child is not that strong, you should have various chairs into which he or she can be transferred (a high chair, a wheelchair, a potty, the couch, etc.), since your child will sit differently in each location.

It may also be good to have a nap time in the afternoon, when your child can lie down after you have taken off appliances and the skin has time to "breathe."

Air space for large body surfaces (when lying down or sitting) can be created by using sheepskins or a variety of flotation devices. Sheepskins not only insulate the body in cold but aid in ventilation during hot weather since the body on sheepskin does not contact a solid surface. Synthetic sheepskins can easily be washed in your machine at home. They are almost as effective as real skins and much cheaper. Waffled foam pads provide ventilation when placed under the sheets, since not all of the body contacts the hard, solid surface of the bed. More elaborate (and expensive) measures include the use of air (or water-flotation) mattresses in which air (or water) circulates through coils, providing a constant shift in pressure without moving the child.

Much experimentation is being done on wheelchair cushions. If your child has pressure sores, and a plain foam cushion or sheepskin is insufficient, read page 92 and seek professional advice as to the best type of cushion for your child. The price may seem outrageous, but do not try to save money here.

Small bony areas such as heels and elbows can be protected by making or buying sheepskin protectors for these body parts. These can be particularly useful in minimizing the rubbing of your child's heels when in bed.

If your child has to wear an orthopedic appliance daily, prevention is crucial. Any lining you can place between the child and the appliance will protect the skin (and the appliance should be fitted while your child is wearing the underwear or socks he or she will use as lining). For example, a child should wear all-cotton undershirts with sleeves beneath corsets and back braces. For boys, a regular cotton T-shirt is fine.

A girl might want a variety of cotton T-shirts that either blend with the other clothing she is wearing or are cut so low that they don't show. You can cut off the sleeves, leaving a flap underneath the arm to protect the armpit. The first complete line of 100% cotton brace liners has been developed by Brace Mates (PO Box 223, Forest, VA 24551), and their lingerie is covered by most insurance companies when purchased with a brace or corset. Any lining added at home after bringing the completed brace home from the orthotist's shop should be very thin, for thick padding will add more pressure to an area. If a red pressure spot continues for more than a day or two, have the brace checked to make sure it still fits properly; your child may have outgrown the brace.

If your child says something hurts or rubs, take the complaint seriously. Try to locate the problem area and alleviate the pressure immediately. If you wait until you can see where it hurts due to skin breakdown, the damage has been done. The healing process may take a long time, for your child will be unable to put any pressure on that area and consequently may be immobilized. For example, a pressure sore on the buttocks will confine a child to lying on the stomach and sides in bed or on a gurney. If surgery is necessary, the process will be not only long but costly.

To prevent pressure sores, you must keep the skin clean and dry. If the skin is sound, you might consider vigorous rubbing with a towel after baths to help circulation.

Nails

Short nails stay clean longer and are less apt to break the skin if your child has uncontrollable itching or spasticity. If your girl decides on long nails, her opinions should probably be respected, since this may be one of the few aspects of her appearance she can control.

Teeth

All children, especially the ill and the disabled, need regular dental checkups. Using the guidelines in Chapter 2, choose your dentist with care, trying to find one who likes working with children and, if possible, has some experience with disabled children. It is important to begin checkups around the age of two and a half (before your child even needs dental treatment) so your child gets used to visiting the dentist. If you anticipate problems before that age, discuss with your dentist or doctor whether your child should be seen earlier.

Sore teeth and gums are not just a dental problem. They can make any feeding problems even more difficult, for a child may become reluctant to chew fully or even to eat at all if it hurts. Also, any cavity or sore can be a source of infection that can become generalized throughout the body.

If your child has seizures or a strong bite reflex, be careful about putting your finger in his or her mouth. Your dentist can help by making a block to prop the mouth open for cleaning, or you can fabricate one yourself by wrapping surgical tape around three tongue depressors or using a new, clean, wedge-shaped rubber doorstop. Sometimes physical or occupational therapists can offer additional suggestions about how to handle children who are particularly sensitive about having things done in their mouths.

If your child can open his or her mouth only a little, ask your dentist or pharmacist whether an electric toothbrush or a Water Pik might be appropriate.

TOILETING

A disabled or ill child often has toileting needs that must be met.

Diapers

Cloth diapers are far superior to disposable ones. They are cheaper, and they are ecologically sounder since they can be reused.

But washing diapers can be a problem. If you don't have the time, energy, washer, dryer, or clothesline, consider a diaper service, which still is cheaper than using disposable diapers.

If you wash your own diapers, and your child is getting rashes or your diapers impress you as being too gray, try placing the diapers in a pail of cold water as you take them off the child (hot water sets stains), and let them soak. Wash them in the machine with soap, *not* a harsh detergent. Since skin irritation is caused by soap residues and uric acid, be sure to rinse the diapers well. You can run the machine through the whole cycle once again, just with water, to make sure the diapers are well rinsed. If your child has sensitive skin and is prone to rashes, add bleach to the cold water you soak the diapers in and give the diapers the second rinse.

If you have the time and energy, hang the diapers out after washing, for the sun not only leaves the diapers smelling nice but also disinfects them. If you don't have time, use a dryer. (An oversized washer and dryer are helpful if you do a lot of wash each day.)

Putting diapers on can be done in a variety of ways. You want most of the thickness where it is needed, between the legs, positioned in such a fashion that your child does not end up with legs wide apart, waddling like a duck. When using one or two diapers, a good method is to place the diaper, folded to the width of the waist, under the child (fig. 10-6). Then twist the diapers a half turn between the legs before bringing them forward to pin. If you need three diapers, or if your child's bottom might be chafed by the fold, fold one diaper into a narrow rectangle and place it straight between the legs.

Large-size diapers are available from hospital-supply stores or by mail order. Most diaper services carry adult-size diapers. Disposable diapers are also available in larger-child and adult sizes. Incontinent pants are sometimes a good alternative for a child embarrassed about wearing diapers.

Toilet Training

Most "normal" children become toilet trained regardless of the method employed, because as such babies grow they develop the ability to con-

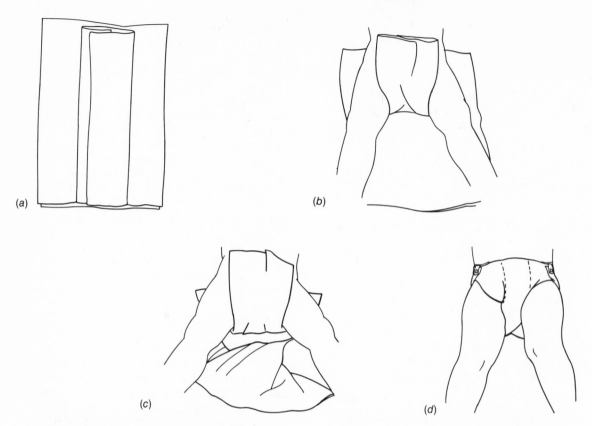

Figure 10-6   Folding diapers: *(a)* lay down 1 diaper or 2 diapers with 1 on top that has been folded into thirds; *(b)* lay your child on the diapers; bring center section of top diaper up in front; *(c)* turn flat diaper over; *(d)* bring up and fasten with clips.

trol urination and bowel movements.

With an ill or disabled child you may need to consider carefully the child's physical, mental, and emotional needs, not only now but as they might change in the future. For example, it might be easiest just to keep your young child in diapers because you don't think you have the time for the long and difficult training process. For little children, diapers are fine. But it is much more convenient for everyone, including the child, if you can get an older child out of diapers.

If your child can be toilet trained, or even if you think this *may* be possible, by all means try. You may have to train yourself so you make sure your child uses the toilet regularly at the appro-

priate times, such as upon waking, after meals, before bed, and periodically during the day. Keeping a record of when your child has wet diapers and bowel movements will also aid you in setting up a schedule.

The following is a reasonable procedure for toilet training. First, help your child get used to sitting on the toilet. At this stage, playing with toys or reading stories may help the child sit still. You may have to strap your child on, if his or her balance is poor or wanderlust great. Since cooperation is vital, have your child sit for only a few minutes. If nothing happens, try again later.

If your child is capable of signaling you, he or she may begin by telling you *after* wetting. You may find this exasperating, but welcome it as the first step in toilet training. Use positive reinforcement and praise your child's every effort. When training your child to stay dry at night, limit liquids before bed if his or her medical condition makes this possible. Make sure he or she urinates before going to bed. Sometimes it helps to get a child up to use the toilet before you go to bed at night. Then be sure to take your child to the toilet as soon as he or she wakes up in the morning, for many children stay dry all night and wet only after they awaken. Girls often train earlier than boys, and even a "normal" boy may have occasional accidents all through elementary school.

If you think your child can be trained but he or she continues to wet the bed, discuss this with your doctor.

Do not assume that once trained, always trained. If your child's condition is progressive, he or she may have to begin wearing diapers again, perhaps only at night, perhaps all day. It is important to understand that such regression can occur. Sometimes it is temporary, as during severe illness or emotional trauma; sometimes it is permanent.

Toilets, Potties, Commodes, Urinals, and Bedpans

Potties are excellent for the toddler and young child. A waist belt helps the child stay put, armrests aid stability, and an optional tray provides a play area. As potties are also portable, you can use them not only in the bathroom but also in other locations, should that be more convenient. If your child needs constant supervision, consider where, besides the bathroom, the potty could be used.

A *children's commode* (fig. 10-7) may be necessary when your child outgrows the infant potty but is too unstable to use the regular toilet. Sometimes the best solution is to modify a standard potty. You can increase the height of the potty by extending the legs or by making a higher seat, which you can cover with vinyl and even pad with foam. Headrests can also be extended with wood or molded plastic. If your child needs chest or head straps to hold him or her in place, you can make these of webbing and

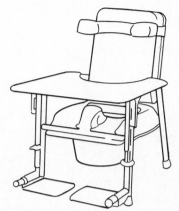

Figure 10-7   Children's commode.

Velcro. A shop that makes orthopedic appliances may be able to make these modifications for you.

A regular toilet can be used by some children. If your child's feet cannot reach the floor, it is important to provide a footrest, for it is *very* difficult to work at having a bowel movement with the legs dangling. Your child will also have a better sense of balance and security if legs are stabilized.

Grab bars, which you attach to the side of the toilet, provide support while sitting and assistance when transferring. Try to find the model best suited to your needs. Some have arms that can be removed or swung out of the way, while on others you can adjust the width between the arms and the height of the legs.

A *raised toilet seat* fits onto the regular toilet and raises it to wheelchair height. An open space in the front of the seat is useful for girls so they can wipe themselves. But unless a boy has a guard in the front of the seat, he may well urinate all over the floor instead of into the toilet. So examine the various models available.

A *padded toilet seat* is more than just a luxury; it is a necessity for a particularly bony child or anyone who has to sit for a long time.

Commodes or commode-shower chair combinations are helpful if your bathroom is not large enough for your child to enter it and transfer from a regular wheelchair. Since commodes are more compact than wheelchairs, they can often be maneuvered into a bathroom and sometimes even wheeled over the toilet. Commodes can, of course, also be used in any other room. Check the dimensions of the commode to make sure you can wheel it into the bathroom, if that is the plan. Also make sure the hole in the seat is small enough to support your child. Some commodes have push-button height adjustments on the legs. Since commodes also come with or without casters, decide whether you want the stability of the plain leg or whether you need the mobility that wheels provide. Some commode chairs have regular padded chair seats, and therefore can be used as a chair to move about the house. When the seat folds up, it reveals a commode seat and can be used as a potty. Since commodes are expensive, try to find one that is versatile, practical, portable, and meets your child's positioning needs.

Urinals are necessary for males who cannot use a commode or toilet (fig. 10-8). These are bottles into which the boy inserts his penis while urinating. Plastic ones with gradations are convenient if you have to measure your child's secretions. Tight-fitting covers help prevent spillage and confine odor. Child-size urinals can be purchased in hospital-supply stores, larger pharmacies, and sometimes even stores with large baby departments. Since there is always a chance that urine will leak out or spill, spread a few sheets of newspaper, a towel, or a piece of waterproof material under your child's perineal area (bottom) before giving him the urinal.

Bedpans come in two basic shapes (fig. 10-8). The contour type is the most widely used; it comes in adult and child sizes. The fracture or slipper bedpans are smaller and flatter and are usually slipped under the patient. Therefore they are easier and more comfortable than the contour type for an immobilized child, such as one in a body cast, and for a child who has unusual difficulty in getting on a bedpan. Emesis (vomit) basins can be used with little girls, but you may want to pad the edges with a washrag or small towel for comfort.

If you are using a bedpan for the first time, here are some hints:

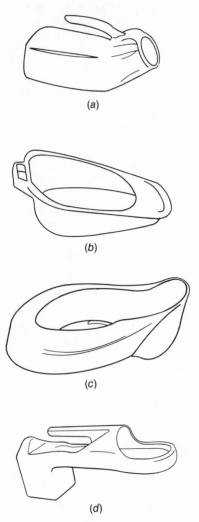

(a)

(b)

(c)

(d)

Figure 10-8 *(a)* Male urinal; *(b)* fracture pan; *(c)* regular bed pan; *(d)* female wheelchair urinal.

- Make sure your child is lying level; if possible even tilt the bed so your child's head is slightly higher than the feet, for it is very difficult to urinate uphill.
- If using a metal bedpan, warm it with hot water and then empty it before placing it under the child.
- If you wet the bottom and sides of the inside of the bedpan by sloshing water about and then pouring it out before use, it will be much easier to empty and clean.
- Place protective padding such as newspaper or a

towel under the child before positioning the bedpan.

- If possible, roll your child onto one side, position the bedpan, and then roll the child back onto it. If your child cannot be rolled you will have to lift him or her.

- Proceed with caution, for it may be difficult to get your child off the pan without spilling the contents, even if you use a fracture pan.

Toileting a Child in a Body Cast

Toileting a child in a body cast extending to the thighs is difficult at best. If your child is not yet toilet trained or is incontinent, cut disposable diapers into pieces about a half inch larger than the hole in the cast, tape the edges with microporous paper tape (available from your pharmacist), and then tuck the diaper up into the cast. Be sure to change it frequently.

Urine-collection devices, plastic bags with an adhesive that sticks to the torso, work better with some children. With boys you can use a condom type urine-collection device. Fecal-collection systems are also available. As the adhesive can irritate the skin, particularly when removing the device, be sure to use an adhesive remover available from ostomy supply houses before hanging devices.

A Bradford frame (fig. 10-9) is used by some orthopedic hospitals for children in body casts. You can construct one of your own, for it is basically a wooden platform on which your child lies with a cutout under the buttocks like the seat of an outhouse. A bedpan can then be placed under the child.

A bedpan, as described above, can be used with toilet-trained children in body casts, but unfortunately this is not easy. If you have time, first tuck a plastic wrap around the edges of the cast and up inside it before toileting to protect the cast from soiling. (Since this plastic is irritating to the skin, it cannot be left in place.) Then slide a fracture bedpan under the child. The real trick is then to remove the pan when full without spilling any of the contents.

Casts will get soiled and you will have to clean them the best you can. Try using Q-tips between the cast and your child's body. On the outside of the cast you can use soap, baking soda, or even Lysol, but use as little water as possible since it will be absorbed by the cast. Do not cover the cast with any waterproofing material, for then less air will pass through the cast to your child's body, causing skin irritation.

Bowel Programs

A bowel program to ensure regular evacuation is vital. Work with your doctor or other health-care professional to develop a program that works for your child.

Constipation is a common problem. The colon (large intestine) can become sluggish if a person has a poor diet, is dehydrated, is in poor health, or is inactive. If food stays in the colon too long, the body keeps absorbing moisture out of this food residue, slowing the passing of waste and hardening the stool, thus constipating the patient.

Preventive care is best. Be sure your child drinks plenty of liquid, preferably water. While clear juices are all right, milk, which contains fat and protein, does not classify as a liquid. Liquid should be taken continually during the day. Half a glass of water every hour is much more benefi-

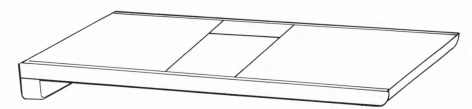

Figure 10-9   Bradford frame.

cial to the body than eight glasses consumed at one time.

If your child can eat solid food, roughage—the fibrous part of plants that is neither digested nor absorbed—is important. Roughage absorbs water, keeping the stool moist and providing bulk, which helps the intestine move its contents along. Plain bran is most effective in providing bulk and much more effective than what are advertised as "bran cereals." Bran can be sprinkled on any food, is tasteless, and will probably be eaten if used sparingly. It is extremely dry and should be mixed with sufficient liquid or moist food such as yogurt, applesauce, etc. Two tablespoons are a sufficient supplement for most adults: ask your doctor how much your child needs. (More information about roughage in the diet is given in Chapter 12.) Drinking hot liquids can also stimulate peristalsis (the rippling movements in the colon and rectum to expel the stool).

Finally, activity, or at least changes in positioning, helps. If your child can move about, encourage sufficient exercise. If your child cannot move unassisted, change his or her position frequently. (See Chapter 7 for more information on changes in body position.)

If your child is constipated despite preventive steps, appropriate external aids can be used. However, these should never replace the preventive measures. Although it is desirable to avoid frequent use of any external aid, some severely disabled or ill children may need to use at least one additional measure daily.

Discuss your child's problem with the doctor and decide upon an approach. It may take experimentation to find out what works best for your child, and as his or her condition changes further modifications may be necessary. Constipation can be treated in the following ways.

Bowel programs can take advantage of the peristaltic action of the stomach occurring after meals. The normal peristaltic movements can often be triggered by digital stimulation, the stimulation of the anal sphincter with your finger. Cut your nail short, put on a disposable plastic glove if desired, lubricate your finger (usually the smallest one for children) with K-Y Jelly and insert it one inch up the rectum. If you feel no feces inside, your child is probably not ready for a bowel movement. If the stool feels soft, this stimulation may cause the bowels to start moving.

Glycerin suppositories can be used if you can feel a normal stool that doesn't move. When inserting the suppository, make sure it is in past the sphincter muscle. Hold the buttocks together so the suppository has time to melt before it is expelled. (See pages 52–53 for insertion of suppositories.) As it melts, the glycerin lubricates the mass of stool in the rectum. If you use a glycerin suppository on a hard stool you may get a defecation reflex, but passing a hard stool will be painful. Preliminary softening should be considered.

An oil enema can soften the stool. These enemas can be purchased in prepared form from a pharmacist or can be made of corn oil. Six to eight ounces is normal for adults; ask your doctor what amount to use for your child. You can use an empty Fleet enema bottle for this. When putting any liquid into the rectum, your child should be lying on the left side so that the liquid will follow the normal contour of the descending colon, running in by gravity. Give the oil very slowly, over a 15-minute period. Otherwise it will fill the rectum and come right out again. A good time to give oil enemas is when your child is in bed, just before going to sleep. Then the oil is more apt to stay in all night and soften the stool. Evacuation will probably be possible in the morning, if necessary with the help of digital stimulation.

Regular enemas cause massive peristalsis, which irritates the bowel and forces out even hard bowel movements. These are painful and to be avoided if possible. If you do have to give an enema, use the prepared types such as the Pediatric Fleet Enema because you will have to insert much less liquid than with a home water enema. Although you may have heard of using soap in an enema, this is not recommended, since soap is irritating to the bowel.

Laxatives come in four basic types:

1. A stool-softener contains detergents designed to break surface tension and keep the stool moist.
2. A bulk-former absorbs water, keeping the stool soft.
3. An irritant stimulates peristalsis.

4. A purgative is a stronger irritant and is often used to empty the bowel before testing or surgery. Purgatives should be used only if nothing else works. Because they are so strong, they leave the bowel relatively paralyzed for a number of days, creating the impression of constipation and the need for more laxative. This kind of use can lead to what is called "the laxative habit."

Whereas some laxatives contain only one of the above ingredients, many contain combinations of them. If your child must use a laxative, ask your doctor which type will be effective and not harmful. For example, if a person has kidney damage, anything containing magnesium (such as milk of magnesia) can be very harmful. You will probably have to experiment with dosages, measuring the amount in cubic centimeters very carefully. (Read pages 47–48 for guidelines on measuring medication.) You may find there is a *very* fine line separating too little and too much. If the prescribed laxative doesn't work, discuss this with your doctor.

Enlist your doctor's aid in establishing a bowel program for your child to ensure regular evacuation. Hospital enterostomal therapists are especially trained in this field and can give you helpful advice. Your pharmacist is also a valuable resource person if you want to gain a greater understanding of what laxatives are available and how they actually work.

Diarrhea is an intestinal disorder characterized by frequent soft or watery bowel movements. It is often a symptom rather than a disease. Diarrhea presents the obvious difficulty of keeping the child clean and preventing accidents. But it is also important to understand that when we have diarrhea, liquid normally reabsorbed into the body during the passage of feces through the colon is passed into the bowel movement. This loss of liquid can lead to dehydration. The smaller the child, the more serious this water loss can be. Do not delay in getting medical attention, particularly for infants. Since this liquid is not just water but contains electrolytes (minerals and other compounds necessary for normal cell function), the fluid loss can also lead to electrolyte imbalance, which upsets the total body chemistry.

Mild diarrhea can be controlled by a diet con-

sisting mainly of clear liquids such as apple juice and the gradual addition of foods like bananas, rice, applesauce, and toast—known as the "brat" diet (see page 34). The lactose in milk and milk products may aggravate the problem. In case of severe diarrhea, your doctor may have to prescribe oral medication or even give an injection to stop it. Lost electrolytes can be replaced with a solution such as Pedialyte. However, since electrolyte imbalance can occur from having too many as well as too few electrolytes, never use an electrolyte solution without first consulting your doctor.

Management of the Neurogenic Bowel and Bladder

Children with defective development of the spinal cord or with spinal-cord injuries have special needs. An understanding of the function of the sphincters and abnormal elimination mechanisms is vital for parents of children with such impairments.

Management of the Neurogenic Bowel and Bladder, is clearly written and provides useful information (see Appendix 3, "Suggested Reading," for a full citation).

A bladder program must be established for your child with professional consultation. Catheters are necessary if your child no longer wants to wear diapers or cannot otherwise urinate.

External catheters can be used for incontinent boys. Discuss with your doctor whether diapers or an external catheter is more appropriate. Usually, incontinent boys wear diapers until about the age of five. For the severely retarded or ill child who is cared for at home, diapers may always be more appropriate. But if your son will be going to school, he may think diapers are babyish and prefer using an external catheter.

The penis is first wrapped with a foam strip that has adhesive on both sides. With small children, sometimes more than one layer is used to build up the circumference of the penis. A urinary collection device (or condom catheter), which looks like a condom with a drainage tube at one end, is placed over the penis; the tube drains into a collection bag, which is fastened to the leg with Velcro straps, or into a bedside drainage bag when the child is in bed.

You may need to experiment to find a device that fits well. A poor fit around the top of the condom can cause leakage. If the external catheter is molded correctly to fit the tube, there is less chance of the tube twisting and crimping, which can cause backflow into the condom. Backflow, in turn, can cause leakage and skin irritation or even prevent adequate emptying of the bladder, which can cause bladder infections. If your child's penis is irritated by the adhesive or urine, look into specially made skin preparations to protect the penis.

Internal catheters are used by incontinent girls and those boys who cannot empty their bladders with external catheters.

Intermittent catheterization (every six to eight hours) is usually preferred to leaving in a permanent catheter, since the foreign body in the bladder often leads to infections that can damage the kidneys. You can learn to catheterize your child; he or she may even be able to learn to do it alone. Your doctor will give you specific instructions.

Colostomies, Ileostomies, and Urostomies

These can be either temporary or permanent. More ostomies have been done than mastectomies, and most ostomates (persons with ostomies) come to lead normal lives. If your child needs such surgery, don't panic. Contact a member of the United Ostomy Association in your area or the enterostomal therapist if your hospital has one and ask for help. *These Special Children* is an excellent book written especially for parents of ostomates. *The Ostomy Book* also provides detailed information, although it is written primarily for the adult ostomate. Both books are included in Appendix 3, "Suggested Reading."

Obtaining information, assistance, and supplies. Enterostomal therapists, employed by more and more hospitals, are excellent resource persons and can be contacted by phone. Some equipment manufacturers will give you information on the phone about their products. Companies that carry a complete line of such products often advertise in the journal of the United Ostomy Association. Many of them have tollfree telephone numbers and employ enterostomal therapists who can give you invaluable advice on the variety of devices available and can try to help you solve equipment problems. But be sure to contact your doctor first if your child has any difficulty urinating or defecating.

It is best to discuss with your doctor in advance what signs or symptoms of urinary or bowel problems your child may have so you can call the doctor if you think your child is ill.

MENSTRUATION

Menstruation usually begins sometime between the ages of 10 and 16, although it can be delayed or irregular due to serious illness. Although sexuality is discussed in more detail in Chapter 15, it is crucial to note here that children are sexual beings just like the rest of us. It is up to you to give your child a healthy attitude toward the human reproductive system.

Your child should know the basics of menstruation and reproduction before puberty. Most younger children are much more interested in the mechanics of reproduction than in sex. If sexuality is handled openly, children will learn as they grow and will gain information when appropriate occasions present themselves. If they see a tampon or sanitary napkin and ask about it, answer them honestly and in a matter-of-fact way. When your children gain knowledge in this way, over time, you won't panic when you see puberty rapidly approaching and feel you must sit down and give a "birds and bees" lecture. When your daughter is nearing menstruation, have a discussion with her, reviewing the information she has learned over the years. Give her the actual sanitary napkins (pads) and tampons she will need when her period does begin and show her how to use them.

Pads are best for regular use, especially to avoid the possible danger of toxic shock syndrome (TSS) associated with tampon use. Toxic shock syndrome is the result of a staphylococcus aureus (staph) infection that enters the bloodstream and becomes systemic. It is thought that TSS can occur in women using tampons because the tampon absorbs much of the vagina's natural moisture, causing it to dry out. Since the tampon is a foreign object, it can irritate and abrade the lining of the vagina. If there are staph bacteria present in the vagina, they can pass through these small wounds into the bloodstream. Although TSS is uncommon it can be fatal.

To avoid risk of toxic shock syndrome, consider the following:

- Use tampons only when you feel your child really needs them, as when flow is heavy or pads might show, leak, or smell. Since tampons are more convenient if your child is incontinent or in a body cast, you will have to use your good judgment.
- Use only the less-absorbent tampons such as "regular" or "small." *Change them at least every four hours.*
- Do not use tampons at night since they mustn't remain in place for more than four hours.
- Alternate between pads and tampons.

- *Never* use tampons if your child has a staph infection, such as impetigo or boils, on another part of her body.
- Stop using tampons and notify your doctor immediately if any of the following symptoms of toxic shock syndrome occur:
    a. Sudden onset of high fever (102° F or higher) during or just after the menstrual period.
    b. Vomiting, diarrhea, or muscle pain.
    c. Rapid drop in blood pressure, often resulting in shock.
    d. Sunburnlike rash followed by skin peeling.

If your child has a physical or mental handicap that means she will need help during her period, she should still know what will happen to the best of her ability to understand. While many retarded children will not comprehend the intricacies of the reproductive system, they should be told about menstruation.

11

How and in What to Dress Your Child

Clothing a disabled child can be a complex problem. Ideally, your child's garments should not only look attractive but should also be comfortable, easy to put on and take off, and easy to maintain. Think about how and in what to dress your child, as well as how you can involve your child in selecting clothing and in getting dressed and undressed.

Dress your child in street clothes during the day and keep pajamas for sleeping at night. What we wear both influences and reflects our self-image, and children are affected in these same ways, although they may not be able to verbalize this. Thus a child who is kept in pajamas will be seen, and may see himself or herself, as an ill or disabled child rather than as, for example, a five-year-old boy named Alex. Even if a child is ill and staying in the house, getting cleaned up in the morning and dressed in clothes helps to emphasize living rather than being ill.

Cleanliness also influences the way one feels. If your child gets dirtier than most because he or she crawls, spills food while eating, or drools, try not only to select fabrics that camouflage the dirt but also to accept the fact that your child and his or her clothing will need to be washed frequently.

Tidiness is still another factor to consider. If your child can't move independently and you position your child, take an extra minute to see that clothing and hair, as well as your child's body, are positioned correctly.

Your Child's Participation in Selecting Clothes and Getting Dressed

A "normal" child who is old enough to dress alone usually selects what to wear for the day. If your child cannot get dressed unassisted but is mentally capable of choosing what to wear, he or she should be given the opportunity to do so. This may be one of very few areas where your child can make choices and be independent.

Your child may decide to try to camouflage some of the more visible signs of an illness or disability. A girl, for example, may want to wear slacks or long dresses to cover skinny legs and braces. If this is the case, it is important to respect her wishes rather than to ignore or make light of them.

Your child can gain independence not only by helping to choose what to wear each day but also by having a say in the purchase of new clothes, even if this requires extra effort on the part of those who care for the child. This isn't to say that your child should have anything he or she wants and should always get the most extravagant item. But if your child does need new clothes and is not mentally disabled, discuss together what you think he or she needs. Looking through a large mail-order catalog may give you ideas of styles and prices. By using the yellow pages of your phone book, you can determine without leaving home which stores carry what you want.

Getting such preliminary information is especially important if your child fatigues easily or has trouble getting about; otherwise, shopping can become an ordeal and it will be tempting to take the easy way out and just leave your child at home. But do take him or her with you, since it can be a valuable experience—and getting out is always important.

Once you are at the store, give your child some choice in what you buy. If, for example, you have decided together that your son needs a shirt in a certain price range, and the desired shirt is available in both blue and green, let him choose, even if your choice would be different.

Almost any child can become involved in the dressing process to some degree. If a child is extensively paralyzed, he or she may never be able to dress alone but can come to understand the procedure. Begin by explaining to your child what you are doing as you dress him or her.

Teach your child to dress independently if at all possible. It is easiest for a child with some mobility to learn first how to get undressed. You see this with babies who at a certain age delight in stripping. A disabled child may be unable to strip, but you may begin to notice that your child tries to cooperate with your efforts to undress him or her. In this case, praise and encourage this cooperation.

Positioning can be very important. If a child has a problem with balance and has to worry about capsizing, it is impossible to concentrate fully on undressing unless he or she feels secure. It is easier to undress some children if they are sitting in a chair with arms for body support or in a wheelchair with the brakes locked. For other children, undressing while lying on the floor, table, or bed, sometimes using the headboard or pillows for props, may work better. Experiment with various positions to find what works best.

Practice one dressing technique over and over again before adding another. Too many different sequences may confuse your child.

As you undress your child, give clear, concise, and consistent directions, such as "Lift up your right foot" or "Out comes your left arm." This way you may teach not only how to undress but perhaps also such concepts as front and back, up and down, left and right. Begin by helping with each step, putting your child's hands, arms, and feet through each motion. Then as your child gains skill, slowly withdraw your assistance. You may have to help longer with certain steps, particularly if they involve fasteners, but any gains in independence are well worth the effort. Your child may prove more capable than you thought if you provide a chance to learn in a peaceful, encouraging, and unrushed atmosphere. Praise every effort and accomplishment however small it may be, and don't dwell on what the child can't do. Every step learned is a step toward independence.

It is not only harder to get dressed than undressed, but often there is less time to teach this skill, as in the morning, when you are trying to get people fed and off to work or school. Nevertheless, if your child is at the stage of learning to dress, try to arrange the morning so you have a little extra time to help. Your child can select in the evening what to wear the next day. If your child can get the clothes out of the closet or drawers, make them readily accessible. Some children will be greatly aided if their clothes are always in exactly the same place. If your child learns to put his or her clothes away, it may help if you check what he or she has done. For example, if your child is retarded and can't tell if the clothes are inside out, but can dress if they are hung up correctly, check the closet after he or she hangs up the clothes. If anything is inside out, just rehang it so your child can dress the next time.

Occasionally you may have to reevaluate your child's ability to dress and undress, taking into consideration your child's mental and physical capabilities. It is very easy to get in the habit of helping a child because it is faster and you aren't sure he or she can manage alone. But your child may be able to do so and, if allowed to, will surely gain in self-esteem.

If you think your child can learn to do more without supervision than he or she is doing (or if someone suggests this to you), ask for help. If your doctor has no experience in this area, a pediatric physical therapist or occupational therapist may be able to assist you.

While there may be no way for your child to

become independent in dressing and undressing, suggestions from professionals and experimentation and practice at home will help you see what your child can learn to do alone. If you never try, your child may never learn to do more than at present.

What to Look for in Clothing

Self-help skills in dressing may, of course, be influenced by what your child wears. The following guidelines may help you choose the appropriate clothing.

The fabric of a garment influences comfort, durability, and ease of care.

Comfort is determined by the fibers the material is made of and how they are woven into fabric. If your child has trouble regulating body temperature, he or she may feel more comfortable in loosely woven natural fabrics such as cotton and wool, which "breathe," allowing air and perspiration to pass through, or in loosely woven blends with high percentages of natural fibers.

Since clothing traps a layer of air beneath it, in warm weather choose loosely woven garments with wide neck, arm, and leg openings so body heat can easily escape. Then in cold weather choose clothing that fits closely around the neck, wrists, and ankles, yet fits loosely enough around the body so some air can be trapped, acting as an insulator. The more layers, the more insulation, but also the more bulk and items to take on and off. If you need warmth but are trying to avoid bulk and weight, consider wool or a compact synthetic insulator such as Thinsulate.

The amount of stretch in a fabric can also influence how comfortable a garment is, for stretch fabrics expand somewhat so clothing does not bind. Such fabric also springs to its original shape after stretching, so there are fewer wrinkles, which may cause discomfort as well as look untidy. (However, many stretch fabrics do contain synthetic fiber.)

Antistatic finishes and antistatic agents in fabric softeners reduce the amount a fabric clings to the body or other fabrics, particularly in cool, dry weather.

Durability is an important consideration, especially if your child is hard on clothes. The tighter the weave or knit, the stronger the fabric. Generally, synthetic fibers are stronger than natural fibers. If you know your child wears out a certain item of clothing, you might want to get it with a higher synthetic fiber content. Usually, wovens are better than knits for surviving the wear and tear of braces or other orthotic appliances.

Easy-care fabrics mean less work for you in keeping your child clean and tidy. Most synthetic fabrics can be machine-washed and dried. Cotton can too, but it may need ironing; wool can often be machine-washed but cannot be dried in a dryer. Remember too that cotton shrinks.

Synthetics have the advantage of "memory." This means that even if a synthetic garment stretches while being worn, it will return to its original shape after laundering.

Prints, textured, and dark fabrics usually show stains less than light, solid-colored ones. Therefore, if you know your child's clothes get dirty due to movement, play, drooling, eating, or toileting problems, consider buying clothes that hide the dirt.

Some fabrics now come with soil-release finishes, which make stain-removal easier. And antibacterial finishes help eliminate odors due to perspiration or incontinence.

The construction of an article of clothing is important, especially if your child is hard on clothes.

The cut may influence whether your child has enough room to move comfortably without putting undue strain on the fabric and seams. Many people using wheelchairs or crutches favor tailored clothing, since extra material gets in their way when they try to move. However, people who can walk with ease may favor a fuller-cut garment that camouflages deformities.

Seams are often the first thing to break. The strongest seams are double-stitched. Usually, the raw edges are enclosed in the seam and the seam is stitched more than once to give a "flat-fell" or "welt" seam. If your child often splits seams, the extra cost of a well-constructed garment with flat-fell seams may be worthwhile. If the garment has single-stitched seams, seam allowances stitched together are stronger than those that open flat. If the seams are opened flat, edges overcast by machine stitching are less apt to ravel or tear than raw edges.

Double-stitching or rivets at pocket openings help prevent tears.

Reinforcing with double fabric on areas that receive heavy wear may greatly increase the life of a garment. Many boys' pants are made with double knees. Sometimes you can find sweaters and jackets with reinforced elbows. If you know your child's clothes wear out in certain places, it may well be worth the effort to sew patches of reinforcing fabric to the garment. These can be sewn either on the inside or on the outside as decorative patches. If your child has sensitive skin, sew the patches on the outside so they won't rub.

Fastenings are often the greatest problem for the physically or mentally disabled child who is trying to learn to dress independently.

Buttons require considerable finger dexterity. The larger the button, the easier it is to grasp and to fasten. Flat or concave buttons slip through holes more easily. Sometimes it helps if the button is sewn on so it stands up from the surface of the garment on a slightly longer piece of thread called a shank. Buttons are easier to manipulate when they are in front. If you teach your child to start buttoning from the bottom up, it may be easier to line up the buttons and holes correctly.

Zippers are easier than buttons for children who have the strength and coordination to pull them up. Adding a piece of fabric or leather, or a ring or other decorative object, to the pull may make it easier to grasp. Larger-toothed zippers are easier than the standard type. You can replace a standard zipper with one of these. Usually a zipper is easier to fasten if the bottom is held taut.

Hooks are very difficult to manipulate unless they are large and sturdy.

Velcro requires minimal dexterity to open and close, although your child will have to learn to position the sides correctly before pushing them together. The pile on Velcro weakens with use or if lint or dirt gets into it. Therefore, be sure to close any Velcro fasteners before laundering and brush the lint out of the pile with a nail brush if necessary. If the Velcro no longer holds well, the pile will probably need replacement first. Fabric, and often camping-supply, stores carry Velcro. Quality makes a huge difference, and expensive Velcro holds quite well. Some garments now come with Velcro closures. If your child has trouble with zippers or buttons, you can replace them with Velcro.

Choosing Appropriate Clothing for Your Child

The clothing needs of children vary greatly and are influenced by any physical disability a child may have. Consider the following points with the commonly worn articles of clothing.

Clothing for premature infants may need careful consideration. For complete information, see *The Premature Baby Book* by Helen Harrison, listed under Chapter 3 in Appendix 3, "Suggested Reading."

Underwear is crucial for your child's comfort, especially if he or she is physically disabled. You may have difficulty locating diapers or special underpants that work well for a child who has outgrown toddler sizes. Most ostomy- and urinary-supply companies have tollfree phone numbers and salespeople well qualified to discuss which product might best meet your child's needs. Your insurance may pay for some of these items if they are required due to a medical condition.

Diapers are undoubtedly the first thing your child will wear. Most diaper services carry adult-size diapers. Read page 141 for full information on diapers.

Waterproof pants, often called rubber pants, come in snap-on and pull-on styles. Which style to use is a matter of personal preference; buy some of each and try them out. As the pants usually wear out before your child outgrows them, it pays to buy better quality.

When your child outgrows the toddler size, you need to buy what are often called "protective undergarments." It is important to choose protective pants for the incontinent child with care, because accidents are embarrassing. Also, a wet, smelly child is not easily accepted and may even be rejected by other children in school. Such pants not only need to fit well, and be adequately absorbent for your child's output, but should also be nonirritating to the skin and comfortable to wear. Some protective pants come with liners. Others can be used with child- or adult-size diapers. Disposable liners are similar to sanitary pads with strips of adhesive on one side so they attach firmly into snug-fitting underpants. While liners are not as absorbent as diapers, they are much more absorbent than sanitary pads and may be sufficient for children with limited urinary output. Most of these pants open flat with snaps or Velcro tabs, although some pull-on types are made.

Underpants come in cotton, man-made fibers, or blends. Synthetics wear better, but cotton and the synthetic fiber Olefin draw the moisture away from the body. This is particularly important when buying panties for girls. Synthetics do not allow evaporation of moisture and thus are apt to cause vaginal infections, for the bacteria flourish in warm, deep, moist environments. Many synthetic panties come with cotton crotches, but this is not good enough: they should be all cotton or Olefin. And white is best, since dye can irritate the moist area around the vagina.

Boys can wear boxer shorts or briefs. The latter may be more comfortable for prolonged sitting because there is no excess fabric to wrinkle and crease. But it may be easier to transfer in boxer shorts, since skin is more apt than smooth fabric to stick on transfer boards. You can sew Velcro to the waistband of boxer shorts and pants so that the two garments can be attached to each other and pulled on as one.

A boy who has weak arms or limited use of his hands may prefer boxer shorts with a snap opening in front, for these will be easier to get on than underpants with fully elasticized waistbands. If he can't manage the snaps, you can replace them with Velcro.

If your child wears braces, you may have to experiment. Braces may wear out underpants, so you may need to add a piece of reinforcing material of the same fabric to the garment in the area of greatest wear. Be sure to stitch the extra fabric to the outside of the pants so there will be no rubbing or chafing of the skin.

A child wearing long leg braces attached to a low-back support system will either have to pull the underpants on over the braces or you will have to modify pull-on underpants and make a drop-front by cutting through the front crotch seam and sewing in a Velcro fastener.

Some physically disabled adults have so much trouble dressing independently that they are willing to dispense with any unnecessary article of clothing, and that includes underpants. A child who does not have accidents and thinks underpants are not worth the hassle may be right.

Undershirts help keep a child warm. Styles include armless vests, T-shirts and V-necks (for boys), and short-sleeved wide necks (for girls). Obviously, the more your child is covered, the warmer he or she will be. But the smaller the neckline, the more difficult it will be to get the undershirt on and off. You can make a shirt easier to get on and off by cutting open the neck seam and sewing in Velcro, thus enlarging the neck opening. All-cotton undershirts are best, especially if a child has a temperature-regulatory problem or wears a chest brace. If the brace comes up to the armpit, buy undershirts with sleeves and have your child wear the shirt under the brace. In summer, you can always cut off the sleeve, leaving a flap underneath the arm to protect it from rubbing against the brace. The undershirt should be long enough to reach beyond the bottom of the brace. Brace Mates (PO Box 223, Forest, VA 24551) has a complete line of 100% cotton brace liners. Their products are covered by insurance companies when purchased with a brace or corset.

Long underwear is good for children with poor circulation who get cold easily. Most is made of cotton-polyester blends. Underwear containing wool or silk is warmer but harder to launder and more expensive.

A bra can be difficult to fit. If so, try to find a lingerie store or a women's store with a large lingerie department that has a wide selection and a saleswoman who specializes in fitting bras. Front-opening bras are easier to put on and fasten, especially for those with limited range of motion or weak hands. Sports bras with no fasteners may be appropriate if your daughter has involuntary movements in the arms and shoulders and, consequently, has trouble keeping the straps in place. Posture bras, with wide straps and stretch panels across the back, provide back support and posture control and can be good for large-busted girls.

Slips are really necessary only under clothing made of clinging, sheer, or scratchy fabrics, or for a girl who needs an extra layer to keep warm. Half-slips usually have more fullness through the hip area (good for braces) and are easier to get on, but they may ride up or get caught in other clothing. A camisole top to be worn under a see-through top may eliminate the need for a full-length slip, which is convenient if your child has limited movement from the waist down. Bra-slips or bra-camisoles also reduce the number of garments needed.

Footwear may be difficult for your child to take on and off alone.

Socks provide difficulties for many disabled or retarded children. No-heel tube socks eliminate the need for correct positioning and precise fit. Since they are longer than regular socks, they also provide higher protection under braces. Cotton and wool socks breathe better, but man-made fibers last longer.

Wool or thermal knit socks may provide additional warmth if your child gets cold feet, as many children who can't walk do.

If your child has trouble grasping socks firmly enough to pull them up, you can sew loops on the tops of the socks.

There are also devices to hold the socks open if your child has trouble getting them on. (See *Clothing for Handicapped People* in Appendix 3, "Suggested Reading.") If your child has trouble getting socks off, pulling them off inside out may be easiest.

Tights or knee socks help keep a girl's legs warm and will hide skin blemishes or scars, if that's important to her. Tights are also good if your daughter has to be lifted by others when she gets older, for then underpants don't show.

Shoes come in a variety of styles. Consider what will best fit your child's needs. If your child has problem feet, try to find a qualified salesperson who has a large selection of orthopedic styles and is willing to work with you. If the best fitting shoe you can get still doesn't fit perfectly, the salesperson may be able to adapt it by either

stretching the shoe or padding with adhesive foam the places that rub. If your child's feet are of different sizes, you may have to buy two pairs, using one shoe from each pair. Naturally, if your child is willing to keep wearing the same style, when he or she outgrows one pair you simply have to buy a larger size, using one larger shoe and keeping the other until your child grows into it. You might also consider contacting an odd-shoe exchange (see *Clothing for Handicapped People* in Appendix 3, "Suggested Reading").

Custom-made shoes are necessary for the foot that is impossible to fit. Such shoes are very expensive, but if they are necessary you may be able to find a service organization to help you pay for them. However, first try to fit your child in regular shoes, bearing in mind the following factors.

A standard leather shoe may be needed for support. If your child needs high shoes, ankle-high work boots or hiking boots may be more acceptable and just as effective as orthopedic shoes. Usually, there is a direct correlation between cost and quality in shoes. If your child tends to wear out shoes because of his or her gait or braces, expensive shoes are worth the cost. If your child wears out the toes of leather shoes, try adding toe taps to act as bumpers.

You can also cover the toe of the shoe with a layer of dental acrylic, which dries to a smooth, hard surface. To avoid white toes, use universal tint (available at your local paint store). If you don't add too much, the acrylic will still harden. The toe caps stay on longer if you first roughen the leather with sandpaper and then paint on a layer of the acrylic solvent. Your dentist should be willing to order one bottle each of dental acrylic powder and solvent for you to use to repair your child's shoes at home.

Stores carrying jogging shoes also sell a liquid adhesive you can apply to shoes to build up or mend worn areas. This doesn't look lovely, usually drying to a dull beige, but if looks aren't important you might try applying this to worn spots to increase the life of the shoe. It dries to a more rubbery surface than dental acrylic, so when used on the sole it may impede your child's gait if his or her feet drag when walking.

Cloth shoes, such as tennis or jogging shoes,

are much more pliable and easier to get on and off than leather but offer less support. They can be worn with leg braces, if the braces are made with a plastic shoe insert that fits inside the shoe rather than stirrups that attach to the outside of the shoe. Many people who can't get about on their feet anyway find cloth shoes more comfortable. They are also usually cheaper than leather.

It is often very difficult for retarded and physically disabled children to learn to tie their own shoelaces. Jogging shoes with Velcro closures may be suitable. Elastic laces may be helpful for children who have trouble lacing and unlacing shoes, for then tying and untying is no longer necessary. You can also get toggles like those often found on sleeping-bag stuff sacks; then the laces can simply be pulled tight and released quickly with one hand. If you can't get shoes on and off easily, and looks are not a consideration (as with shoes used with night braces), consider dispensing with laces altogether and just have your shoemaker or orthotist sew a Velcro closure on the shoe. If you feel like something more radical, have the orthotist cut out the front of the shoe so the toes can be positioned with ease.

Boots are necessary in cold climates and, again, the style you choose depends upon your child's ability to put them on. Lined boots designed to be worn directly over thick socks may be easier to get on and off than boots meant to go over shoes. What are sometimes called "ski-doo" boots are easy to get on and off. These are nylon outside, with rubber soles, thick removable felt liners, and a big zipper. An insulated boot of synthetic materials worn inside all day long will probably lead to hot and sweaty feet. A child who wears such boots to school may have to take shoes along and change during the day.

Sandals can be difficult for a child who walks with difficulty but may be appropriate in hot weather for a child who can't walk yet wants something on his or her feet. Sandals give the feet a chance to feel the air and sunshine in summertime.

Dress shoes may not seem necessary, but at some point most children want them. Girls often want patent-leather Mary Janes. It's an expression partly of wanting to look pretty, partly of wanting to look like other children. If you can afford it, buy a pair, even if they are worn only for special occasions. If your child can't walk and shoes are simply something to cover the feet, save some money by buying as large a size as looks respectable so your child will fit into those infrequently worn shoes as long as possible. Since such stiff shoes are often hard to get on, buying a large size may help.

Boys usually don't ask for dress shoes until they're teenagers. But for the boy who can't walk, the same problems mentioned above apply, since dress shoes are expensive and often hard to get into.

Slippers are easy to slip on and off, which can be an advantage for those who have trouble getting footwear on and a disadvantage for those who have trouble keeping it on. For the latter, slipper socks may be a good solution. If your child gets cold feet, consider booties insulated with down or synthetic fiber, available from camping-supply stores. You may be able to avoid slippers completely with little children if you buy them footed pajamas with skid-resistant plastic soles attached to the feet.

Sleepwear should be comfortable and adequately warm. Federal regulations require flame resistance for sizes 0–14.

Pajamas are good for boys or girls. Your child's particular disability may influence the type you buy. Rib-knit bands or cuffs around the neck, arms, and legs make the pajama warmer but also harder to get on and off. Front-opening tops may be easier for your child to get on if he or she needs help. A child who has trouble with fastenings may be more independent with a pullover style.

Bottoms with elastic all around the waist eliminate the need for fasteners but may be harder to pull on than bottoms with elastic in back and a fastener in front. A front fastener can be replaced with Velcro.

Heavyweight one-piece sleepers with skid-proof soles are the warmest and may eliminate your child's need for blankets when in bed and for slippers when up.

Nightgowns or nightshirts eliminate the need to struggle with pants. Large neck openings or long front plackets make it easier to get in and out of the gown.

Shirts come with a variety of openings, fasteners, and sleeve styles. Muscle strength, coordination, and range of motion all influence which shirts are best for your child.

Full-front openings can be better for children with limited range of motion or muscle strength, particularly if they are dependent upon someone else to help them get dressed.

Pullover styles are good for children with limited use of their hands, for often they can use the muscle strength they do have to pull a shirt on, thus helping them gain independence. Some paralyzed people learn to bite clothes to hold them as they pull them off and on.

Shirt pockets may be handy for children in wheelchairs who can't reach pants pockets.

Cuffs, as mentioned with regard to pajamas, can cause problems. Ribbed cuffs are difficult to get on and off. Some weak people learn to use their teeth. Others just avoid them.

Button cuffs are standard on many long-sleeved shirts. Your child may be able to slip a hand through the cuff without opening it. If your child can't and the buttons cause problems, you can make a stretch cufflink by sewing matching buttons on either side of the cuff and connecting them with elastic thread, leaving at least half an inch between buttons. You can also move the button to the hole side and make a Velcro closure, or you can decide your child will just need help with that step and stick with the standard button and hole.

Shirttails easily come untucked, especially on children who use crutches or have involuntary movements of the upper part of the body. Try to find shirts that can be worn with their tails out or that have long tails. If a girl doesn't care about pants, a dress may be a better solution than a shirt and pants. If she wants to wear a shirt and pants, boys' shirts, which are usually cut longer than girls', are a solution if she doesn't mind the tailored look. The only visible difference between boys' and girls' shirts is the direction of the front lap. Since boys' clothing is generally made better and is frequently cheaper, it is usually a better buy for girls too. If you get desperate in your efforts to keep tails tucked in, you can sew Velcro to the waistband and shirt back, or you can make a body suit by attaching panties to the blouse, opening the crotch seam and sewing in fasteners.

Seams frequently pop with children who use crutches or who use their upper extremities to transfer. If this happens with your child, try to find a shirt that is adequately full through the shoulder. Gathers or pleats across the back help. If you buy shirts in woven fabrics, try to find those with the flat-fell seams (see page 152). Knitted shirts have more stretch.

Full-length sleeves can present some difficulties for children in wheelchairs, because they pick up dirt from the wheels, or for children who use Canadian crutches, because the sleeve is hard to insert into the crutch cuff. Depending on the climate, you may decide to sacrifice warmth for convenience.

Pants are great for girls as well as boys and are available in many fabrics and styles. Their advantages over dresses are that they don't fall into the toilet when a girl is in the bathroom, and they will protect her modesty when transferring. As always, take your child's needs into consideration when buying them.

Smooth-woven fabrics are easier for transferring than rougher materials like corduroy. The higher the synthetic-fiber content, the longer the pants will last, which may be a consideration if your child wears pants out fast. However, some synthetics, especially polyester knits, snag badly. So these may be inappropriate, depending on how your child gets around.

Stretch fabrics are easier to get on and off. Warm-up suits have a lot of give and are so fully cut that many people like them for daily wear. They usually have some synthetic fiber in them.

The waistband can fasten with buttons, zippers, Velcro, a drawstring, or elastic. An elastic waistband may make the pants easier to get into than front fasteners and may also provide greater comfort for prolonged sitting. However, some people in wheelchairs find that elastic waistbands let pants ride down in back. If your child has trouble getting pants on, you can sew loops into the waistband to allow for a better grip. If your child has weak arms, front-opening pants may be easier to get on.

Fastenings are often difficult to manipulate. If side openings would be better for your child, you can open the seams of ready-made clothing and insert zippers or Velcro. Some clothing especially made for the disabled has this feature. You can replace any zipper with Velcro. If your child has trouble getting his or her feet through trouser legs, buy pants cut wider through the leg. If necessary, you can sew in a Velcro insert.

Overalls and jumpsuits are easy to get on and keep up, and they solve the problem of untucked shirttails. Overalls for a child in braces with a low-back support can be easily expanded through the hip region by opening the side seam and sewing in wide elastic. A proper fit in trunk length is important with overalls and jumpsuits, for if they are too short they will bind and be uncomfortable through the crotch area. If the legs are too long, it may be difficult for your child to walk. Toileting can be a problem with such clothing unless the pants have snaps in the inside seam of the leg (frequent only in sizes for little children). You will have to weigh the benefits of one-piece jumpsuits and overalls against any difficulties in toileting.

Dresses that hang from the shoulder and do not have fitted waists often look better on physically disabled girls. It is usually better to let your daughter pick the dress in which she feels good rather than make her wear the one you think is more flattering.

Long dresses cover the legs, keeping them warm and hiding any braces. While it may be almost impossible for some girls to go to the toilet alone in such a garment, young girls often love long dresses so much that it may be worth it to help your daughter in the bathroom so she can wear one.

Outerwear is an important consideration, especially if you live in a cold climate. The fiber content, construction, and thickness of the fabric help determine how warm a garment will be.

Sweaters should be both warm and comfortable. Bulky loose knits provide warmth but are apt to get caught on crutches and wheelchair wheels. Sweatshirts and velour don't snag. Lots of sportswear is available today, much with zippers or Velcro closures. Hoods provide extra warmth and eliminate the need for hats and scarves.

Coats and jackets can be difficult to get on and off if they are heavy. If your child cannot move with ease, select lightweight fabrics that give warmth without weight, such as synthetic fiberfills or even down, rather than heavier and bulkier pile. Smooth, slippery, synthetic linings, particularly in the sleeves, make a coat easier to get on and off. Some jackets come with Velcro fasteners, large zippers, or toggles, all of which may be easier to manipulate than buttons.

Sleeves always present a problem for children using Canadian crutches. Try to avoid bulk and buttons. Your child will have to experiment to see if he or she can best get the arm into the crutch cuff by sliding in from the top or by pulling the arm across and into the crutch cuff.

The wrist opening of the sleeve may also affect how easily your child can get into the jacket, especially if your child has arm braces or a prosthesis. If necessary, you can slit the sleeves to the elbow and reengineer them to close with Velcro.

Capes may be good if your child has limited arm or shoulder movement. However, they tend to get in the way of a child using crutches or a wheelchair.

Snowsuits come in one-piece styles for little ones and often in two-piece styles for older children. For ease in dressing, the longer the zippers and the more of them the better.

Leg sacks, which are like short sleeping bags, can be helpful for a child in a wheelchair who gets very cold legs and feet. How cold your child gets will determine how warm the sack must be. A lightweight sack could be made of quilted cotton. A very warm sack can be had by just using a child's sleeping bag. You can, of course, just wrap your child's legs in a blanket, but a sack will stay in place better and keep your child warmer.

Mittens are usually easier to put on than gloves. They are also warmer.

Swimsuits are generally made of stretch fabric, which makes for a good fit. When buying a suit, try to find one that will not be too hard to get off when wet. For girls you can sew a one-piece wrap-around suit of stretch fabric. Bikini tops can be modified to open in front, bikini bottoms to open at the side. Boys' swim trunks can be adapted by sewing Velcro down the side seams so the suit opens flat.

Home-sewn clothing may be the solution if you can't find what your child needs or if he or she is hard to fit.

If you aren't able to sew for your child yourself, you may have friends who would be willing to do so. Or you may be able to find someone in your community who sews for others for a reasonable fee. Sometimes managers of fabric stores can suggest such persons to you. Your child can help pick out the pattern and the material. If an older child has the ability to sew, it might be worthwhile to teach your child yourself (if you know how) or even have your child take lessons.

12

How and What to Feed Your Child

While it is relatively easy to meet the nutritional needs of a "normal" child, many ill or disabled children need carefully planned diets that should be worked out with their doctors or dieticians. (See Appendix 3, "Suggested Reading," for books on nutrition.)

PLANNING YOUR CHILD'S DIET

The Basic Food Groups

Using figure 12-1 as a guide, and preparing a variety of foods out of each basic group from day to day, you can provide a balanced diet for a child who can eat regular, soft, or bland foods. If your child finds it hard to eat meat due to difficulty in chewing or swallowing, sufficient protein can be had from grains, dairy products, fish, and eggs. Children go through phases of eating or refusing to eat one thing and then another, but as long as the foods they eat are nutritional, very young children usually balance their diets, even if left to their own devices.

Monitoring Your Child's Diet

It is important to check regularly to see that your ill or disabled child is eating a balanced diet with the appropriate number of calories. This is particularly true with an over- or underweight child.

The overweight child adds excess weight to any other medical problems. The more limited

MEAT, POULTRY, FISH	1–2 servings.
GRAINS, LEGUMES, NUTS, SEEDS	4 servings of whole grain bread, cereals, beans, nuts, or seeds.
(Vegetarians, omit meat and eat 6 grain servings for recommended daily protein allowance.)	
MILK AND DAIRY PRODUCTS	3 or more glasses for children, 2 or more glasses for adults. (Other dairy products may be used to meet part of milk requirement.)
EGGS	Up to 4 *per week.*
VEGETABLES	3 or more servings, including 1 yellow and 1 dark leafy green, such as romaine lettuce, spinach, or chard.
FRUITS	1 to 4 pieces, including a raw source of vitamin C, such as citrus fruits, cantaloupe, strawberries, or tomatoes.

Figure 12-1   The basic food groups: suggested daily servings.

your child's mobility, the easier it is to consume more calories than he or she burns off. Extra calories are converted to fat, making it harder for the child to get around independently or to be moved. Also, diets restricted in calories are more difficult to balance, since each calorie is important. It is similar to being on a budget: if money is tight, every dollar must be used wisely. So if your child is overweight, consult with your doctor to work out a low-calorie, nutritious diet that will meet your child's needs. At home you can help your overweight child by having tasty food that is low in calories available not only to your child but to the whole family. It is not fair to serve sweet desserts or highly caloric fast foods to the rest of the family and then tell your overweight child to pass.

Once your child loses weight, you must continue to monitor his or her diet carefully. It is actually physiologically easier for a person who has been overweight in the past to become overweight again at a later time.

The underweight child also needs a carefully planned diet. Some ill or disabled children look skinny due to lack of muscle mass. You shouldn't try to fatten up such a child if the additional pounds would take the form of fat rather than muscle.

Other children are underweight because they either metabolize food poorly or eat with great difficulty. In such a case your doctor may want you to encourage your child to gain weight.

Be sure to monitor how much food and liquid actually gets into your child's stomach. Milk that drools out of the side of the mouth or food that your child massages into his or her hair, or spills on the floor, or vomits up cannot be counted as caloric and fluid intake. You will have to compensate for the food and drink lost by a child who has difficulty eating.

If your child has a progressive condition, you may think that weight loss or a decline in general responsiveness and alertness is due to the medical condition. But a child may become unresponsive and seem to fade because of insufficient caloric or fluid intake. While it might seem unlikely that parents would be so naive as not to realize that their child was starving or becoming dehydrated, it is easy to make this mistake.

If your child is underweight, consider if you can prepare food in a form that is easy to chew and swallow. Your child may be working so hard at eating that he or she becomes exhausted long before enough calories and nutrients have been consumed. If you feel your child should not be losing weight on the diet he or she is receiving, discuss this with your doctor, since weight loss can be a symptom of a new medical problem.

Special Diets

A soft diet can aid the child who has difficulty chewing and swallowing. However, such a child should receive only as much help as necessary in getting food to the right consistency. Begin by chopping the food into small pieces. If this doesn't work, use a food grinder. Baby stores carry small portable manual food grinders that you can use right at the table. You can easily grind very small amounts, like ten peas, then a quarter of a potato, then a bit of chicken, keeping each food and flavor separate. The food will still have some texture.

The next step is to use a food processor or blender. If you are going to be blending many meals, the construction of the blender cutting blades is important. If the blender has four blades and a smooth bottom, you may find food sticking and jamming. A blender with six blades on a cone-shaped base with two blades pointing up, two level, and two down (such as the Bosch) is the most efficient type for blending small quantities. If you blend different foods together, be sure to taste your combinations yourself. One can get caught up in the fervor of good nutrition and forget that the appearance and taste of food are also important. (If you had similarly flavored brown mush three times a day every day you might lose interest in eating too.) It may be easier to put all the bits of the meal together and give them a whirl, but the resulting concoction may be anything but appetizing.

Even a child who can swallow only mush may yearn for the taste of certain solid foods. For example, a child who loves potato chips but can't swallow them might push them up to the roof of the mouth, probably licking the salt off in the process. After about five chips, the parents would have to pry the lump out of the child's mouth so there would be room to keep "consuming" potato chips.

Nutritionally it makes no sense to feed a child in this way, but it is important to remember that the taste buds are working, even if chewing and swallowing are defective. However, if your child yearns for certain foods, you should weigh the pleasure against any risk of choking.

A liquid diet is necessary when your child can no longer get enough calories from soft foods alone, or when the difficulty in swallowing has reached the point where he or she can consume only liquid. When this happens, it may be necessary to abandon the four food groups and start thinking simply in terms of calories and necessary proportions of proteins, fats, carbohydrates, vitamins, minerals, and water. Work out an appropriate liquid diet for your child with your doctor or dietician.

Commercial powder or liquid preparations provide a balanced diet. The powders are more economical per serving and can be stored longer after opening the package than the premixed liquid formulas, but any undissolved lumps will jam your syringe, if you are feeding that way (see pages 167–168). The premixed liquids are lump-free but are more expensive and have to be used within a given period. Some preparations are especially high in protein. All of these formulas are more expensive than "real" food, and any natural food they contain has gone through extensive processing. If you let taste be your guide, you will most likely discover that commercial liquid diets cannot be classified as tasty.

Homemade liquid preparations may be an alternative. Discuss your child's nutritional requirements (calories as well as the proportions of fats, carbohydrates, and protein) with your doctor to see if you can devise a liquid preparation.

Milk-based preparations may be appropriate for your child. In addition to milk-based ingredients (acidophilus milk or yogurt is sometimes recommended for children on antibiotics), these may contain egg, sweetening (sugar or honey), and spices or syrups for flavoring. Protein powder can be used to increase the protein content, but it will make the liquid thicker and harder to swallow.

Vegetable and fruit juices or juice-based preparations are another possibility. Freshly made juices contain more natural vitamins than the frozen, canned, or bottled kinds, so if you are trying to make a liquid diet as nutritional as possible, consider using a juicer to make your own juice.

If you make your own juice, try to make combinations your child finds tasty. While spinach-celery-beet-carrot-watermelon juice might contain a wider variety of vitamins and minerals than straight watermelon, if your child prefers the latter it might be better to serve that. Egg and/or protein powder may be added, but both will alter the taste.

Experiment with different kinds of drinks if your child is on a liquid diet, but if you find that he or she likes certain drinks best, consider providing these regularly and augmenting them with a good vitamin-mineral preparation.

Other special diets may be needed by children with specific disorders. Often the appropriate organization dealing with the disorder can offer general guidelines on how to plan your child's diet. But you must always discuss your child's specific dietary needs with your pediatrician or dietitian. With just a little ingenuity you can develop a diet individualized to meet your child's needs.

HOW TO FEED YOUR CHILD

Breast-Feeding

Breast-feeding has many advantages. Nutritionally it is beneficial since human milk is created especially for humans, whereas cow milk is created for calves. It is difficult to convert cow milk into the nutritional equivalent of human milk, as is attempted with formulas, and the ideal match has not yet been made. Scientists are continually discovering new differences between cow milk and human milk. Most ill or disabled children would benefit from the superior nutrition breast milk supplies.

A breast-fed baby rarely develops allergies to mother's milk and is much less apt to suffer from allergies later than is the bottle-fed baby. Breast milk is well tolerated even by immature digestive systems, and nursing itself helps good tongue and jaw development. The stimulation received from the mother's closeness and from actual suckling can also aid respiratory functions and, consequently, the oxygenation of the blood.

A child's immune system can also be bolstered by breast milk, which contains antibodies from the mother.

The convenience of having a constantly available supply of warm, sterile food makes breast-feeding, for many people, the easiest way to feed a baby.

Mother-baby bonding, which is the term for the mother and baby coming to know and love each other, may also be enhanced by breast-feeding. This bonding may be especially important with a baby who has come into your family under not exactly ideal conditions. Since it takes time to get to know anyone, nursing your child throughout the day is a marvelous way for this mother-baby bonding to occur.

Most sick or disabled babies can be breast-fed, even the retarded and those with a harelip or cleft palate.

If your baby is in the hospital, explain your desire to breast-feed to your doctor and the nursing staff and elicit their cooperation. You may have to be experimental in finding ways to nurse your child, especially if he or she is immobilized due to traction, intravenous feeding, or an oxygen tent. Some mothers have even found ways of getting into the crib (once it was found to be strong enough to support their weight), much to the amusement of the nursing staff. If the hospital wants to limit visits (and consequently nursing), try for rooming-in or at least try to get your doctor to write onto your child's chart that you have unlimited visiting privileges because you breast-feed. If your child cannot be taken out of an incubator or if you cannot always be with your baby and there are times when he or she must be fed with a bottle, you can express your milk so your baby receives human milk and you keep up your milk supply for the time when you can nurse at home.

Problems with breast-feeding can occur. If they do, experienced nursing mothers can be very helpful. You can get free advice day or night by calling your local La Leche League, which has qualified mothers who are committed to helping others successfully breast-feed their children. If you do not find a local chapter of the La Leche League listed in your phone book, call La Leche League International (see "breast-feeding" in Appendix 4, "Helpful Organiza-tions") which will put you in phone contact with someone who can help you.

Dorothy Brewster, in *You Can Breastfeed Your Baby—Even In Special Situations* (see Appendix 3, "Suggested Reading"), gives helpful suggestions for nursing babies with a variety of disorders and shows how most physically disabled, retarded, and ill babies can be breast-fed.

If you want to breast-feed your baby but have never breast-fed or have not done so for some time, you can reestablish your milk supply. This supply is produced by hormones that are normally given off at birth but that are also stimulated by feeling motherly while handling and caring for your baby. Also the stimulation of the milk ducts by sucking promotes milk production.

If you find you must supplement what your child gets from nursing, remember that bottle-feeding provides such an easy means of sucking that a baby may reject the breast. An alternative to the bottle is the Lact-Aid (Box 6861, Denver, CO 80206), a bottle with a feeding tube coming out of the nipple. When nursing, you tape the tube on your nipple so when your baby sucks on you he or she stimulates your milk supply and gets some of your breast milk supplemented by milk from the tube.

Bottle-Feeding

Although it might be nutritionally better to breast-feed your baby, you can provide the love and closeness your baby needs with bottles, particularly if you take the time to hold your baby that a breast-feeding mother must spend.

Certain children may never learn to eat solid foods and may, if they have difficulty drinking from a cup, need to be weaned from the breast to the bottle or simply be bottle-fed for years. With such a child you may want to develop your own liquid diet (see page 162). Consider enlarging the nipple holes with a hot pin to increase the liquid flow.

One note of caution for bottle-feeding: if you let your child fall asleep with a bottle in the mouth, the sugar in the milk or juice may cause cavities. These are unpleasant for a "normal" child but particularly difficult to fill with most disabled children.

Feeding Your Child Solid Food

Children gain a great deal of independence if they can feed themselves, and it is important to encourage them to learn how. The disabled or retarded child may need help with the various steps involved, and it may take years to master the skill. But if you think there is any chance that you can teach your child to self-feed, you should try.

Discuss any specific feeding problems with your doctor. Occupational therapists, who are trained to help with all phases of daily living activities, can also be of great help. For example, if your child has an eating problem, an occupational therapist can not only help teach your child maximum use of the muscles involved in chewing and swallowing but can also help your child learn to use his or her hands most effectively for the special utensils or other assists that may be required. Speech pathologists may also be able to help.

Seating is important. You must have a chair in which your child can sit comfortably. The head and trunk must be stable in order for your child to be sufficiently balanced. Then the hands are free and the child does not have to worry about capsizing. Head, chest, or foot straps can aid in positioning if necessary. (See pages 85–102 for a fuller discussion of seating.)

It is important for the morale of a child to be able to eat at the table with the rest of the family. High chairs are appropriate for a young child. If an older child needs to sit in a special chair, such as a wheelchair, see to it that the chair is at the right height relative to the table. If the table is too high, you can raise your child with a seat cushion or with blocks under the chair legs. If the child's seat is too high, you can raise the table with blocks under the legs or with new legs. If you increase your table height other children may need to sit on stacks of newspapers or high chairs, and adults will have to learn to accept the convenience of having the plate closer to the mouth.

Finger foods such as crackers, raisins, and pieces of cheese can be good starters for the child learning to feed himself or herself. Most children can learn to put things into their mouths. With a retarded child you may have to help develop the two basic skills of grasping the food and lifting the hand to the mouth. Place your hand around your child's hand, pick up the food, and then guide the hand to the mouth.

Avoid food that is hard to grasp as initial finger foods. Sometimes the way you prepare foods may help. For example, broken banana pieces are much less slippery than slices. You can break a banana into bite-size pieces if, after peeling it, you push your finger from the tip down the middle of the banana to the other end. It will divide into thirds, which can then be broken into pieces. Or instead of simply scrambling an egg, cook it flat like an omelette over low heat until it is firm and then cut it into pieces. Just a little innovative thinking can make meals much easier for your child to eat.

Eating utensils are necessary for the child who has mastered finger foods but cannot yet use standard cutlery.

Spoons should have bowls that fit your child's mouth (fig. 12-2). If a spoon is too large, you will have trouble getting it into his or her mouth. If it is too small, you get too little food in each bite. A fairly shallow bowl makes it easier to get the food off the spoon, especially if you have to pull the spoon upward as you take it out of the mouth so the food is scraped off the spoon by the upper teeth. This will *not* work if your child has a bite reflex.

The child who begins self-feeding needs a handle that he or she can grasp with ease. A long handle can be held with the whole hand rather than with just a few fingers. A wide spoon handle is often easier to grip. You can purchase stainless-steel eating utensils made with resilient vinyl-plastic handlebar-type handles with finger-grip knobs. However, these are more apt to fit an adult than a child hand.

Rehabilitation centers have facilities to mold the handle to the shape of the child's hand. If you have no rehabilitation center near you, you can try using a plastic resin material such as Cold Set to build up the handle. You can also insert the handle of the spoon through a hole in a rubber ball or rubber grips for bicycle handlebars. As a

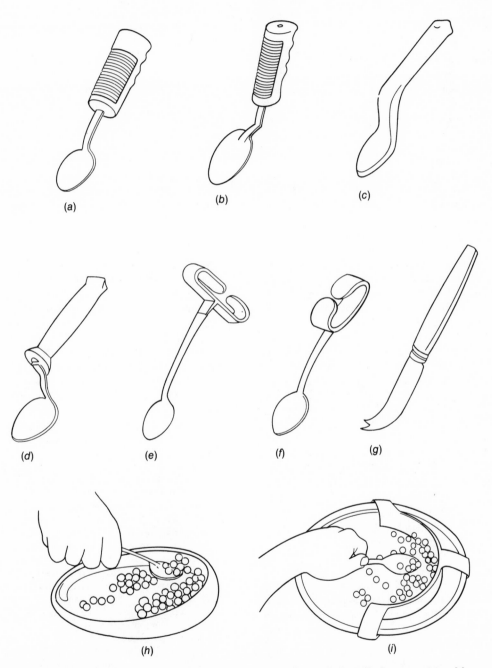

Figure 12-2   Eating utensils: *(a)* spoon with built-up grip; *(b)* angle-handled spoon; *(c)* rubber spoon; *(d)* self-leveling or swivel spoon; *(e)* vertical palm-handled spoon; *(f)* horizontal palm-handled spoon; *(g)* rocker knife-fork combination; *(h)* scoop dish; *(i)* dish with snap-on plate guard.

temporary measure, pieces of sponge (as from hair rollers) or washcloths wrapped around the handle and fastened with rubber bands may be used.

If your child has limited use of his or her hands or arms, you can get angle-handled spoons, as well as self-leveling spoons that permit the spoon bowl to remain level even though the handle is rotated as the child lifts the spoon to the mouth. A child with a very weak grasp may need a custom-made strap or cuff to hold the spoon in the hand.

Forks can be modified in these same ways. For some children forks are easier to handle than spoons. However, you must take care that involuntary movements do not make forks dangerous.

Knives for one-handed cutting have curved blades so cutting is achieved by rocking rather than sawing. Rocker knives with fork tines on the end are a good fork-knife combination for persons with only one hand available for self-feeding. Again, take precautions if your child has involuntary movements.

Plates and bowls can be chosen to meet your child's needs. Plastic dishes do not break. Suction cups on the bottoms of dishes or a skidproof mat made of material such as Dycem help prevent falling dishes. Dishes with reservoirs for hot water keep food warm for the slow eater. And it is obviously easier to scoop the food onto the spoon or fork if the dish has sides or if a plate guard is attached to a regular plate.

Cups and glasses are more stable if they have wide bases. A weighted cup or heavy glass is less apt to tip than a light plastic one, but the latter is of course easier for a weak child to lift. One or even two handles make lifting easier. When a child is just beginning to drink from a cup, it is helpful to put very little in the cup or use a lid with a spout that controls the rate of flow. Some children can manage drinking better through a straw. Especially wide straws can be purchased in 18-inch lengths and can be cut to the required length. The longer the straw, the greater the effort to suck.

Breaking the feeding process into stages is helpful in teaching an activity as complex as self-feeding. The following is a logical breakdown.

1. Pick up the appropriate utensil.
2. Cut the food if necessary.
3. Get the food onto the utensil.
4. Lift the food to the mouth without spilling.
5. Chew the food.
6. Swallow the food.

This breakdown not only helps you see how you can teach a child the necessary steps one by one; if feeding problems arise, it also helps you to determine the step with which your child is having difficulty. Once you understand where the problem lies, it is easier to get suggestions from professionals.

Teaching chewing and swallowing may be part of teaching your child to self-feed. Again, you can best help your child by breaking the process down into steps. It can be extremely valuable to have an ongoing consultation with a therapist (usually an occupational therapist) who is experienced in working with children who have problems with lip closure, bite reflexes, tongue thrust, tongue mobility, or chewing, or who have a slowed swallow or an insufficient gag reflex. The therapist will evaluate the problem and work with you and your child to teach you techniques to overcome or, at least, decrease the problem, if possible. General tips to consider are:

- Seat your child upright with the head slightly forward. If he or she tips the head back for what is called "bird feeding," it will be more difficult for your child to learn to swallow correctly. There is also a greater chance of aspiration (food in the lungs rather than in the stomach).
- Slowly thicken the consistency of the food from a soft puree to semisolids as swallowing improves, since thin liquids are the most difficult to swallow. (Powdered agar flakes—available at health-food stores—are a tasteless thickening agent.)
- Use crunchy foods that soften quickly in the mouth (such as soda crackers) to help your child learn to chew, since he or she may associate the crunch with chewing. If your child does not yet chew well enough, the food will soften enough in the mouth so it can be swallowed.
- Make sure a child with a tongue-thrust reflex, which pushes the tongue forward out of the mouth, has the tongue in the mouth before food is given. You can walk the tongue back with a rubber-coated spoon by touching the tip, pushing down and back,

then slowly repeating the process as you move toward the middle. Or you can push down on the
center of the tongue as you put the food in. Or try
inserting food from the side rather than from the
front of the mouth.

- Before eating, massage the sides (not front) of the
  gums of a child with a bite reflex. If a metal spoon
  hitting the teeth sets off the reflex, use a solid hard
  rubber spoon or a plastic tongue blade.
- Place the food into the mouth from the side, rather
  than the front, to aid your child in moving the food
  from side to side in the mouth for chewing.
- Control the movement of your child's jaw or lips
  with your fingers. Sit in front of your child and
  place your middle finger under the chin to help you
  control the jaw. Put your thumb on the front of the
  chin so you can help your child close lips and control the jaw. Place your index finger along the side
  of the cheek to control your child's head.

When you are working on specific eating skills
like this, it may be easier for your child to concentrate if he or she eats in a quiet place before
the rest of the family eats and then joins the
family for companionship and nibbling on some
favorite foods at mealtime.

Syringe-Feeding

Syringe-feeding is necessary when your child
needs a liquid diet and cannot easily drink from
a cup or a straw (fig. 12-3). Syringes are used to
squirt the liquid into the back of the mouth.

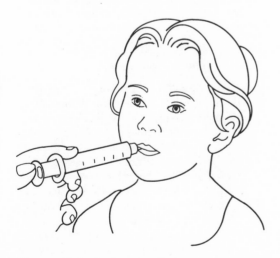

Figure 12-3 Syringe feeding.

The syringe that works best for feeding is a
glass, non-Luer-lock, metal-tipped 10-cc syringe.
Plastic disposable syringes may be necessary if
your child has a bite reflex, but the plunger is
usually not strong enough to use for a whole
meal. If your pharmacy does not carry a glass
syringe, it can order one for you. When you start
feeding regularly with a syringe, it pays to buy
a number of them because you are sure to break
some. Since the barrels and plungers are inter-
changeable, if you break one part you can continue to use the remaining section. Glass syringes are expensive, but they should be covered
by your insurance.

The procedure for syringe-feeding may seem
so awkward the first time you try that you will
feel it is one of the messiest ways of feeding ever
invented. But you can learn how to use syringes
effectively if you keep the following points in
mind.

- Keep the liquid in a mug rather than in a tall narrow glass.
- Hold your thumb on the plunger, or else it will fall
  out of the barrel, getting liquid all over and possibly
  breaking the plunger.
- Start by using two hands; with time you will master
  holding the syringe between your first and second
  fingers and pulling the plunger up with your
  thumb. This gives you a free hand for a napkin or
  tissue to catch the drips en route to the mouth and
  to wipe your child's mouth after every squirt.
- Have your child keep his or her mouth closed, then
  insert the tip of the syringe into the corner of the
  mouth pointing toward the molars. In this way the
  teeth prevent the liquid from being squirted down
  the throat.
- Do not ask a child with swallowing difficulty to
  open his or her mouth, because if you squirt the
  food hard to the back of the mouth your child is
  very apt to choke. Thin liquid may run down the
  esophagus so fast that the epiglottis can't close to
  prevent food from entering the trachea.
- Liquid at room temperature may be easier than
  cold liquid for a child with swallowing difficulties.

Since the barrel and plunger of the syringe
have a very close fit, food particles easily jam
them. To avoid this, strain any liquid that may
contain jamming particles, such as undissolved

protein powder or fibers in vegetable or fruit juice. Keep a glass of plain water on the table whenever feeding with the syringe and give a small squirt of water after each squirt of food. This not only helps to keep the syringe from jamming but also aids in providing adequate liquid intake.

If a syringe starts to move with difficulty, put it into the water and move it up and down a few times. If it still jams, leave it in warm, soapy water overnight. Proceed with another syringe. (Sometimes soaking will not help a jammed syringe. Call your pharmacy and ask if they have a device to unjam it. You may have to phone your way through the yellow pages to find a pharmacy that carries one, but if you do find one that does, the pharmacist can make your jammed syringe functional again.)

Small squirts of less than 10 cc may be necessary for a child with serious swallowing difficulties, especially when he or she is sick. *Learn from your doctor what to do if your child chokes.* (See page 39 for advice on what to do in case of choking.)

Tube-Feeding

If your child is not getting enough nourishment from a liquid diet, you will have to move to tube-feeding for dietary supplements or even for complete feeding if your child cannot swallow liquid from a bottle or syringe. Do not panic if your doctor prescribes tube-feeding.

Tube-feeding can be done at home, for it is not extremely difficult; your child can survive on tube-feeding for years. However, *do not tube-feed your child until you have been thoroughly instructed, supervised in each step of the procedure, and approved by your doctor.* This caution is necessary because the tube must go down the esophagus into the stomach and not down the trachea into the lungs.

While information on tube-feeding is given in Appendix 2, this is *not* to replace working out the procedure with your doctor but rather to give some written guidelines that you can modify with your doctor to meet your child's specific needs. Remember, *tube-feeding is dangerous if done improperly,* so proceed with supervision and great care. But if you decide to tube-feed

your child, remember that other parents have learned how and you can too.

Other Modes of Feeding

Other modes of enteral nutrition are possible if your child cannot eat by mouth or requires tube-feeding on a long-term basis. Your doctor may recommend the surgical placement of a tube into the esophagus (esophagostomy), into the stomach (gastrostomy), or into the small intestine (jejunostomy). Placement of these tubes is usually done in the hospital but is a minor surgical procedure. The prescribed diet can be given by syringe, by drip feeding, or by feeding pump. You and your doctor will have to work out what is best for your child.

Parenteral nutrition means feeding directly into the veins. Such intravenous (or IV) feeding may be necessary if your child is unable to tolerate any type of feeding using the gastrointestinal tract. IV feeding may consist of short-term delivery of water, dextrose, and electrolytes if your child is unable to eat because of surgery or illness. But IV feeding can also consist of long-term delivery of all nutritional requirements by vein due to a more chronic condition. Parenteral nutrition is usually done in the hospital, but if your child needs it for an extended period of time, you can learn how to do it at home. This is a very specialized procedure and requires training from professionals.

The Reluctant Eater

Many ill and disabled children simply don't like to eat because eating is difficult for them. Others have problems because they like the wrong kinds of food. So while understanding what constitutes a balanced diet may be one thing, getting that food into your child may be another.

It helps if mealtime is calm. Pleasant atmosphere and conversation not only aid digestion but help keep the unwilling eater from focusing on the food to be consumed.

Although you should try to make the food as tasty and attractive as possible, there may be no fast and easy way to feed your child. Diversion is often the best tactic: if you have time at breakfast and lunch you might play games, watch an educational television show, eat outside in the yard, or have school with the home/hospital teacher. Dinner, eaten with the whole family and any guests, could then focus on conversation. Patience and perserverance are best; threats and anger will just put a child off eating.

Try not to feed your child alone in the bedroom. If your child has to spend a lot of time in bed, coming to the dining room or kitchen for dinner not only provides a healthy change of scene but also a change of position, which is beneficial to the respiratory and digestive system. If your child is too weak to sit, even if strapped into a chair upright or semireclining, you can provide a place where he or she can lie and eat in the same room as the rest of the family. If your table is large, a small immobile child may actually be able to lie on one end so you can see each other.

Mealtime atmosphere is important, not only for the reluctant eater but for your entire family. Psychologically it is helpful if everyone in the family washes his or her hands (and faces if necessary) and dresses tidily for meals. While you may bathe your child before dinner and put him or her into pajamas, at a certain age your child may want to dress for dinner. Even though this may mean extra work for you, it is important to respect such wishes.

PART 3

MEETING YOUR CHILD'S EDUCATIONAL AND SOCIAL NEEDS

13
Play, Recreation, and Travel

PLAY AND RECREATION

Play is one of the most important ways children learn and is therefore a crucial part of their development, to be fostered and encouraged by parents. Children not only gain coordination and endurance through play, but through use of their lively imaginations and keen powers of observation they also work to make sense of their world. A great deal of children's play is imitation or variation of the behavior of the adults in their lives. Children learn at least as much from what we do as from what we say, and as much from our attitudes as from our words. Indeed, this is the crux of the problem of creative play for the disabled or ill child: our attitude toward our children, the expectations and limitations, both psychological and physical, that we impose on them, determine the kinds of opportunities we provide for the all-important growth through play.

For example, it is easy for parents of a disabled child to become overprotective. Of course, reasonable precautions are important. But within sensible limits you must provide opportunities for all sorts of other experiences and challenges. You must teach your child to try—and, in case of failure, to get right up and try again—and give your child the courage to try by conveying your faith in his or her ability. Disabled children especially need the self-confidence gained by successfully meeting new challenges.

On the other hand, it is also common for the parents of a disabled child to deny their child's disability and to impose unrealistic expectations on their child, pushing him or her too far. This leads to inevitable failures and often to a poor self-image.

It is often difficult to gauge the influence of such thoughts and feelings. But we must remain aware that we teach by example and that our child reads our feelings through our actions as well as our words.

Providing Opportunities for Play in the Home

All parents help expand their children's horizons, but the parents of a disabled or ill child have a much larger role in helping their child grow through play. You do not need actively to play with your child every waking moment; you can have much contact with your child just by being in the same room, offering verbal attention while you continue with your work, and providing physical assistance as needed. But there is much to be said for spending "prime time" with your child, when your child knows that he or she has your undivided attention, even though this involves setting priorities.

How much direction and involvement in your child's play you need to provide depends on your child's condition. If he or she has a permanent disability, or if there are certain types of play you feel are especially beneficial to your child's development, you may want to provide certain play opportunities within your daily routine. And anytime a child undergoes a drastic change of condition you may have to be much more involved than usual in creating innovative play activities until your child is able to amuse himself or herself again. Whenever a change in physical condition is involved, it is very important that you discuss with your doctor what your child can and cannot do. Do not assume anything. Often parents are overly protective simply because they don't really know what their child can do. When such a major change occurs, the more your child can be involved in the activities of the family, the home, and his or her usual play, the happier your child will be.

In addition to looking at commercially available toys for your child, you may want to consult catalogs of special-education materials that list toys, games, and learning materials for children of various ages and disabilities. Your local special-education department may have catalogs you can borrow or look at in the school (see Appendix 3, "Suggested Reading").

Specially arranging a room or positioning your child to provide for the exploration of items that he or she may not contact or understand alone is vital. If, for example, your son is immobile and cannot move his head, position him in a room so he can easily see most of the action, and have young and old alike try to stay within his sight. Bring things to him and put them near him or on his wheelchair tray so he can touch, feel, and observe them closely. If, on the other hand, your son is blind but can move about, provide him with opportunities to smell, touch, feel, hear, and be told about that which he cannot see. Each child has special needs. Try to imagine what your child's world is like, and then think about what play experiences would expand your child's horizons.

Communication is crucial. Speech or nonverbal signs, signals, and symbols greatly enhance your child's exploration and understanding of the world. Talk to your child, even if he or she is not old enough, or able, to talk to you. Talk about what you are seeing, thinking, and doing. Your child may understand more of what you say than you think and will definitely learn about the use of language.

Of course, you can do more than report to your child on what you are doing. There are an infinite number of verbal games, stories, and conversations to be had with and without toys—activities that you and your child can do together

even when your hands are busy with other tasks.

Remember that when you talk to your child your tone of voice is very important, especially if your child cannot understand everything you say.

If your child is nonverbal or can communicate only with difficulty due to a speech or hearing problem, it is important to encourage and develop other means of communication. Read pages 125–133 for information on communication for the speech- or hearing-impaired child. If your child has difficulty speaking, the sooner your doctor examines him or her the better, for communication is vital to child development. Of course, words aren't everything, and nonverbal communication can be very rich.

Music can provide stimulation and enjoyment even to a very young child. Lullabies, in addition to soothing, provide a sense of rhythmic continuity and speech patterns that may aid a child in approaching language. As a child grows older, he or she can come to make "music" vocally and with rattles, bells, drums, pots and pans, or almost anything that will make a lively sound. While all this may seem like noise to you, to a child it has meaning.

Children also enjoy listening to records and tapes, which you can either buy or borrow from the library. If you lose interest in hearing a certain children's record again and again, you can give your child earphones. Remember that any sounds in the house, even if in the form of good music, may make it harder to hear your child's calls for help.

Arts and crafts are especially important for disabled children because they aid in the development of fine motor skills, hand-eye coordination, and the perception of spatial relations as well as other important functions. The joy is in the making, and it is probably only through the influence of the adult world that children get so concerned about what is a "good" or a "bad" creation. Working with arts and crafts gives a child the opportunity for self-expression and for depicting the world as he or she perceives it. You can learn about your child's perceptions of self and of the world by asking your child to tell you about what he or she has drawn or made. If your child has limited use of his or her hands, consider providing the opportunity to try using his or her feet or mouth.

Drawing can be done with crayons, markers, pencils, or pastels. Offer a variety of mediums so your child can experiment.

Painting can also be done with various mediums. Water colors are the least messy for the bed artist. Oils smell, and spills are difficult to remove. Finger paints are a bit messy but great fun to use. They add tactility to the other senses at work while painting.

Paper can be used not only for drawing and painting but also for cutting and pasting pictures and making chains, snowflakes, and a variety of objects, as any good crafts book will show. If your avid young artist uses up much paper, he or she may be willing to use paper that already has writing on one side. You can get end rolls of newsprint rather inexpensively from your local newspaper, and some print shops will give away odd-sized sheets of paper.

Cloth can be used to make such items as doll clothing, beanbags, pincushions, and wall hangings. While cutting and pasting material is faster and easier, an older child may get interested in sewing or embroidery. The occasional lost pin is dangerous only if your child lacks sensation in part of his or her body. With other children the hazards of sewing, even in bed, are far outweighed by the advantages of having a happy, productive child. A child who has good hand coordination may want to learn to sew his or her own clothing, learning to make adaptations indicated by any disability (see Chapter 11).

Weaving is neat, clean, and easy to do while confined to one position, especially if your child has some hand or foot dexterity. You can progress from potholders to weaving on simple looms, which are relatively inexpensive and easy for handy people to make.

Clay provides valuable tactile experience. Pinching, pulling, stretching, rolling, joining, cutting, kneading, and pushing clay into shape is often as important as pride in the completed object.

Construction and manipulation toys can be used not only to gain manual dexterity and to develop the sense of three-dimensional spatial relations but also to make objects for imaginative play. Usually, these can be taken apart and used again and again. Such toys include blocks with smooth surfaces as well as blocks with interlocking surfaces such as Bristle Blocks. Construction sets such as Lego and Lincoln Logs are more elaborate. Sets can contain objects to sort, stack, or string, such as beads. If your child cannot work on a horizontal surface, try magnetic boards or peg boards.

Models come in various degrees of difficulty. The easiest are snapped together; more coordination is needed for gluing. Making models can be an expensive hobby because you can make a model only once. While making models may give a child the opportunity to learn to read and follow directions and to develop manual dexterity, it is often less creative than some other forms of play. And you must be careful about inhaling fumes from the glue.

Board games can help develop a variety of skills such as counting, memorizing, and vocabulary-building. They also require varying degrees of manual dexterity. While games are usually designed for a given number of players and are targeted for specific age groups, you may have to adjust those figures to your child's degree of mental or manual dexterity. Games afford a time of companionship for a child and other family members. Children often love to play the same game again and again. While they usually want to play the whole game, you can speed it up. For example, if a game involves dice, by rolling six dice each time instead of just two, Peter Rabbit (or whoever) can hop along at quite a rapid rate (and your child may learn to add beyond 12).

If your child is an avid game player but you don't have the time or interest to play for hours, consider teaching your child to play against himself or herself, an imaginary friend, or a doll.

The rules, the intricacies, and the fun of a game are often better learned by playing with an adult, who can convey all this more clearly than another child. You can't just buy a game and expect your child to enjoy it. But if you spend the time to get your child enthusiastically involved, he or she will then often play for some time without you, even if against a teddy bear.

Magnetic-board games can be tilted and jiggled a bit. Many popular games such as Scrabble, chess, and checkers come in magnetic travel editions.

Electronic games are handy for play in bed, in the hospital, or while traveling—anytime it's better to have a self-contained toy with no pieces to lose that can be played even while lying down. Some memory games with tonal patterns can also be played by a blind child.

Literature opens a whole world to children. Most children enjoy being read to from an early age. Any long medical or therapy procedures that require a minimum of physical activity are good times to read to your child (see Appendix 3, "Suggested Reading").

When your child starts to look at picture books or to read alone, learning to turn pages can be a real art. If your child is coordinated enough to turn pages, you may want to begin with sturdy books with cloth or cardboard pages and then progress to books with paper pages.

Electronic page turners are available, but before you purchase one test it on the type of book your child is most apt to read and see if it will really work.

Talking books are wonderful if your child wants to hear more stories than you have time to read.

Anyone who is unable to read regular books due to a visual, perceptual, or physical disability can borrow free tapes and records from two sources. The National Library Service for the Blind and Physically Handicapped of the Library of Congress has a wide variety of materials available. The Recording for the Blind of the American Foundation for the Blind has primarily a collection of recordings of textbooks and literature used in academic classes (see "education" in Appendix 4, "Helpful Organizations"). In addition, your public library may have records of children's literature. Your child can listen to records using a headset, which has the advantage of giving you some peace and quiet. The disadvantage is that, if you don't hear the stories, you will be unable to discuss them with your child.

A variety of literature is good for a child so he or she can learn about the thoughts and actions of others, real and imaginary. It may be helpful to see how others have used courage, determination, perseverance, and often humor to overcome difficulties. Reading about successful disabled people such as Helen Keller, Franklin Roosevelt, Beethoven, or Ray Charles, about great men and women such as Gandhi, Martin Luther King, Jr., or Florence Nightingale, and about the heroes of the fairy tales and myths of old can provide valuable role models for your child.

Improvised stories that you or your child make up are also fun. Your child will relish stories you invent. The great advantage of telling your own stories is that you can do so while your hands and eyes are busy doing something else. Improvised stories also give you and your child an opportunity to verbalize in an indirect way ideas that have been concerning you.

Dramatic play is a natural activity for young children. While children may read about others, they also want to act out different lives as they imagine them. That is what playing house, at being a fireman, or at having a store is all about. To act out one's thoughts often requires a certain amount of dexterity: don't be limited in imagining how this can be done. If, for example, your daughter cannot use her hands, she may give lovely tea parties, pouring and serving all her dolls with her toes. Some children like to use puppets and dolls, others simply act the parts of their imaginary characters themselves. You can either make or buy dolls and puppets with physical disabilities, should you think your child would profit from having a little friend just like himself or herself. If a child becomes disabled suddenly, having a friend with whom to identify may be valuable. However, in play, as in dreams, many a disabled child is no longer disabled.

Children go through phases with their play, enacting events important to them and in that way gaining some understanding of them. Sometimes a child will play the same thing over and over again until you are bored and wonder why he or she isn't. Unless the play indicates some deep fear or anxiety (in which case you may want to discuss the matter with your doctor), let the child imagine freely. Your child's interests will change with time.

Television is a decidedly mixed blessing. There is some truly fine educational programming, but much programming is not at all elevating. In addition, viewing television is a passive activity. Reading or listening to radio drama or records at least requires imagination to "see" what is going on. Particularly if your child is immobile, it may be tempting to turn on the television to amuse him or her. Avoid this unless there is something truly of value to watch.

Children learn by example, and your child's viewing habits may be greatly influenced by your own. If you have the television on when you're not watching it, or if you watch programs out of inertia rather than genuine interest, your child will probably want to do the same.

Watching good educational programs can be a family activity. Listener-supported public television stations have some excellent programs. Commercial stations also have some good programs, but then your child is subjected to all the commercials. Many metropolitan areas have one station broadcasting educational programs for the school district. Since this is usually *not* mentioned in *TV Guide*, you may have to locate the station by flipping through the channels during school hours or calling your school administration. Once you have located the channel, you can write and ask for its program guide. You should never feel the need to watch every good program that is shown on television or you won't have time for other activities. So choose what your child watches with care. If you view a program with your child, you can also discuss it together afterward. If you can't stand to watch what your child is viewing, consider whether he or she is learning anything from the program. If not, your child's time may be better spent doing something else. A little carefully selected television can be a good thing, but better too little than too much.

Certainly, a television set in the bedroom is about the last thing an ill or disabled child needs. What could be a more effective way of passively isolating your child from the rest of the family?

If your child is bored and doesn't know what else to do but watch television, the responsibility is yours and your child's to think of something.

Household chores may well not fall into the play category for you, but if you consider that play is the way a child learns you can understand why he or she may find it fun to help. Helping with household chores can also develop a sense of responsibility in your child. With a little ingenuity you should be able to think up tasks that give a sense of accomplishment even to the most physically disabled. Your child might, for example, dip a piece of cotton in linseed oil and polish wooden items such as egg cups; or help you fold diapers as you pick up his or her arm and run it over the folded cloth. Such "help" doesn't speed your job, but your child's involvement in your duties can make them more fun for both of you. After all, you have jobs to get done, so why not do them together? Another factor to consider is that even a mentally able child who will never have the strength or coordination to accomplish certain household tasks alone, should know the procedures involved in order to supervise any attendants he or she may have when grown up and living away from home. There are "environmentally deprived" young adults who have never been taught the basics of running a household, which anyone must learn in order to live away from home.

Cooking not only provides opportunities for learning basic skills but also gives a child the chance to eat the results of his or her efforts. Many children are happy to help with the many steps involved in preparing meals: washing vegetables, chopping, stirring, kneading, and so on. While sharp knives and hot stoves can be dangerous, rather than ban your son or daughter from the kitchen, teach your child good safety habits like always sitting at the table when using a knife, keeping pot handles turned in, and so on. Often you can avoid some of the mad before-dinner rush by doing some food preparation such as fixing salads, desserts, or casseroles in the morning when you have more time and your child would like to play chef.

While cooking you also have the opportunity

to teach your child about nutrition, which can be important for a child who has dietary restrictions or needs to watch his or her weight. Cooking can afford you and your child a creative opportunity to find ways of making what your child has to eat taste good.

Pets provide companionship and help instill a sense of responsibility in a child. You will probably have the ultimate responsibility for supervising the care and feeding of the birds and beasts. But it is worth it, since pets are important for children. They can be dear companions from which your child learns not only the meaning of life but also something about the meaning of death. Especially in families where there is a possibility that a child will die, that child and his siblings can learn from having pets. If an animal dies, they have the opportunity to see and discuss what has happened and then bury it with a brief ceremony. This will aid your children in understanding that, while we love and care for those who live with us, death is inevitable and final, though we can always remember the joy the departed brought to our lives.

Opportunities for Play Outdoors

There is so much to do, see, and learn out-of-doors. Most babies are happy if they can just be outside in a playpen or buggy, listening to and watching whatever is happening. A mobile child can get into the grass and dirt, make mudpies, collect dandelions, and so on. An immobile child can still sit or lie outside as you bring the world —snails, earthworms, flowers, leaves, and so on —to him or her. Walks are adventures to be undertaken in any weather. If you live in town, it is an adventure to go to the country or at least to a wooded park. Your child may see these places only if you take him or her there.

If going out is difficult because of your child's condition or the climate, you can do many things to bring the outside in. You can observe insects in the kitchen, arrange flowers, and press autumn leaves. Mudpies and snow ice cream can be made in the kitchen or even in bed if necessary.

"Normal" children get their share of bumps, scrapes, and falls playing outside, and these are generally accepted as part of growing up. If your ill or disabled child doesn't have the occasional mishap also, you are probably being overly protective. Do not be too fearful of the occasional minor accident. You may have to make certain adaptations to help your child play outside. For example, if your child is visually impaired, you may have to yell "Stop" if he or she is running and playing and is about to bash into or trip over something. Your child can also learn to play with special balls that have bells or beepers inside. Your child might even learn to climb trees by feel, testing every branch to see if it will bear his or her weight.

Even if your child is in a wheelchair, there is no reason not to go outside and play. While there is a minimal danger of a chair capsizing, that doesn't happen often before a child learns what can and cannot be done in the chair. A child in a motorized chair can get stuck if the motor malfunctions, but if he or she knows how to ask a friend for help the problem can be solved. A travel chair can capsize relatively easily, especially if pushed by young children, so you may have to supervise if, for example, a sibling or friend wants to push your disabled child.

If your child can jump and climb and explore, provide opportunities to do so. If you have a yard, consider making or buying a fort or swing set. Climbing and swinging, riding tricycles, scooters, bicycles, or skateboards all help develop coordination and gross motor skills. If your child can't move much alone, he or she can still enjoy the thrill of swings, merry-go-rounds, and slides while riding on your lap, or of climbing a jungle gym while in your arms.

If you live in a colder climate, you can bring outdoor toys like swings inside. This can help amuse your child and preserve your sanity when it is too cold for your child to be outdoors.

Sports for the Disabled

The human body functions best if it is exercised, as discussed in Chapter 8. While physical-therapy programs are designed to help disabled children, this exercise is often seen as work. It can be complemented with sport, which not only aids physical development but is also fun. There are many opportunities for a disabled child to participate in sports.

The need for athletic activity is particularly great among previously athletic children who became disabled due to an accident or illness. For such people, one problem of adjustment to their new condition is the feeling of being cut off from the sports that were so important to them before. Of course, sports are also important for children with congenital disabilities: all children profit not only from the much-needed exercise sports provide but also from the joy of participating in the activity, from the comradeship, and from the feeling of accomplishment that comes from doing one's best. Sports also help a child gain in gross motor skills, which aid mobility in daily life, and can teach a great deal about interacting with other children. Furthermore, a child who participates in athletic events held between schools of neighboring communities has the opportunity to travel, to learn to manage on his or her own, and to ask for assistance from others when needed. The determination and self-confidence developed through sports programs are often evidenced years after the experience.

While it may take a conscious effort on your part to find, support, or even start appropriate community athletic activities for your child, such efforts are well worth the trouble.

There are organizations to promote most sports for the disabled, including, but not limited to, archery, bowling, golf, horseback riding, skiing and winter sports, swimming and water sports, tennis, and track and field events. While you may have to live in a metropolitan area to get enough children in wheelchairs together to form a wheelchair basketball team, you need only two to play table tennis or tennis, and your child can engage in many sports, such as archery, bowling, track and field, and weightlifting, alone or with an able-bodied friend. Most children can participate in some sort of adaptive sport program, and most can do more than we think. Blind children and amputees can ski, children with cerebral palsy can ride horseback and do karate, paraplegics can swim. Most likely there is some sport your child can do.

Swimming and water sports are especially notable. For if a weak person doesn't have to confront gravity, it is much easier to move. Some children will always need support and assistance in the water but will greatly enjoy the experience anyway. Children with any ability to move unassisted should, if possible, be "drownproofed," which entails teaching them to float face-down in a dangling position, with their heads beneath the water, propelling themselves upward periodically for air by performing an easy, modified version of the breast stroke. In this way they use their natural buoyancy to advantage, conserve energy, and control their breathing. A professional swimming instructor should teach your child this technique. Drownproofing can be learned by children over the age of four, even if they are disabled and cannot swim. Water holds a special attraction for children and can be dangerous without proper precautions.

Many communities have adaptive physical-education programs that include swimming instruction. If your community does not have such a program, check with local public and private pools (such as the YMCA or any private athletic clubs) to see if they can recommend an appropriate swimming instructor to you. If the local public pool is inaccessible or inappropriate due to the severity of your child's disability, you might want to check with your doctor or friends to see if there is someone in your community willing to share his or her pool with your child.

When you have an idea of what kind of athletic activity your child could and would like to do, find out which activities are available in your community. Physical-education teachers in schools, particularly in those with adaptive physical-education programs, and your local recreation department will be able to tell you of present programs. Local athletic organizations or private clubs may offer programs or be willing to start one with your encouragement and support. If nothing appropriate is available for your child's specific needs, you may have to work with other parents to get an appropriate adaptive sports program started. For information on how someone with your child's disability might be able to participate in a particular sport, see Appendix 4, "Helpful Organizations." Magazines such as *Sports 'n Spokes* (PBA Publications, Phoenix, AZ) are also very informative.

Your child will probably have preferences regarding which sport to participate in. Often parents project their own interests and desires onto their child, failing to realize that the child may have interests quite different from their own. You may like swimming and have difficulty seeing the point of weightlifting, but if the latter interests your child encourage him or her to pursue it. On the other hand, your child may not be interested in sports at all. As long as your child is getting enough exercise in other ways, there is no point in pushing sports.

Playing with Friends

It is very important for children to be involved with their peers. They not only learn how to relate to and cooperate with others, but they also expand their world by interacting with other children as they slowly develop independence and start loosening family ties. A "normal" child interacts with other children in structured classroom situations as well as during recess and often plays with other children on the way home from school or on weekends. The older a child gets, the more of this he or she arranges independently of parents. In contrast, a disabled child often lacks social contacts, and the child's physical or mental disability may indicate the need for you to help organize opportunities for play.

For example, since preschoolers are often happy to play with teenagers, you might arrange for students from a local service group to come and play with your child every Saturday morning. Then in elementary school when your child wants to play with children of the same age, you can call parents of your child's friends and arrange for the children to come over, perhaps even to spend the night. (Don't worry if you must give your child medical treatments every morning or night; the friend will gain a greater understanding of your child's disability if he or she is present during your child's medical treatments. Simply tell the friend's parents, so if their child asks them about what he or she has seen they will not be surprised.)

Organized youth groups give a child the opportunity to meet and interact with a number of children. A large city may have special groups for disabled children, but for a child with normal intelligence there is an advantage to being mainstreamed in a group of able-bodied children, such as Boy Scouts, Girl Scouts, or Camp Fire. Your local city recreation department, YMCA, church, or synagogue may also have youth groups. The advantage to becoming involved with a group whose membership remains constant throughout the year is that your child and the others will have the time necessary to get to know each other and to establish friendships.

Phone other parents and organizations such as those mentioned above to find out about what programs exist, as well as something about the children and leaders involved. While it might be nice to find a leader who has worked with a child like yours before, it may be more important to find a respected leader who has a group in your neighborhood so your child has the opportunity to play with the children at other times during the week. If your child cannot function independently and will need much help, you cannot expect the leader to care for your child. You will probably have to go to the meetings with your child. Think through in advance what kind of help your child may need and how best to get it. Of course, you should help your child become as independent as possible, but you must be realistic and plan ways for your child to get the assistance he or she needs without placing a burden on the leader.

Once you have decided which group would be best for your child, contact the leader. If you have a friend who knows both you and the leader, this individual may be willing to make the initial contact, telling the leader about your child and giving the leader the opportunity to raise questions that he or she might feel uncomfortable asking you as the child's parent. After all, it is important that the leader fully understand your child's needs.

Camps provide opportunities to spend time out-of-doors with other children away from home. Some service organizations and private agencies run camps for disabled children at minimal cost. Check with local organizations helping your child about camps they or affiliated organizations run. For more information about how to find out about camping opportunities, see Appendix 3, "Suggested Reading." Children with minimal disabilities can often be mainstreamed into regular camps.

Ideally, camp offers a learning opportunity for the child and a respite for the family. Unfortunately, some camps are poorly run and inadequately staffed; some parents send children to camp to get them out of the way; some children, although they might like to spend a few weeks in camp, value the leisure time summer provides and would prefer to spend the time at home playing with friends. Yet while camp is not the best summer activity for all disabled children, it is appropriate for some. If both you and your child think camping would be a good experience, find out what camps exist in your area. The camp director will tell you the advantages of his or her program. Talk also with other campers (past and present) and their parents to get their impressions.

Another important way to learn how a camp is actually run is to spend a day observing the program.

If you are mainstreaming your child, make sure the camp director understands your child's disability and is willing and able to provide for any special needs.

Going Out into the Community

In any community, there are many activities of interest to a child. Many children enjoy accompanying their parents when they go shopping and run errands. While it is often easier and faster to do errands alone, try to take your child with you when possible. A disabled child may grow up environmentally deprived because the parents think it is too much of a hassle to take their child along. It is not very exciting for you to go to the bank, the post office, the supermarket, the department store, or the gas station. But these can be fun outings for a child as well as a way to learn about places and services in the community that he or she will have to utilize as an adult, either alone or with help. Your child's specific disability may indicate the need for certain kinds of experiences. For example, a blind child may learn from handling objects, not only in self-service stores but also in shops where such articles are made, the process involved in creating the completed article. Speciality stores sell-

ing crafts, musical instruments, sporting goods, or pets are all very interesting to a child. City or county facilities such as the fire department or the airport may not be regular tourist attractions but can be of great interest to your child. Often you can phone to arrange a special tour. Your community may also offer cultural activities such as concerts, plays, exhibitions, or story hours at the public library.

Outdoor events such as parades, fairs, zoos, or other tourist attractions in your area are possibilities, as are recreational facilities where you can participate or just observe. You might also classify as outings the various trips to medical facilities. When a health-care professional has time to talk, your child may be fascinated to learn more about the work he or she does.

Restaurants delight children. There is joy not only in eating out but also in being able to order whatever (within reason) you want. Your child may be quite unable to eat most dishes on the menu. If so, take his or her special meal along and let your child nibble at what he or she orders. You can eat the unfinished portion. Actual food consumption is only one part of the experience.

Seating in a restaurant can usually be arranged. Many restaurants have high chairs. Larger children can sometimes be propped in the corner of a booth. If your child will be eating in a wheelchair, you might take along four cans of tuna so that, if necessary, the height of the table can be increased by slipping these under the legs. Blocks of wood with identations to secure the legs work just as well, but if you don't do woodworking yourself tuna cans are a resourceful solution.

While some children have the patience to wait until their food is served, others get wriggly. If waiting is a problem, consider dining out when a restaurant isn't crowded, such as on weeknights or early on weekends. If your disabled child eats very slowly, take books and toys along for siblings. In spite of this, someone may still end up walking restless siblings outside while their brother or sister finishes inside.

When you take your child out, people may stare and ask questions, which usually spring from curiosity and interest. Be ready and willing to respond politely to such questions, for they provide an opportunity to teach others about the disabled.

TRAVEL

Take your child out of your community if possible. For a child it can be a real advantage to take a train or bus to the next stop down the line, even if someone has to drive down to bring you home. You might be able to visit a friend in a neighboring community. Just being in another home with friends is very interesting for your child, a nice "mini-vacation" for you, and inexpensive. Another possibility is spending a weekend in a hotel or motel nearby.

If you are not sure that travel farther afield is possible, make trial runs. For example, to see if a cross-country plane trip would be possible, take a half-hour plane trip to a nearby city. If it is a success, take the train back home to practice for the longer plane ride. If all goes well and your child enjoys the experience, you are ready for the real trip. On a trip of any length, an accident or mishap can happen. But you can also fall out of bed at home. Again, try not to be too fearful or overprotective.

Plan your trip realistically. While there is no point in planning a trip that is too long and exhausting for you and your child to enjoy, it is equally bad never to try to go anywhere because you think it might be too difficult. With proper planning you can take reasonable and enjoyable trips.

Your child may also have to travel to a medical facility in a different city for treatment. In that case you must determine the best (which is usually the fastest) way of getting there. For information on traveling with a severely ill child, see pages 184–186.

Medical considerations vary from child to child. Some factors to consider are:

Your child's energy level. If your child is very weak or tires easily, trips closer to home or destinations you can quickly reach by air are better than long car rides, unless it is possible for your child to rest adequately along the way. If he or she hates being confined and needs to move about, this could also affect your choice of travel mode.

Tolerance for infections. If your child has lowered immunity due to a medical condition or treatment or can become seriously ill from common germs that are not a hazard for most people, limit your travel to modes that expose your child to fewer germs. Obviously, you are most self-contained in a recreational vehicle, have more contacts if you travel by car and utilize restaurants and motels, and have the most contacts if you use public transportation. You may want to plan a trip for a time of year when there are fewer infectious diseases around—like summer instead of winter, when more people have colds or the flu.

Tolerance for temperature changes. Obviously, if your child freezes on cool days in Southern California, don't go to Alaska; if your child gets too hot on warm days in Maine, a summer trip to Florida would be inappropriate. Some children have difficulties with their temperature-regulatory systems, and changes in climate seriously affect them.

Tolerance for air pollutants or pollens. If your child has severe respiratory or allergy problems, this may be a consideration.

Motion sickness. This is unpleasant for most children but a serious hazard for anyone without a gag reflex, who could aspirate. Therefore ask your doctor which preparation for motion sickness to purchase for your child and whether you should give it to your child before he or she even *begins* to feel strange.

Medication. Take along a third more medication than you or your doctor think your child will need on the trip. Carry at least a 24-hour well-labeled supply of your child's medication with you in your purse or totebag in case you get separated from your luggage. (Some people pack half of their medication in the luggage and carry the rest with them.) Take along written prescriptions for medications and eyeglasses, so you can get refills if necessary. When traveling abroad, take extra prescriptions with the generic names of the drugs in English and in the languages of any countries you plan to visit. Before departure on a long plane trip, discuss with your doctor how to adjust medication dosages to account for jet lag.

Medical equipment. Keep with you any machines your child will need immediately upon arrival. This also applies to any delicate machines, which might get damaged in the baggage compartment. Even planes will let you carry on such equipment if you explain why you must keep it with you.

Buses, trains, and ships may allow you to bring your own portable supply of oxygen, but planes will not. The latter may provide oxygen for a fee when given advance notice and after consultation between your doctor and the airline's medical staff. Arrangements for oxygen en route should be initiated when you first make your reservation. This oxygen is usually preregulated for flow delivery at two to four liters per minute and is not humidified. The tubing and fittings are often different from those used on your personal portable tanks, so check this in advance if you plan to use your own oxygen mask or nasal cannula. If you will need oxygen at your destination, arrange for this service prior to departure. This is particularly important when traveling overseas, for the "pin" configuration and yoke fittings are often different in other countries, making it difficult to refill your own tank.

Portable suction machines can be carried with you and are vital if your child may need suctioning. If your child needs to be suctioned regularly, you may want to carry a 60-cc catheter-tip syringe, which works well with a whistle-tip catheter in an emergency. See pages 66–68 for more information on suctioning.

Your child's medical records. Always carry a concise record, including your child's diagnosis, present treatment, and medication, in case your child needs medical attention away from home.

A doctor away from home. If you think there is a good chance your child will need to see a doctor, particularly in an emergency situation, it is best to contact a doctor *before* you leave home or at least as soon as you reach your destination. If you are visiting friends, their doctor may be your contact. Otherwise ask your doctor for suggestions as to how to proceed. Remember, once an emergency has arisen is not the time to start looking for a doctor and the appropriate medical facility.

Toileting can be a problem with any mode of travel if bathrooms are not wheelchair-accessible. If you can carry your child, with a certain amount of ingenuity and acrobatics you can get him or her undressed and seated on the toilet even in cramped quarters.

When using public transportation on a longer trip with a larger, heavier child, you may want to check to see if the restrooms are accessible. If not, see if the company will provide small wheelchairs that can be used in the aisles. If toileting is a major problem there are three alternatives. You can purchase and keep with you your own travel-stool on wheels designed for just such situations; you can use diapers; or you can dehydrate your child or limit high-fiber foods before departure and during the trip. But this can be dangerous with some conditions.

Food should be thought of before you leave home. Traveling is much more pleasant if your child has favorite foods available when he or she is hungry. This means traveling with snacks, even if you expect to be served meals or stop at restaurants. While an adult may not mind eating something new and different an hour or two later than usual if an unexpected delay occurs, a hungry child wants something he or she likes to eat right then. Children can get grouchy, tired, and generally unpleasant if not fed when they are hungry. Take liquid along also.

Clothing can also influence comfort while traveling. Comfortable clothing that hides dirt and wrinkles is best. It is wise to carry a change of clothing for your child in your totebag in case of a toileting, eating, or vomiting accident. When using public transportation, dress your child in lighter-weight clothing and bring a sweater or jacket so your child can be made comfortable if the vehicle becomes too warm or cool.

If your child will want to take his or her shoes off, you may want to bring along some slippers.

Travel information is available from travel books for the disabled available at your public library. The Moss Rehabilitation Hospital Travel

Information Center (see "travel" in Appendix 4, "Helpful Organizations") has a free service providing information to disabled people on all aspects of travel such as accessibility, modes of transportation, and so on. Most guidebooks for the general public contain specific information for the disabled traveller, so check these as well.

Travel agents can be most helpful, especially with plane, cruise, hotel, and sometimes also with train reservations. The Society for the Advancement of Travel for the Handicapped (see Appendix 4, "Helpful Organizations") maintains a current file of cooperating concerned travel agencies and tour operators familiar with the needs of the disabled. But any reliable travel agent in your community should be able to help you, particularly if you explain your specific needs.

Air Travel

For ease in traveling by air, request the most direct flight with the fewest number of stops and transfers. Also try to avoid traveling during holidays or at particularly busy times during the week. When your agent makes your reservation, ask for assigned seats. You may, for example, want a window seat in the nonsmoking area, with easy access to restrooms and exits. The first row (called the bulkhead) in coach and the emergency-exit rows provide more space in front of the seat. It is difficult to take in the view below if you are seated over the wing. If your child cannot sit up during takeoff and landing, most airlines require that you buy extra seats either in first class or coach, which is very expensive. If you think your child can sit up at least during takeoff and landing, a shorter child could lie across you and his or her seat for the rest of the flight if the seat arms can be lifted. For a taller child, you might want to buy one more seat so he or she can stretch out. Some special diets can be ordered. This is best done when you make your reservation and must be done at least 24 hours in advance. Your agent will also be able to advise you if you need any travel insurance.

Airplane accessibility. Access to the Skies Program, an offshoot of Rehabilitation USA (see Ap-

pendix 4, "Helpful Organizations"), is working to make airliners more accessible for the disabled by encouraging removable or foldup aisle armrests to make wheelchair-to-aircraft-seat transfers easier; access improvements to restrooms; and the development and use of onboard wheelchairs to transport a disabled passenger to and from restrooms during the flight. This organization can give you the latest information on the accessibility of different aircraft.

"Meet and assist" service is provided by most airlines. With this service, someone meets you at the airport and assists with boarding, deplaning, and any flight connections. Wheelchairs, motorized carts to take you between airlines, special lifts to help you board at airports without jetway facilities (corridors linking the inside of the terminal with the aircraft) are all services available upon request; have your travel agent notify the airline that you need this service when making your reservation. As most disabled persons are boarded first, be sure you know how much prior to departure time you should arrive at the airport. *Access Travel: Airports* (see Appendix 3, "Suggested Reading") provides invaluable details such as design features, facilities, and services for 472 terminals in 46 countries. This information is also included in *The Official Airline Guide Travel Planner and Hotel/Motel Guide*, which your travel agent should have.

Before departure make sure the airline has contacted any personnel needed to assist you in deplaning. If your flight is delayed, ask the stewardess to phone ahead and see if your connecting flight can be held until your arrival.

Air travel with a severely ill child. It may be necessary for an ill child to travel to or from a medical facility. While the social worker there should be able to assist you in making travel arrangements, you should also have a complete understanding of any medical problems your child may have while traveling and how to take care of these. Discuss this thoroughly with your doctor.

Atmospheric changes (pressurization and depressurization) are not tolerated well by some children. Your doctor may suggest using a decongestant prior to takeoff and again after about six hours during a particularly long flight. Some children feel better if they chew gum or suck on hard candies. Others can learn to pinch their nostrils while trying to blow their noses, forcing air into nasal cavities.

Checked luggage. Extra precautions should be taken to make sure your luggage arrives with you. Clearly label each piece inside and out, with your name, flight number, destination address, and phone number. The agent who tags your bags at check-in will attach baggage-destination tags to your luggage and give you the stubs as claim checks. Each tag has a three-letter code and flight number to indicate on which plane and to which airport your luggage should go. Check the tag and flight number *before* your bags go down the conveyor belt to help ensure that your luggage ends up where you do. You can use tape to write your initials on your luggage so no one will take it by mistake.

Wheelchairs. The rare airline may allow a small child's wheelchair or travel chair in the storage compartment of a cabin, but most do not. Sometimes an airline will let your child use a chair until close to departure time. While this is handy, you do run the slight risk of the chair being left behind. Therefore, it may be better to ask for "meet and assist" to provide a chair for your child's use in the airport. Also check the airline's requirements for transporting batteries of electric chairs when making your reservation. The airline should be willing to accept the battery, if you have secured it to the chair, disconnected the terminals, taped the cables and terminals, and tightened the battery caps. Before checking a wheelchair, remove any loose parts, such as cushions or totebags, and take these with you. Lock the arms. Tape your name, flight number, destination address, and phone number to the chair. You may even want to add a note such as:

Attention: This chair is very important to a physically handicapped child. Lift by grasping the front bumper and under the back end. Please handle with extreme care and do not drop. Thank you.

Most airlines hold themselves liable for only a limited amount of the cost of lost or damaged baggage (including wheelchairs) per ticketed passenger, not per bag. Therefore you may wish to purchase "excess valuation insurance," which you can get at the baggage counters for about $.50 per $100 value declared.

Hand luggage should be used to carry the medication, clothing, food, and toys you need while traveling. Plan this carefully. To keep your hands free, use a shoulder bag or, if you aren't carrying a child in a backpack, consider getting a travel backpack, which can be worn like a pack or converted to a suitcase that will fit under the seat. As mentioned before, any delicate medical equipment should be carried onto the plane and stored there. If you need to carry on a great deal you may have to be persistent, but if your needs are understood your requests should be honored.

Medical clearance. If your child has severe problems, your doctor must submit a travel request to the airline's medical staff for approval. Carry copies of your doctor's letter and the written approval, in case anyone questions whether your child should be allowed to travel. The initial request for any special help should be realistic but not overly dramatic, for an airline does have the right to refuse travel to anyone deemed incapable of surviving the journey. As only a limited number of disabled persons are allowed on each flight, submit your request as soon as you know you will be traveling.

Regular travel on a commercial airline is the cheapest way to fly if your child can sit up during takeoff and landing. Remember, if you think your child may need to lie down part of the time but is too long to lie across your lap and his or her seat, you may purchase an extra seat.

Stretcher service is provided by many airlines if you have proper medical authorization from a doctor. But you have to pay for the number of seats required by the airline, such as four in first class or nine in tourist. You also have to arrange for an ambulance crew to assist with boarding and deplaning. While airplanes have blankets, be sure to bring a sheet along to cover your child, especially if he or she may need to use a bedpan.

Patient-assistance-and-service companies (also known as medical-transfer-assistance companies) were originally developed to help international corporations get appropriate medical care for employees taken ill abroad. These companies now perform the same services within North America and should be able to:

- Determine the nature of your child's condition and travel needs through consultation with your doctor.
- Determine how to get your child to a facility and back home as economically as possible. Often it is possible to arrange travel with a commercial airline, even on a stretcher. Otherwise air-ambulance service will be arranged.
- Arrange to have any necessary medical personnel (doctor, nurse, or paramedic) or equipment fly with your child. (If you can provide for all your child's needs except oxygen, you can arrange that yourself, as indicated on pages 184–185.)
- Arrange ambulance assistance at both ends of the journey, as well as any plane transfers en route.

Such services can be invaluable if your child will need more medical assistance during the flight than you can provide yourself.

Even if you think you can provide for your severely ill or disabled child while traveling, you may want to consider purchasing a service agreement for the duration of your trip; then if your child does become ill away from home this will help defray the costs of medical transportation and will augment your personal insurance. If you think you may need sophisticated patient-assistance-and-transfer services, be sure to deal with an established, reputable firm such as International SOS Assistance, Inc. (P.O. Box 11568, Philadelphia, PA 19116; 800-523-8930).

Air-ambulance companies are the most expensive way to travel, costing up to four times more than a patient-transfer service. And air ambulances do not necessarily provide better flights than commercial planes, which refuel less frequently and can fly faster. Since air ambulances are not yet regulated by FAA standards, examine very carefully the credentials of any company you are considering and compare its services with what a patient-transfer service provides in terms of such factors as the length of the flight, medical personnel and equipment available during the flight, and cost, to determine whether chartering an air ambulance would in fact be better than having a patient-assistance-and-service company arrange the appropriate travel on a commercial flight or on an air ambulance.

Dealing directly with an air-ambulance company presents two difficulties. First, it is very difficult for you to determine if the type of flight, medical equipment, and medical personnel are really appropriate for your child. And second, since all an air-ambulance company can sell is its service, it is more apt to tell you your child needs an air ambulance than a patient-assistance-and-service company, which is committed to getting your child transferred safely via the least expensive appropriate means.

If your child is sick enough to need such sophisticated assistance as an air ambulance it may be wisest to use a patient-assistance-and-service company that is experienced in all aspects of travel and has an established reputation for carefully dealing with all details involved in such travel.

Train Travel

Travel by train is possible for the disabled with most large railroad companies such as Amtrak. *Access Amtrak* (included in Appendix 3, "Suggested Reading") describes services available to the disabled. Before making your reservation, discuss your child's disability and requirements with an employee qualified to advise you to be sure your child can be accommodated. Stretcher-borne persons can sometimes be boarded through a removable window into a private bedroom, but if your child is that disabled you will probably want to fly to get where you're going as quickly as possible.

Bus Travel

Major companies such as Greyhound and Trailways allow the disabled to have an assistant travel at no additional cost if the disabled has a letter from a doctor indicating that he or she cannot travel alone. Before departure, make sure you know when and where the bus will stop and if you will need to change buses or terminals.

Car Travel

Travel by car is often the most convenient for short distances, but long car trips with any child can be trying. When planning a car trip, consider how long your child can travel with ease. If a long trip is necessary, consider whether your child will travel better in the day or at night and which food and toys you should bring along for your child's nourishment and amusement. Be sure your child has and uses a good car seat (see pages 86–87). It is also wise to establish certain rules for car behavior. Particularly when driving alone, if your child needs disciplining or help of any kind, pull the car over to the side of the road and stop. It is very hard to concentrate on the road and your child at the same time, and a minute's inattention can cause a bad accident, as anyone who has had one will tell you.

With a certain amount of stamina, flexibility, patience, resourcefulness, and a sense of humor you will find that travel with your disabled child is possible.

14

Teaching and Educating Your Child

To assume that education is limited to classroom learning is seriously to limit your child's education and opportunities to learn and grow. The word "educate" comes from the Latin *educare*, meaning "to draw out," implying that everyone has some potential that, if fostered and encouraged, may be realized.

From the moment of birth, a child is learning, and we as parents are the most important teachers. Moreover, our children learn physically, emotionally, mentally, and even spiritually. Education, in other words, concerns not just the ability to add and subtract or the size of a child's vocabulary but the attitudes, habits, and values that will shape our child's character and remain with him or her throughout life.

Such an expansive conception of learning has special significance for an ill or disabled child. Academic achievement may not be important for your child, and holding to such a goal can be frustrating if your child will never perform at grade level. To think of learning in terms of what the "average child" can do at your child's age is futile, because there is no such thing as an average child. It is more valuable to think of your child as a unique individual, knowing and accepting that he or she may be able to learn some things and not others, yet helping your child to develop to the fullest.

HELPING YOUR CHILD LEARN AT HOME

You may feel that you have so many medical problems to take care of that education is a low-priority item. But you cannot concentrate on the physical problems and ignore the rest of your child. Your child learns from you whether you are consciously teaching or not, and you must use the learning process to help your child develop as fully as possible, to become as independent as possible.

Parents of "normal" children naturally expect, from the birth of their child, that their son or daughter will grow up to be independent, living away from home and from direct parental influence. But the parents of an ill or disabled child may lose sight of the necessity of helping their child develop to his or her highest potential and become as independent as possible. If your child is physically disabled, there may come a point when, although you can toilet, bathe, dress, and feed your child faster than he or she can do these things, your child must be taught as many of these skills as possible or he or she will never learn to be independent. When a retarded child learns to tie his or her shoes, it is a step toward independence; when a blind child learns to eat unassisted, it is a step toward independence; when an immobile child asserts individual preferences as to what to wear, it is a step toward independence.

Most ill or disabled children can work toward and obtain some measure of independence and self-reliance. To help your child learn the necessary skills and attitudes, it helps to set goals. Think through what would be best for your child to learn and then set challenging but realistic goals toward which you both consciously work. Your goals may range from learning to read to learning to wash the dishes to learning to say please and thank you.

How Do You Choose Goals for Your Child?

Looking ahead to your child's future vocational employment will help you set realistic and worthwhile goals that you can work toward now. Children are often asked what they want to be when they grow up. Their answers to this question may change as they learn, grow, and gain new perceptions of themselves and the world. Taking into account your child's disability and present level of functioning, ask yourself what your child could do when grown and what he or she has to learn now to be qualified to do it.

If you question whether your severely disabled child will ever be gainfully employed, ask yourself what self-help skills your child can learn. The more skills learned, the easier and more enjoyable it will be to care for your child now and the greater will be the number of possible living arrangements when he or she no longer lives with you.

Also, consider more than goals of an academic or self-help nature; ask yourself what humane qualities and behavior you would like to see your child develop in order to be cherished and valued as a friend. Achieving these important humane goals may also require mastering specific skills. For example, to help develop a sense of responsibility toward others, your child could learn to set the dinner table every day.

Your goals should be neither too simple nor too difficult, which means you must find a balance between unrealistically high expectations that lead to frustration and goals that are so low that a child may be protected from failure but will never be challenged. To help you organize your thoughts about your child's potential and future so you can set realistic goals, take some time to consider the following questions. Get a pencil and write down your answers. Keep them so you can refer to them periodically to assess your goals and your child's progress. (You can make them brief; there is no need to write a series of essays.)

- What is my purpose in caring for my child at home? What skills, attitudes, and behaviors would best help my child develop to the highest potential?
- What skills and behaviors do I feel my child is ready

to learn now? What goals or objectives would I like my child to reach in the next year? Consider such areas as academic or vocational development; self-help skills (bathing, toileting, dressing, eating, involvement in his or her own medical care); how he or she interacts with the family, with friends, and in the community; how he or she spends leisure and recreational time.
- Are these goals realistic for my child? Do they meet my stated purpose in caring for my child at home and having him or her go to school? Change your list of goals if you wish.
- Which goals are *most important* for my child to learn this year? Put a star beside those goals. Explain *why* you think they are the most important.

How Can You Help Your Child Attain the Goals You Have Set?

Give your child ample opportunities to learn and to succeed. For example, if one of your child's goals is to learn to feed the dog every day, you must be patient and willing to help your child master the task. You may well be able to feed the dog much faster yourself, and you may wonder, when your child needs reminding, spills the food, or steps on the dog's tail, whether it is all worth your effort. But if the goal is realistic (which does not necessarily mean easily attainable), your child can learn if you persist in teaching and assisting in the task.

Break down tasks into short-term objectives or sequences of skills to be mastered. Most often it is best to master each step involved in the task before proceeding to the next. Obviously, the more ambitious the goal, the greater the number of steps in the sequence and the greater the importance of evaluating whether each step has been mastered. It is not necessary that every task be broken down into its component parts. But if your child has difficulty learning to do something, teaching that task may seem overwhelming until, perhaps with the help of the appropriate professional, you break it down into sequential steps. Read the information in Chapters 11 and 12 on how to teach your child to dress and eat independently for examples of how you can break a task down into its constituent steps.

Provide appropriate motivation. Motivation can be both internal and external.

Internal motivation is most effective. Ann wants to write her name because she sees that her older brother and sister can. With such strong internal motivation she will probably continually ask for help and practice until she can. Do what you can to ensure that your child really wants to master the task he or she is learning.

External motivation may take the form of rewards that reinforce positive performance. There are four major types of rewards you can use with your child:

1. *Social rewards* involve your behavior as you give your child praise, smiles, or attention.
2. *Primary rewards,* such as bits of food or candy, provide instant reinforcement of correct behavior. These are important for any child who cannot understand the meaning of a reward unless it is given immediately after correct behavior.
3. *Token rewards* such as points or gold stars can be accumulated and exchanged for other objects or activities (see below) a child really values. This works well for the child who can understand delayed reward.
4. *Activity rewards* are activities your child would like to engage in when he or she has finished a task or mastered a skill. These may include playing a game with you, playing outside, or a special outing.

To make the most of your rewards, bear in mind the following major points:

- *Reward immediately* when teaching a new task.
- *Reward every correct response* in the early steps of learning a task. As the behavior becomes more proficient, you may require more and more correct responses before you reward.
- *Reward improvement,* or steps in the right direction, rather than insist on perfect performance on the first try. Then little by little you can require more perfect responses; this is called "shaping" behavior.
- *Reward appropriately.* This means not only giving a reward your child values but also one commensurate with the task.

It is dangerous to rely too heavily on the external reinforcement provided by rewards, for what you really want is for your child to perform the task—and he or she shouldn't perform only if there will be a reward. Don't forget that the goal should ultimately be that successful completion of the task is itself the reward.

Part of a good self-image and a willingness to try to learn comes from recognition that we can do things well. We may sometimes think we are helping by pointing out to a child what isn't quite right yet, figuring that he or she would like the opportunity to improve, like going over the one word our child missed on the spelling test and not offering congratulations on the rest, which were right. But a child who doesn't feel that he or she can succeed may, with time, begin to lose faith and the willingness to try. There are times, of course, when consequences for incorrect responses are necessary; these may be a frown, a harsh word, a slap on the wrist, or taking back rewards your child has won. But you must strike a balance. Do not forget how important and valuable positive reinforcement can be.

Learn how much and how fast your child can learn. You will find out what this is only when you try to teach your child something. If you pick a realistic task, break it down into sequential steps, and work regularly with your child, you will see what and how quickly your child can learn. If you're not making any progress after a reasonable amount of time, reexamine not only what you want to teach but also how you are teaching it. Sometimes input from the outside (a friend, a relative, or a teacher) can help you evaluate your methods.

Periodically assess your child's present skill level. This will help you determine what skill he or she can or needs to learn next.

Of course, some skills will take much longer to master than others. Just keep up your faith and persist in your efforts. For example, it may take a retarded child not days but weeks, months, or even years to learn how to eat without assistance.

Help your child remember what he or she learns. Retaining what one has learned is vital, and practice obviously aids retention. If you move too fast, your child may not remember what he or she learned yesterday. When Ann writes her name correctly for the first time, her parents may be so delighted with her progress that they proceed to teach her the names of everyone else in the family; by the end of the week she has written them all but can remember none. On the other hand, you can be so worried about retention that you pound a skill into your child's skull to the point where he or she is bored or annoyed. If Ann has to write her name 100 times a day, she may finally learn to do it—but she may never want to write it again. You need to find the right balance between progression and practice.

With time you will discover what kinds of things your child has difficulty in retaining so you can give appropriate practice in those areas. For example, certain simple skills are automatically used in more complex ones.

Addition is used in certain multiplication problems. Consequently, it is automatically reinforced as your child continues to learn math. But understanding how to use πr^2 to find the area of a circle is an isolated skill that requires specific goals and objectives for maintenance, such as doing problems using πr^2 periodically.

Help your child use what he or she has learned in a variety of situations in life. After your little girl learns to wave "bye-bye" when her sister leaves for school, you will then want her to learn to wave good-bye whenever appropriate. After your son can count to four on his fingers, you will also want him to be able to count out four spoons when he sets the table. We adults rarely need to write out a list of spelling words, but we do have to transfer this learning to situations where it is needed. Try to help your child do the same.

Whatever you attempt to teach, try to keep the learning process enjoyable and in perspective. Spending every waking hour in the frenzied training of your child can be just as bad as deciding it's hopeless to try to teach him or her anything. What your child needs is love, encouragement, and intelligent care and supervision in a stimulating environment.

YOUR CHILD AT SCHOOL

If and when your child attends school, learning about the available educational opportunities will help you work with the teachers to provide the best possible education. Today you are not only encouraged to observe and help in the classroom but you are given the opportunity to help plan an individualized educational program for your child, should he or she have special needs. In order to do this effectively, it is helpful if you:

- Know the educational rights of your child, as mandated by federal law PL 94-142 and state laws.
- Know how an individualized educational program (IEP) is developed, in case your child needs one.
- Know how to work with your school system to provide the educational opportunities and any special services your child needs.
- Understand how you, the parent, can work with the schools to help your child develop to his or her full potential.

This is not as complicated as it sounds.

What Is PL 94-142?

In 1975, the United States Congress passed the Education for All Handicapped Children Act, Public Law (PL) 94-142. The law is designed to give all children equal access to educational opportunities, and states must comply with it in order to get federal funding for education. In addition, each state has its own regulations, which must meet federal requirements. PL 94-142 focuses on the child, establishing four major rights and two important protections for *all* children with exceptional needs. The four rights are:

1. Free and appropriate public education (FAPE).
2. Placement in the least-restrictive environment (LRE).
3. Supplementary aids and services.
4. Fair assessment of learning needs.

The two protections, designed to ensure that all handicapped children are afforded these rights, are:

1. A process for developing and implementing an individualized education program (IEP).
2. Due-process procedures in case you disagree with the recommendations or actions of school personnel at any point in the process.

It is essential that you understand your child's educational rights and needs in order to work with the schools to provide the best possible education for your child. Translated into nonlegal terminology, PL 94-142 is easy to understand. Remember, *these are your child's rights.*

Free and appropriate public education is the most fundamental and important right, for it mandates that an appropriate educational program be available for each child. After an educational program has been designed to meet a child's unique learning needs, if no public school can provide the program, a private school or individual instruction must be provided at public expense.

Least-restrictive environment means that each disabled child must be educated in a program that allows the most beneficial amount of contact with nondisabled children. This has become known as "mainstreaming." A school district must make available the maximum variety of programs and placement alternatives possible. No placement is forever. As a child's learning needs change, so should the type of placement. *The school must have your consent for the initial placement and for any changes.* Possible alternatives can be diagrammed as follows:

1. Regular placement
2. Regular placement with:
   a. Supplementary materials or equipment
   b. Consultation services
   c. Support from specialists
   d. In-classroom tutors
3. Regular and special-education placement
   a. Part-time placement with resource teacher
   b. Any designated special services such as physical or speech/language therapy
   c. Part-time special day class
4. Special placement within regular school
   a. Special-education class
   b. Special-education class and home instruction
   c. Special-education class and special day school
5. Out-of-regular-school placement
   a. Special school
   b. Residential
   c. Hospital
   d. Home

Supplementary aids and services must be provided to assist the ill or disabled child to benefit from his or her special-education program. The specific aids and services are not spelled out in the law but are determined by federal regulations that designate how the law is to be implemented. Such supportive services may include:

- Speech and language services
- Special readers
- Braillists, typists, and interpreters
- Physical and occupational therapy
- Mobility trainers for the visually disabled
- Vocational counseling
- Other therapeutic services
- Social work services
- Consultative services
- Supportive institutional services
- Counseling
- Psychological services
- School health nurses
- Parent counseling and training
- Resource centers
- Medical services for evaluation and diagnostic purposes

Other services may be needed, such as adaptive physical education, appropriate instruction in music, art, and home economics, and other nonacademic subjects that children in your school receive. Sometimes these services will be provided by other agencies in the community, creating the need for close communication among the school, the agencies, and the parents. Remember that federal regulations can be changed and weakened so not all these services are provided. Public (including parental) protest at any attempt to weaken the intent of PL 94-142 is an important and effective means of preventing this, as was seen in 1982 when public protest caused the Secretary of Education to withdraw proposed revisions of the regulations that would have seriously weakened the implementation of PL 94-142. It is equally important, however, to tell Congress, the Department of Education, and the President that you appreciate their work and to encourage them to continue their efforts to carry out the intent of PL 94-142.

Fair assessment means that an educational assessment must be conducted to identify a child's learning needs and to determine whether the child requires special education. It must also designate what type of special education is needed. The parent must be notified of the school's plans to conduct an assessment and must be informed of the methods to be used. The school must obtain the written consent of the parent for such an assessment to be made. This assessment must be conducted *before* a child is placed in a special-education program or an IEP is written. *There must be an annual review of the IEP and a formal reassessment every three years or sooner if necessary.* If you are not notified of plans for an assessment, remind the school that it is time. If you would like a review before a year is up, or a reassessment before three years, you can request one.

You should fully understand the purpose and nature of the proposed assessment *before* giving consent. Schools must not use tests that discriminate on the basis of race, cultural background, or the child's disability (like testing a deaf child by purely auditory methods). All assessments must be conducted by appropriately trained and certified persons.

Placement in a special-education program may not be based on one test alone. The assessment must be comprehensive, taking into account the child's development and performance in several areas. The test scores and results must then be interpreted by a team of professionals who are knowledgeable about the child *and* the assessment methods. Parents must be informed of their right to obtain an independent assessment (a second opinion from a qualified person at their own expense), and the school must consider the independent assessment results in planning the child's program and placement.

Don't be too affected by test scores. For example, an IQ test does not measure creativity, motivation, the ability to adapt to new situations, or the ability to solve problems, all essential features of how well your child functions now and as he or she matures. The Freedom of Information Act gives you the right to see all documents pertaining to your child, including test scores.

The four rights guaranteed by PL 94-142 are protected in the following ways:

Protection #1: The individualized educational program is the formal written plan of your child's educational program. This is where you enter, where your carefully thought-out goals become so important. The IEP should include the following information:

- A statement of your child's present level of functioning in assessed "need areas." This might include your child's general ability (IQ), academic performance, language functioning, social and emotional status, motor abilities, health, and vision or hearing factors.
- Your child's planned educational program, including specific information about in which classroom(s) and by whom your child will be taught as well as any necessary supplementary aids and services.
- The anticipated date for initiation and the expected duration of each program and service.
- Annual goals for your child in specific areas.
- Short-term instructional objectives, which define the smaller steps to be taken to reach a particular goal.
- Specific evaluation procedures and a schedule for reviewing your child's progress throughout the school year to determine to what extent the educational objectives are being met.

The IEP is the key to receiving appropriate services. It shows where your child stands now and gives an individually designed education plan for achieving new learning goals.

The team that develops and reviews the IEP each year includes:

- You, the parent.
- Your child, if appropriate.
- Your child's teacher, if your child is already in school.
- A representative of the public school, other than your child's teacher, who is qualified to provide or supervise your child's educational program. This is the head of the IEP team.
- Any other person(s) who took part in the assessment of your child.
- Other persons, of the school's or your choosing, who have a current educational interest in your child, such as an audiologist or speech therapist for a deaf child, a physical therapist or a special-class teacher for an orthopedically handicapped child.

The advantage of the team approach to IEP development is that persons with varied skills are involved in the decision-making process, including individuals actually assessing and teaching your child as well as you, the parent.

Your school must advise you of meeting dates and times. While the school may proceed without the benefit of your input if you do not want to participate, it must also reschedule meetings so you can attend if you want to and have a time conflict. Needless to say, if you are to be involved in your child's education, you must be involved in the IEP development. Even if you choose not to be involved in the actual IEP meeting, your written consent is needed for any special-education placement.

Protection #2: Due-process safeguards protect the rights of the student, the parents, and the school staff, ensuring that each is treated fairly. While the specifics may vary slightly from state to state, basically this protection states that parents must be given written notice requesting consent for the school to conduct an assessment to determine if their child has any special educational needs. Within a clearly defined length of time the assessment results must be shared and an IEP developed.

You or anyone you delegate has the right to attend the IEP meeting to discuss assessment findings and program-placement recommendations. You are allowed access to any records used. *You may request additional assessment by the IEP team before you give your permission for placement, or you may request an independent assessment,* unless it is determined at the IEP meeting that the public assessment was adequate. *If you disagree with the IEP decision, you have the right to a fair and impartial hearing within a specified amount of time.*

Is Your Child Covered by PL 94-142?

PL 94-142 covers all children from three to twenty-one. Some districts have early-intervention programs available to children with special needs from birth to age three. Such young children profit from stimulating environments and direct teaching, which aid their development. Parents benefit from specific instruction on how best to work with their children, as well as from the overall emotional support that such a program can provide. Even if early-intervention programs are not mandated by your state, school personnel may know of other programs or services in your area that could assist you until your child is three. If your district has programs only for children over three, it may consider taking a child a bit early, should it appear that the child qualifies for and would benefit from the program.

How Can You Get the Appropriate Educational Placement for Your Child?

Your first step in placing your child in the right program is to let the school district know your child exists by phoning your school district's director of special education and discussing your child. In a very large district, the special-education director may have special personnel who work with parents of incoming students. In a small district, the superintendent may be the one to contact. In any case, make contact as soon as you feel your child may have special educational needs. (School administrators work all year long so you may be able to reach someone even in the summer.) If your call is not returned that day, call back and leave your message again the next day. Persist until you reach the person you need.

When you reach the appropriate person, make an appointment to discuss your child's educational needs. It may be helpful to give some information by phone about your child. Also ask if you should bring your child or any specific information with you to the initial meeting.

The initial meeting will not only give you some idea of what school programs and other services are available for your child but will also enable you to indicate what you perceive your child's needs to be. And you will have the opportunity to get to know and establish rapport with the school personnel, who will be working with you to provide the best possible educational opportunities for your child. Such a meeting is a variation on the theme of visiting the doctor (see page 10). *Before* the meeting, think through what information you would like to share about your child and what questions you have.

After you have discussed your child's needs with the appropriate members of the school staff, together you will consider how appropriate assessment can be made. The assessment may be a moment of truth for you, particularly if significant difficulties are diagnosed. Accepting a child's learning disabilities can sometimes be as hard as accepting a medical disability, because even if you have a nagging feeling something is not right it's different when it is laid out before you in black and white. Of course an assessment is not 100 percent foolproof and cannot be used to foretell the future, but it should give you a realistic picture of your child's strengths and weaknesses.

While PL 94-142 mandates that a district create a program for your child if the appropriate one does not exist, you must have realistic expectations. A Holy Grail search for a better prognosis, a better teacher, a better school, and so on can lead to frustration as well as to loss of time, money, and energy that could often be much better spent helping your child progress. Unless you feel the assessment is absolutely incorrect, in which case you have to request reassessment, try to use the identified weaknesses to help you formulate goals, and use the strengths to give you clues as to how to approach instruction for your child in a positive, productive way.

To review, an IEP should answer the following questions:

- *Why* does your child need special education?
- *What* does your child need to learn?
- *How* is your child going to learn it?

The *how* is very important, for that tells what your child will actually be doing throughout the school day.

By the time the IEP is formulated, you should know:

- *Which school will your child attend?*
- *How and by whom will your child's special services be provided?* Do the personnel have experience in these areas?
- *Where will your child be instructed if he or she cannot be taught in the public schools?* This could be in a private school, at home, or in the hospital.

Although a school is not required to provide the following information at an IEP meeting, it is helpful if you also learn:

- *Your child's daily schedule.* Which classroom(s) will your child be in and for how long? Which subjects will be taught when? When will special services be provided? If these are provided during the school day, which subjects will be missed? (If so, ask whether a full academic program *and* additional services would be more appropriate.)
- *Your child's teacher(s).* Who will teach each class? Has the teacher worked with children like yours? Will he or she be working alone or with an aide?
- *Your child's classmates.* How many children will be in the class? What are their disabilities and levels of functioning? When, during the day, are these children mainstreamed?

These six points are very important, for you need to know how, where, when, and by whom your child actually will be taught.

It is helpful if you visit the classroom(s) for which your child is being considered *before* the IEP is written so you get some idea of what learning environments are available and which might be most appropriate for your child. Your assessment person should be able to arrange such visits for you. Try to spend at least two hours, if not longer, in each classroom so you can get an accurate impression of the class. Beware of making quick judgments for the wrong reasons. For example, you might be more impressed with a classroom of higher-functioning students than with one of slower ones, but that doesn't tell you where *your* child would get the type of instruction he or she needs. Or you might see that the neighbor boy, Sam, is functioning very well at home since he has been in a specific classroom. But your child's needs may be very different from Sam's. Educational comparisons of children can be as unhelpful as medical comparisons and may cloud your ability to evaluate what you see. However, while you need to be realistic, you can learn a great deal by visiting classrooms.

First, you will get some understanding of how your child may spend his or her day. Your impressions of how your child acts at home and, consequently, how he or she would function in the classroom may be helpful. Second, you can learn something about individual teachers. Most schools are not apt to be very responsive if you just say you like Mrs. Jones better than Mr. Smith. However, if you can give specific reasons for requesting a certain placement, based upon your knowledge of your child's needs, the IEP team will (or at least should) be interested in what you have to say.

For example, from observing in the classroom you may see that one teacher is very free and easygoing in attitude and teaching style, while the other is much more structured. If you know your child is a bit "scattered" and has trouble getting organized, it can be helpful to point out specifically why the latter teacher might be better. On the other hand, if your child is a bit rigid and hesitant to try new things, the former might be better. The teachers' genders and ages may also be factors to consider. You may have still other reasons why your child might respond better to one teacher than another.

Your assessment person would much rather know of your opinions and concerns *before* the IEP is finally written and placement has been made. Sometimes you may have specific requests and good reasons for them. At other times you may not fully understand what the placement possibilities are. But if you don't ask questions, you won't get answers. Sometimes an educator will slip into jargon. If it sounds like so much alphabet soup and you don't understand, ask. If you don't understand why the educator thinks something is necessary, ask. If he or she doesn't mention something you think is necessary, ask about that. You can work together only if you understand each other. With cooperation and good communication you should be able to develop an IEP that is appropriate for your child.

Before the IEP meeting, consider *together* with the educator what your child needs to learn (the goals) and write enough specifics into the short-term objectives so that they are relevant for your child. For example, it is easy to say your child should learn to read or to eat with a spoon, but the challenge of an IEP is to divide the goal into enough measurable pieces so you not only know which step-by-step (sequential) skills must be taught but also if your child is actually learning them and moving toward the goal.

While the teacher may have more experience in different ways of teaching a specific skill, you know your child and can contribute what you have tried, how it worked or didn't, and what might be tried in the future. Writing a good IEP depends upon the goodwill of everyone involved. This preliminary work will help the IEP meeting go well.

This all sounds easy, but as with anything, there are snags. First of all, your child in flesh and blood may be very different from what he or she seems on paper. It is simple to move from A to B to C in writing, but it will take time, hard work, cooperation, and good cheer on the part of you, the teacher, and your child for your child actually to make those moves. Second, there may still be disagreement about which placement would be best for your child. Third, although PL 94-142 mandates a free and appropriate education, it takes careful planning to get the funding and personnel to staff the program best suited to your child's needs. This is particularly true if your child has unusual needs and there is no existing program like the one that should be proposed for your child. A school district may tell you it doesn't have unlimited financial and staffing resources (and that may be true), but *it still has an obligation to your child.* In such a situation you may have to be very actively involved in making sure the appropriate program and teacher materialize before placement. While PL 94-142 requires your local school district to meet your child's needs, exactly what the program should be is open to interpretation, and a district, because of lack of commitment to or funds for special education, may try to provide only the minimum necessary to meet PL 94-142 requirements. Therefore you may have to be vigilant in your efforts.

If in spite of all your careful groundwork and sharing of information the members of your team have differing opinions, your input at the meeting is crucial. In this case, both you and your spouse should attend the meeting. If you are a single parent, or if only one of you can go, try to bring a friend to share information or just listen and offer moral support. You may also want to call on education or health-care professionals to clarify your child's needs. The IEP meeting is not the time to introduce a lot of new material, but a concise review of relevant material by an outside person may be indicated. If you do decide to bring extra people to such a meeting, phone ahead and tell the school who your guest(s) will be. If you think it would be valuable to tape the meeting (perhaps for your spouse, who may be unable to attend), inform the school of your desire to do so. Legally you can do this. But some people are less willing to speak openly if the conversation is being recorded; some may also feel that you are trying to "nail" them.

Try always to be informed, polite, and forthright in your efforts to work with the system for the good of your child. Marching into an IEP meeting in a business suit with a bevy of support persons, a tape recorder in one hand and your annotated copy of PL 94-142 in the other, would set a tone of aggressive confrontation. Being a mousy little wallflower, exclaiming that an understanding of the development of an IEP and of your child's legal rights are totally beyond the scope of your weak brain, is equally unhelpful. You are your child's best advocate, and by seeking the cooperation of all parties involved in his or her education and care you will be doing your child the most good.

It is hoped that careful planning and cooperation result in an IEP the whole team agrees upon at the first meeting. If during the meeting, however, you feel there are areas needing further consideration, ask that the meeting be adjourned to a specified later date. If no agreement is reached, and the IEP is implemented without your signature, you have the right to due-process proceedings (see below). But these should be the last resort, for they are costly in terms of time, money, and energy, and often bring no better results than could have been achieved with strong cooperation and commitment

throughout the formation of the IEP.

Once an acceptable IEP has been written, you progress through a cycle that looks like that in figure 14-1. Of course, since learning is not static, the cyclic process depicted by this diagram will be repeated annually as your child progresses in what might be seen as a spiral, in which he or she learns and moves upward toward realizing full potential.

Does Your Child Really Need an IEP?

While PL 94-142 is designed to make sure that the special-education needs of all children are met, your child may have been in a regular classroom until an accident or illness. If you hope your child can return to the regular classroom, you may wonder if an IEP is necessary. It is best to contact the special-education director in your district to discuss this. The advantage of being identified as disabled is that your child is eligible for any special services he or she may need. However, if you think your child can be mainstreamed again and needs no special services, be sure the teacher fully understands your child's present needs.

How Can You Work with Your Child's Teacher?

Like doctors, teachers come in all shapes and sizes—with an equally wide range of personalities and abilities. What they have in common is a commitment to providing the best education for children. Consider the following suggestions to aid in effective interaction between your child and his or her teacher.

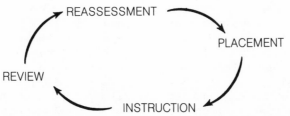

Figure 14-1　The special-education assessment cycle.

Help the teacher come to know your child. It is best if your child's teacher knows as much as possible about your child before the first day of school, especially if your child has special needs and is mainstreamed. If an IEP has been written, be sure the teacher has a copy before school starts. If your child is not a special-education student, make sure the teacher understands your child's condition. Factors to share with the teacher *before* the first day of school may include:

- Any significant changes in your child's condition since the IEP was written.
- Specific information about your child's present condition and how it is being treated.
- Treatment or medication your child is taking, when it is given, and what the potential side effects are, including those that may affect appearance or behavior.
- Approximate schedule of upcoming treatments, procedures, and tests that may result in your child's absence from school.
- Limitations, if any, on your child's activities.
- What your child knows about his or her illness or disability.
- What your child's classmates should know about the illness or disability and how they can help. This can be particularly important if a child looks "normal" but has a disability such as hemophilia or epilepsy.
- Your suggestions as to how or by whom this information should be shared. Especially at the elementary level, a parent may provide the teacher with necessary information, help with a class discussion, or arrange for someone else to do so.
- What your child should be able to do alone and when he or she will need help.
- Any problems that you anticipate might occur in the classroom.

The greater the teacher's understanding of your child *and* your child's disability, the greater will be his or her ability to meet your child's special needs. Sometimes it is helpful to share pertinent written information rather than assume a teacher knows everything. For example, if your child has cancer, you might share one of the excellent pamphlets for educators published by the National Cancer Institute. You might also want to arrange for the teacher to talk with your child's doctor to discuss any exceptional needs.

Communicating such information is often much easier in an elementary-school setting, where your child spends most of the day with only one or a few teachers, than at the secondary level, where larger classes and a greater number of teachers may make it necessary to have one person in the school maintain contact with the family or medical staff and disseminate information to all teachers involved with your child. Such ongoing contact is particularly important at the beginning of each semester or if your child's medical condition changes. A liaison person who has good rapport with your child can also discuss your child's academic progress and social interaction with your child, keeping lines of communication open and referring to the appropriate person any problems that may need attention.

Inviting your child's teacher to your house may help him or her understand your home environment and how your child functions there. You might invite the teacher to dinner, if not before school starts then at least in the fall. Dinner is good because you all have something to do (eat) and talk about (food) if the conversation is slow in getting off the ground. The teacher can also see what self-help skills your child has and how he or she interacts with the whole family. Keep such dinners *very simple* so you can all enjoy the evening and get to know each other. You might invite the teacher to bring his or her family, because not only is this fun but your child can also see that the teacher is a real person with a family too.

If this would be difficult because of your child's medical needs in late afternoon or because your house is too wild that close to dinner, suggest an evening visit or a daytime visit during the weekend.

Alternatively, talk sometime within the first week of school. You can make an appointment to meet with the teacher at school to discuss your child's needs. The end of the first week is none too early to contact the teacher and ask which afternoon it would be convenient for you to come. If it's easier for you to consult by phone, call the school and leave a message for the teacher to call you. You may want to ask about your child's daily schedule and consider how this compares with what was planned on the IEP. And you may have specific questions about your child's work or behavior.

Following through at home on teaching done at school is one way you can help the teacher. If your child is learning academic material, such as addition and subtraction, you can buy flashcards to review with your child at home. If the teacher is working on teaching your child to tie his or her shoes, you can help by following the same method and giving your child the opportunity to do so also. If the speech therapist is working on the *th* sound, find out how you can reinforce that learning at home. If the teacher is working on certain types of behavior, try to carry through with those efforts at home. It is important to help your child's teacher to move your child toward the established goals.

Homework is another area where you can help your child. While you shouldn't actually do your child's work, you can provide a quiet work area at a time of day when your child is most apt to work well—before school, after school, before dinner, or after dinner. Show an interest in homework. You can help by quizzing your child on rote learning, explaining any concepts he or she doesn't understand, and helping your child to work regularly on any long-term project.

In spite of efforts such as these, in many families homework is a point of contention. Whereas there are industrious, obedient little ones who do homework willingly and with great relish, there are at least as many children who are unenthusiastic at best. For the recalcitrant, you might establish a "homework policy" with the teacher before any homework is even assigned. Consider what will happen if the homework isn't done. Does it get completed at school during recess, at lunch, or before your child goes home? Will it get marked down? A homework policy doesn't necessarily have to be established for the whole class. Rather it can be an agreement among your child, the teacher, and yourself. Of course, if an assignment seems much too long for one night, it makes more sense for your child to get a good night's sleep than to stay up until all hours. In that case, a phone call or note to clarify the situation should help.

Of course, homework may deal not only with academic skills but also with self-help skills, communication, or behavior. Therefore, close cooperation among you, your child, and the teacher can help ensure that time spent doing homework is as productive as possible.

Preparing to go to school each day can be an important part of the learning process, for the way your child starts the day with you influences the time at school. It is important that your child begin the day as calmly as possible. Lack of organization can make many a reasonable household closely resemble a madhouse as departure time for school approaches. If things get a bit wild at your house, sit down and figure out what you can do to make your mornings calmer. Jobs like packing lunch and school supplies, setting the table for breakfast, and laying out clothes can easily be done the night before.

What If Your Child Can't Go to School? —Home/Hospital Instruction

In a sense school is a child's job, and providing the school-age child with a formal learning situation lends normalcy to the day. Sometimes a child may become ill or have a bad accident so it is necessary to miss a substantial amount of school. And there are some children who are so ill that they will never be able to go to school and in whose lives "school" at home plays an important part. It is for these children, who are temporarily or permanently too ill to go to school, that home/hospital teachers are available.

A hospital teacher is employed by the school district to teach hospitalized children. Often a larger hospital will have a full-time hospital teacher who will work with your child as soon as he or she is well enough to have "school." However, if your child is in a community hospital to which your school district sends a teacher only as needed, you or your doctor will have to contact the special-education director as soon as possible so a hospital teacher can be assigned to your child. Although sometimes a pediatric unit or a doctor will automatically refer your child for hospital instruction, don't assume that this has been done for you. A child can languish in illness and boredom because no one knew that hospital teachers were available or because everyone figured that someone else had arranged for the teacher.

It is helpful to make an exploratory call to the school district's director of hospital instruction to get the eligibility requirements for having a hospital teacher. Some districts require that a child be out of school for a minimum amount of time before providing a teacher since this service is very expensive. This may be at least four weeks *after* the school is contacted to get a teacher twice a week, and at least three months to get a teacher five days a week. While such a program should not be abused, a child sometimes fails to qualify because the parent did not contact the school as soon as the child was hospitalized or the parent and doctor were optimistic about a speedy recovery. This is one case where you and your doctor should consider the maximum length of time needed for recovery. If your doctor estimates it will be 15 days to three weeks before your child is back in school, ask him or her to indicate four weeks so your child will get a teacher. If your doctor reckons it will be between one and three months before your child is back in school and you know a child must be out at least three months for daily instruction, ask him or her to indicate 14 weeks. Optimism should not prevent your child from having daily instruction. What is much more apt to happen with the "wait and see" approach is that no teacher is provided or the teacher comes for only a minimum amount of time and the child does not receive the instruction he or she could so well use.

A child who has been in a regular classroom and has an accident, surgery, or a short-term illness may be given only the minimum services provided by your district. However, if your child has an accident or illness that will produce residual disabilities or if your child has a progressive condition, it may be wise to begin procedures to identify your child as disabled so the district, under PL 94-142, will be able to provide an appropriate education as soon as possible. This could mean a hospital teacher now and a home teacher when your child comes home, as well as any other necessary support services.

The hospital teacher provides a vital link between the child and the classroom. By being in regular contact with your child's regular teacher, the hospital teacher makes sure your child stays caught up not only with schoolwork but also with classroom activities. The hospital teacher also provides invaluable focus on something other than the medical problem: your child may get plenty of attention all day in the form of treatments and procedures to help the body, but the hospital's daily medical routine and the television in the room become boring at best. Hospital teachers are not just there to pound missed school lessons into a child. They also interact with your child on a one-to-one basis, providing some focus on nonmedical things. No child is too ill for school, even if there are times when the teacher merely reads to your child, perhaps for only part of the allotted time.

A home teacher continues where the hospital teacher leaves off.

If your child was at a large hospital with a full-time hospital teacher, you may have to contact the director of home/hospital education again to get a home teacher assigned to your child. If your child was in a community hospital, the hospital teacher may continue to come to your home as a home teacher. In any case, carefully check on eligibility requirements so your child is not disqualified on a technicality.

Some children may need a variety of services. For example, your child may become able to attend school on a part-time basis but still need the home teacher to come for one hour daily to provide the necessary remedial instruction. The home teacher can also greatly assist the classroom teacher provide a receptive environment to which the child can return. After an absence due to severe illness or traumatic injury, it is important not only that the teacher and classmates understand the nature of the child's problem but also that they be encouraged to provide normal equal attention rather than grant special favors that a child's condition doesn't warrant. If your child goes directly back to a full-day program after hospitalization or a stay at home, you may want to work with your teacher to find out how your child might best be reintegrated into the classroom setting.

Permanent home teachers are provided by most school districts for those few children who can never go to school. "Grade level" work is usually irrelevant for such children. Rather, it is important that the child have an enjoyable learning situation where he or she is challenged to do his or her best in a supportive environment. The great advantage of home teaching is its flexibility. Your child can have school in any part of the house or even outdoors. A child too weak to sit up can have school lying down. A child who hasn't had breakfast by the time the teacher comes can be fed during school. This flexibility extends to what your child learns: "classes" can be tailored to his or her condition. If your child is too weak to do much thinking the teacher may simply read stories, or if your child is feeling especially healthy the teacher may take him or her on an outing, with you along as a paramedical aide. School is a very important part of your child's life, offering contact with the outside world and interesting activities you don't have the time to provide. And you should not underestimate its importance in giving you some time off, whether to pay bills, take a nap, or bathe.

If your child is permanently instructed by a home teacher, you can have an IEP written and include in it a formal request for a longer daily period of instruction than is customarily provided by your district for students temporarily instructed at home.

Home-classroom telephone hookups are another way a child can keep in contact with school. Usually a special line must be run from the classroom(s) to the home. Then a "speaker phone," which picks up the voices of anyone speaking in the room, is installed at each location so your child can not only hear but also participate in class discussions. While the connection itself costs only about as much as a private phone line, the installation cost can be quite high. With the willingness to make innumerable phone calls, great patience, and friendly perseverance on your part, a phone company might be convinced to do such an installation as a "public service." Some school districts will pay the monthly service charge. If you think your child could profit from a phone hookup but you can't convince the phone company or the school to pay for it, try appealing to the PTA, local service organizations, or even the school's student-government association for help. No child should be denied beneficial services for financial reasons.

How Do You Resolve Problems with Education Professionals?

If and when difficulties arise with education professionals, it is best to resolve them in a logical, organized, and friendly manner.

Identifying the nature of the problem and even verifying that one exists is the first step. This means talking with the school person closest to the problem. For example, if you are not sure what is going on in a classroom because of reports of your child or your child's friends, or if you question the kind or amount of homework, it is best to clarify the situation with the teacher. Working together on small problems in good faith is the best way to develop understanding and cooperation. Confrontations and accusations are a waste of time and energy that could be much more constructively used in educating your child. Needless to say, moaning to your family and friends is equally unproductive.

There may arise difficulties that do not respond to your efforts at communication and goodwill. First, of course, examine your actions to see if you are being rational, straightforward, and nonjudgmental. Are your expectations for your child, the teacher, and yourself reasonable and realistic? If you see that you have erred, try to correct the situation. If you have constructive advice, try to give it in a helpful manner. Feeling defensive, anxious, negative, or overly concerned can indicate that you are anticipating and may even precipitate conflict. Remember that you are interested in your child's needs—not yours, the teacher's, or the system's. While almost everyone will agree that your child's needs are most important, there may be more than one way of meeting those needs. When conflicting points of view arise, try to brainstorm with the other adults involved to find alternative solutions to the problem. If appropriate, even your child can be involved in this process. Neither teachers nor parents know everything, but if you all share your perspectives on the situation you may come up with a workable solution, or at least an idea of what, when, where, and by whom actions need to be taken next.

Enlisting the help of others may be necessary if the cooperation described above doesn't work. In this situation the most tactful way of proceeding may be to suggest that the teacher's immediate superior (supervisor or principal) be brought in so you can all explore the problem together. If the teacher is unresponsive or opposed to such a suggestion, you must be as assertive, yet as gracious, as necessary and ask for help from the supervisor on your own in the hope that he or she or someone else up the chain of command will be willing to work with you in a reasonable and fair way to provide the educational opportunities your child needs. You can make the best use of the time available to express your concerns if you have thought the problem through in advance in terms of the facts, the options open to everyone, and the actions you are prepared to take on behalf of your child. Goodwill, politeness, calm, and persistence are essential.

You should know how your district is organized and administered, so you know to whom to address your concerns. Although the size of a district will determine its administrative structure, it will probably look something like that diagrammed in figure 14-2. The school board is

elected by the public and is therefore responsive to the opinions of its constituents. The other persons are hired or are on contracts. The teachers are usually the only ones with tenure, which means that they are guaranteed employment if their job performance is satisfactory and if enough jobs exist in their district.

When you decide to take your concerns higher in the system, proceed with tact as well as determination, always keeping your goal—the best education for your child—in mind. Interaction with teachers and principals is usually informal, consisting of telephone conversations or informal meetings. However, when you have concerns or requests that need higher intervention, keep track of what you are doing in writing. You can keep a log of phone calls made and decisions reached, including the date and the name of the person you contacted. Follow up any important phone call with a letter. It can be brief and to the point:

Dear Mr. Martin,
    Thank you for taking time to talk with me yesterday about Mark. I look forward to hearing from you soon to learn how you think this situation can best be resolved.

Of course, it is easy to get in the habit of firing off complaint memos, failing to give credit where credit is due. Therefore you might add to such a note:

District school board

District superintendent of schools

Elementary assistant superintendent	Secondary assistant superintendent	District special-education director
Principals	Principals	Special-education principals
Teachers	Teachers	Special-education teachers
		Other certified personnel, such as speech therapists, nurses, psychologists, etc.;
		Personnel contracted from other agencies to provide special services such as physical therapy

Figure 14-2   School-district organization.

I do want to tell you that Mark is doing very well in school this year, and I am sure much of his progress is due to the efforts of his teacher, Mrs. Smith.

While sometimes it pays to send copies of your letter on up the chain of command, so everyone who could become involved knows of the problem, it is best to carry your problem to a higher level only when you have tried and failed to get help at the present level. Only rarely and after due deliberation should you consider skipping a link in the chain of command.

If you need specific information to back up a claim or complaint, it is usually no farther away than your telephone. Since a school is a public agency, almost all its records (except information about specific students) are open to the public. You can call and find out enrollment in different programs, who staffs them, what the budget is, and so on. Often you may not know specifically what questions to ask and who could best answer them, but with time you will find who knows what and who is willing to share that knowledge. Through conversation you may discover the personnel's perspectives on issues as well as cold facts and figures. Persistence is the key. It may take many phone calls to find out what you need to know. If you can't reach someone, leave a message and then do your part by being home and staying off your phone. If your call isn't returned by the end of the day (or whenever the person will be back in the office), call and leave your message again, and again, until it is returned.

If your problem is a matter of policy, you may have to turn to the school board, whose members make important policy statements and decisions. Occasionally it is helpful to inform the board members of your concern and get their opinions in private before appearing before the entire board.

In order to find out how best to contact a member of the board, call the school district switchboard and ask for the secretary of the board; if there isn't one, ask for the superintendent's office. The person you reach should be able to tell you if a board member would rather you leave your name and number so he or she can return your call when convenient or if he or she is will-

ing to receive calls at a place of business or at home. If you wish to write a letter, you can either address it to a specific board member or request that the school district distribute copies of your letter to all members of the board and any other appropriate school administrators or teachers. Most school boards have a time allocated for community input in case you decide to make a public statement. Be sure you know how long you are allowed to speak. Then organize your thoughts. Speaking extemporaneously from notes is usually more effective than reading a written text. However, it is helpful to have a written statement of your main points that you can hand out to each of the board members, the superintendent, and any representatives of the media before you speak. Providing clear information is often the key to overcoming lack of understanding, lack of appreciation, and ignorance as to the benefits of educating disabled children.

Any statement made by the many on behalf of the many carries more weight than a plea for an individual child. So try to formulate your concerns in terms of which school policy would be best for all children in a given situation rather than what you want for your child.

If major policy decisions are to be made, encourage other parents and interested persons to become involved in circulating petitions, writing support letters, or attending school-board meetings. Making statements as the spokesperson for an organized group, even if you are just informally organized into "Parents and Friends of the Disabled," lends strength to your position. Parents are important in furthering growth and change because they can speak out freely as taxpayers. Teachers and administrators may be less willing to make waves, fearing that it might jeopardize their positions.

If the issue is controversial, it may take much more than a phone call or letter. And it may require attending school-board meetings not just once but for the duration of the discussion of a certain issue. It may require convincing others to attend such meetings too. But if you think an issue is important, you must be willing to put in time and effort.

Whatever method you take in approaching your school board, if you give an organized, succinct, yet polite account of the problem as you see it the board should (and usually will) welcome your input.

Filing formal legal complaints is possible. State and federal laws protect the rights of the disabled. We have discussed PL 94-142 at length; the other important national legislation is Section 504 of the Rehabilitation Act of 1973 (PL 93-112), and its amendments of 1974 (PL 93-516). Known simply as "Section 504," it provides that "no . . . qualified handicapped individual . . . shall, solely by reason of his handicap, be excluded from the participation in, be denied the benefits of, or be subjected to discrimination under any program or activity receiving federal financial assistance." This, of course, includes the public schools.

As we mentioned before, formal actions are the last resort and should be avoided if at all possible because:

- The parent and school district are immediately placed in conflict.
- It takes time to reach a decision.
- Such procedures are expensive in terms of time, money, and energy—for school personnel, for you, and for your family.

The informal approach solves many problems better and more quickly than filing a formal complaint. However, if you decide to file a formal complaint or ask for a hearing, inform the school of your intent as soon as possible. PL 94-142 requires that a district tell you how to proceed. Usually you give your written notice to the person in charge of the program or to the superintendent. This initial written statement is a matter of information, not a threat.

You may then agree to postpone the action for a period of two to four weeks while you and the school continue to work on an informal solution. If progress is being made, you can agree on another postponement or withdraw formal action completely. But if progress is not made, you have taken correct formal action and can request that the district proceed with the formal process. Since due-process procedure is time-consuming and costly, if you decide to take such a serious step you should be willing to accept the decision made. If you do not, you will continue to consume time for your own child at the expense of many others. The request for a hearing is a right, but it should not be abused.

15
Adolescence

Adolescence, which means literally "growing up," is a turbulent period for any child, but it can be especially so for an ill or disabled one. It is a period of remarkably rapid growth, not only toward physical and sexual maturity but toward psychological, emotional, moral, and social maturity as well. In all these areas, the adolescent struggles to become aware of himself or herself as a person with a singular identity. Choosing what beliefs to hold and what humane qualities to embody, the adolescent needs the opportunity to think independently as well as to talk with others about who he or she is, how he or she got that way, and what he or she would like to become. Initially this means at least questioning and maybe even rejecting (perhaps only temporarily) the values, attitudes, and goals of parents.

When your disabled or ill child reaches this tumultuous age, you will need to think about a great deal, including your child's self-image, the development of the skills necessary for independent living as a young adult, your child's social-sexual development, housing alternatives for the time when he or she no longer lives with you, and vocational planning for the future.

Developing a Self-Image

For a teenager, developing a self-image usually involves critical self-examination, including (and sometimes primarily) of one's physical appearance. Adults know that looks are not of primary importance, but a teenager, acutely aware of and often uncomfortable with a changing body, may believe that body, hair style, clothing, and other physical characteristics are most impor-

tant. And here is the rub. Just when conformity, especially in the sense of looking like one's friends, can boost a child's self-esteem and social acceptance, a disabled or ill teenager may be gaining a deeper awareness of the fact that he or she is different and that it may always be that way. At this age "different" from parents and other adults is often viewed by the teenager as good, while "different" from peers (both "normal" and disabled) is viewed as bad. Therefore your teenager may need extra help in achieving self-acceptance. With your encouragement and support, a child who has proved capable of managing in school and at play, with friends and family, may find that being disabled has made a positive difference in the quality of life. Many disabled people have said that being disabled made them think more seriously about what they were doing, where they were going, and why.

Becoming Independent

Teenagers, in their natural striving for independence, want and need to move beyond the family circle. Your ill or disabled teenager too must develop a group of friends outside the family. As parents, it is our job to empty the nest by encouraging our child to become as independent as possible. We must gradually make ourselves unnecessary so our child can learn what is required to become an independent adult. Take the time to think carefully about what skills and habits your child should learn now in order to become as independent as possible later.

This may require that you reorder or modify

what you feel are the most important skills for your child to learn and develop. For example, you may feel that walking is a skill you would like your child to acquire. But if your child cannot walk by age 13, chances are he or she never will, and you need to shift your priorities to emphasize other means of mobility.

Independent-living skills include all the kinds of activities discussed in Chapters 8 through 13. As your child develops psychologically and emotionally, the attainment of these skills becomes increasingly important to the development of a positive self-image as well as to the attainment of independence. A teenager who can but does not develop the ability to look after himself or herself may develop a self-image as more disabled than he or she actually is. So remember, what may be good parental care for a five-year-old may not be good for a 15-year-old. If you are in the habit of doing certain things for your child, it is time to stand back and reassess the situation to see if any changes are appropriate. *Design for Independent Living: The Environment and Physically Disabled People* (listed in Appendix 3, "Suggested Reading") is an excellent book for parents and teenagers alike, because it describes the difficulties physically disabled young adults experienced when they left home, how they worked to overcome their problems, and how they think they could have been better prepared to live independently. While the young adults interviewed commended their parents for their love and support, none felt that they had learned sufficient self-help skills at home.

Devising methods of self-help may require some ingenuity, and you should consider any way that works, even if it is unusual. *Design for Independent Living* and *Housing and Home Services for the Disabled: Guidelines and Experiences in Independent Living* (see Appendix 3, "Suggested Reading") are excellent sourcebooks that can help you.

Learning independent-living skills does not consist solely of learning to perform various tasks. It also means understanding how the tasks are performed in order to teach someone else to help if appropriate. Independence is being responsible for one's own care, even if this means delegating responsibility to someone else actually to perform the chores.

Personal hygiene and appearance are areas where it is important for teenagers to be independent. The ability to care for his or her own personal hygiene may be a high priority for your teenager, who may no longer want to depend upon a parent, especially a parent of the opposite sex, for this. Encourage your child to learn self-help skills in this area.

Since appearance is important not only for your child's self-acceptance but perhaps also for acceptance by peers, allow your adolescent, within broad guidelines you provide, to make independent decisions about clothing and hair styles, areas where independence is possible. Your child may not always choose what you think is most attractive, but allow him or her to make the choice. Moreover, arguments about matters of individual taste in haircuts, style of dress, and so on can distract from other issues, where consistently enforced standards are much more important.

Since the desire to experiment with appearance is common, teenagers who must depend on others for their grooming may find this period very frustrating, for a parent or attendant is likely to be influenced by personal taste in the appearance he or she creates. Try to keep your child's preferences uppermost in your mind.

Mobility includes not only getting around in a wheelchair and transferring but becoming more mobile in the community. Support your child's desire and need for mobility by teaching him or her to use public transportation and by having your child evaluated by qualified professionals to see if he or she can learn to drive (with hand controls if necessary). Even if you are willing to take your child out, the child who can get out independently will gain more freedom and maturity. Spontaneous interaction with friends, so very important in adolescence, is greatly aided by freedom of movement.

Mobility is also an issue for children who can walk but have medical problems. It would obviously be safer to keep at home a child who has seizures, but that child needs the opportunity to be with peers. Your child's friends are probably reliable enough to help if necessary. Allow your teenage son or daughter to participate in decisions about what he or she can and cannot do. Your child needs to be given the opportunity to make such decisions, even if he or she sometimes makes mistakes. While overprotectiveness may keep the body intact, it has a negative effect on the rest of the child. Emotional dependence can be much more handicapping than physical dependence.

Privacy is also essential to your child's growth toward independence. If possible, your child should have the privacy of his or her own room, the privacy to choose (within the guidelines established by your family) how and with whom to spend free time. Respecting this need for privacy is a way of showing your respect for your child.

Assuming responsibility for one's own medical care is a crucial part of growing up and becoming independent. Ideally, there has been an atmosphere of open communication and frank discussion about your child's disorder from the time he or she was very young. As a child gets older, a fuller understanding of his or her medical problems and the implications of not giving the body the care it needs is important. Not taking medication regularly, not doing exercises, not following a diet, not keeping to a bowel program, and so on can all lead to consequences that will complicate life and compromise its quality. It may not be very exciting to do wheelchair push-ups and check for pressure sores daily, but your child must understand that the effort surely beats surgery or spending months lying prone to heal a pressure sore on the buttocks.

Eric, by Lois Lund (see Appendix 3, "Suggested Reading"), offers valuable insight into how the teenager in one family came to assume more and more responsibility for his medical care, working with his doctors on his own and reporting to his parents when necessary.

The more responsible your teenager is for his or her own disease treatment and management routines, the less will be the temptation to rebel against your authority by refusing to give his or her body the medical attention it needs. Involving teenagers in the decision-making process is particularly important when there are pros and cons to initiating or continuing treatment. (This

is discussed in connection with terminal illness in Chapter 18.)

Communication is vital to the attainment of independence. Your teenager needs to communicate not only with you but also (and especially) with peers and friends of all ages. And in the future your child may need to communicate with attendants and medical professionals without your assistance.

When your teenager communicates with you, he or she probably wants you to listen without offering unsolicited advice or judgmental comments. The ability to listen attentively, often with no more than a sympathetic grunt, shows our interest while giving the child a chance to expand his or her thoughts and express himself or herself in words. Especially if your child has difficulty communicating, you will have to be patient; listen carefully and avoid trying to express your child's thoughts for him or her any more than is necessary.

Communication falters in many families in matters of discipline when parents choose to flaunt their power and superiority. It is easy to fall into communication traps such as ordering ("Do it because I say so!" or "Stop feeling sorry for yourself *now!*"), prescribing ("The trouble with you is . . ." or "What you need is . . ."), and lecturing ("What you must understand is . . ."). Whenever our words, tone of voice, or actions indicate that our child has no voice in the decision-making process, that we don't trust our child's judgment, that we have all the power, and that there is no room for discussion and compromise, we may be doing great harm to our child's self-esteem and sense of being able to control his or her life, both especially important to an ill or disabled child. Neither does such an attitude on our part offer our child a positive model.

It is important for everyone in the family to learn, when expressing feelings, to state the facts rather than to accuse. Implementing this, the following steps may be helpful:

1. Note a specific behavior: "When you don't answer my questions about what the doctor said" or "When you don't put the dishes away after you have a snack."

2. Use an "I" statement: "I feel angry" or "I get annoyed."
3. Give a reason: "Because I am concerned about your treatment" or "Because I think you are old enough to assume responsibility for that."

Speaking thoughtfully also demonstrates that, although you may be dissatisfied with a specific action, you still love your child.

While hitting, biting, and yelling are naturally unacceptable, a mobile teenager has the option of leaving a scene of conflict and slamming the door. A nonmobile child can only face the music or retaliate verbally. But rudeness and shouting have no place in adult communication. While your teenager may yearn for total independence, learning that there are limits to acceptable behavior, clearly defined and consistently enforced, will help your child develop a sense of responsibility for his or her own actions. While all children need to learn basic social graces, the disabled teenager particularly needs to develop the ability to explain his or her needs, to ask for help politely, and to express thanks graciously for assistance given.

All teenagers seem to adore the telephone. For teenagers who lack mobility, it can be an especially vital mode of communication, not only for purposes of social interaction but also in case of an emergency. If possible, teach your child to use the phone. If your child is deaf or speech-impaired, consider installing a telecommunications device (see pages 132–133), which is an important means of improving communication skills and not an expensive frill.

Social-Sexual Development

Growing up means developing the ability to share warmth, affection, and approval with others through friendships that may develop into romantic attachments. Your child, whether physically or mentally disabled, is a sexual being. Daily you have the opportunity to teach your child about social-sexual relations in a loving, understanding way, answering questions about sex and interpersonal relations as they arise, offering information when it seems appropriate. Retarded children especially need help in learning

age-appropriate behavior. The hugs and kisses acceptable from a five-year-old give way with time to handshaking and friendly greetings for persons outside the family.

To regard your ill, disabled, or retarded child as asexual might be easier insofar as you would never have to face social-sexual matters, but it is unrealistic and patronizing to think that your child doesn't have the same desires to share love and affection that you have. Many disabled, ill, and retarded people form romantic relationships and many get married—some to other persons with illness or disabilities, some to persons with none. Individuals with mild disabilities often don't need any help, not even from their spouses. Persons with greater disabilities often need help from their spouses or attendants with daily physical care, homemaking, child care, financial support, or even positioning for sexual relations. But none of this diminishes the strength and value of strong interpersonal relations. There is no reason that marriage should have a greater chance of failure for a disabled person than for a "normal" one.

Of course, sexual relations often precede marriage. If your teenager is old enough to be in love, he or she should have the information necessary to love responsibly. Therefore teach your child about contraception before dating even begins. This is necessary for both boys and girls. A teenager who falls in love and does not have the facts and means of contraception may be too embarrassed to ask for information. Pregnancy is a wonderful thing if it is planned, but it can be a personal disaster if it is not. A substantial proportion of all boys and girls under seventeen have sex. You can tell your son or daughter not to do many things, but your child has the power to have sex and risk pregnancy if he or she wants to, even if the motive is simply defiance of authority. If your daughter is already disabled in some way, she certainly doesn't need the trauma of an unwanted pregnancy, and your son most probably does not yet need to assume the responsibilities of being a father. Therefore, *include in sex education information about birth control,* given openly and in a nonjudgmental way your son or daughter can understand. Such information will not cause your child to go out and hop into bed with the first member of the opposite sex he or she can find.

Planned parenthood is, of course, appropriate for young married couples. They should never be told "You could never manage to care for a child" before they have explored whether they might be able to do so with help. And if genetic counseling indicates that it might be inadvisable for a couple to have a biological child, adoption may be a viable alternative.

When an individual or couple decides *never* to have children, sterilization may be the safest way to prevent unwanted parenthood. However, a child should be as actively involved as possible in any decision concerning his or her life, and we have the responsibility to provide information and guidance to aid the child in deciding whether or not to be sterilized. This may be appropriate in the late teens or early twenties. Never sterilize a child without the child's knowledge and consent. Doing so and then having to lie to cover up what has really happened can cause a great deal of grief for both the parents and their child. Honesty, as in all matters, is the best route to take.

It is also sometimes difficult for parents to accept that their child may masturbate. Masturbation is common among all children; it is a problem only when it is accompanied by guilt and anxiety. So deal openly and honestly with masturbation. If a young child begins to masturbate, as by rubbing against the sofa, you can calmly redirect his or her attention to another activity. An older child who masturbates needs to know that there are specific situations or places where masturbation is acceptable, namely, when he or she is alone. Scolding or threats such as "If you masturbate you will go blind, or insane, or get dumber" or that you, the parent, will no longer love your child will not necessarily eliminate the behavior. But they will certainly foster unnecessary feelings of guilt if your child thinks about masturbating or does masturbate again. Often masturbation is just one step in the developmental cycle and, with time, your child may well derive sexual satisfaction from relations with other people.

As your child grows up he or she will probably feel the need for sexual satisfaction. While the purely biological need for sex and sexual stimulation is very small in comparison with other human needs, it is still genuine and should be respected by us as such.

Substance Abuse

Chances are good that your teenager will more than once be offered alcohol or street drugs. And it is important that he or she fully understand the implications of both, *particularly if he or she is taking medication.* Beyond their "desired" effects, street drugs can be hazardous because one is never sure of the quality of the drug and what kinds of additives or fillers it contains. Moreover, alcohol and drugs may interact adversely and dangerously with prescribed medication. Your child should realize that he or she is responsible for decisions in this area and will experience the consequences of the choice. Medical problems caused by the irresponsible use of drugs may create increased dependence at a time when your teenager most yearns for more independence.

Communicate about drugs and alcohol openly and honestly, without panic. If your child is taking drugs regularly, it is probably a symptom of a larger problem. If you think this is the case, you should seek professional help.

Teenage Depression

Teenage depression is an increasingly common problem, and an ill or disabled teenager may be more susceptible to depression than a "normal" one. In addition to the stresses and mood swings of a "normal" adolescent, an ill or disabled child may feel very much alone if the illness or disability causes him or her to feel or be different from other children and if the child therefore lacks others of the same age with whom to associate. Furthermore, by the time an ill or disabled child is a teenager, he or she has come to a deeper understanding of the nature and extent of his or her medical problems; the ability to acknowledge the reality of the condition and accept whatever limitations it imposes will make a difference in how he or she views life. Thus while an illness or disability can help a teenager develop into a thoughtful, considerate person, grateful for the opportunities that life provides, it can also be one more problem with which to cope—and a problem with ramifications for all aspects of life. Especially since some teenagers tend not to talk to their parents, it may be difficult to discern whether your child is depressed. You must be aware not only of what your adolescent says but also of what he or she expresses through behavior. It can be difficult to distinguish between normal teenage rebellion and early warning signs of depression. If rebellious behavior becomes more frequent and intense, lasting for weeks or even months, and if it is a drastic change from the way your child behaved before, you may have reason for concern. Other symptoms of depression may include a serious inability to communicate, negative moods, changes in eating and sleeping habits, losing or breaking ties with friends, hyperactivity, excessive self-criticism, extreme passivity, psychosomatic complaints, weight gain or loss, substance abuse, taking uncharacteristic risks, having accidents, sexual promiscuity, running away from home, and other sudden changes in behavior. One of the clearest signs that something is wrong with your child is if his or her grades in school go down for no apparent reason.

Don't panic if any of the above occur, but try to learn what is going on. If your family has been able to communicate well in the past, consider how you could make your child more willing to communicate with you. Sometimes other children in your child's peer group will let you know something. Since the values of a peer group are indicators of what the individuals within it feel are important, this may give you some clues. Your child's friends may even respond to direct questions if they don't feel your questions are too nosy or judgmental. One of the best sources of information about your child is his or her teachers. A teacher who has known your child well over an extended period of time may be able to tell you in what ways your child seems different now and what the possible causes might be. Even a teacher who doesn't know your child well can tell you how your child's behavior compares with that of the other hundred or so teenagers the teacher sees each day. If possible, talk with each of your child's teachers so you learn

about those classrooms in which he or she functions well as well as those classrooms in which your child (or the teacher) seems unable to cope. It may even help to talk with teachers your child has had in the past, so that you can also consider the perceptions of teachers who knew him or her when he or she was functioning better.

Severe depression may lead to thoughts of suicide. Many teenagers when considering the meaning of life may philosophically also consider the meaning of death, including what it would mean or be like to take one's own life. However, there is a difference between the child who thinks about suicide philosophically and talks to friends about it and the child who brings up the subject with his or her parents, perhaps even indicating that he or she has been considering suicide. An adolescent with a terminal illness may feel that committing suicide is a way to gain control over that illness (and consequently over his or her life). And if a family has had difficulty coping with the stresses and strains of a child's illness, the child may feel guilty, become depressed, and try to get out of the situation by leaving home or committing suicide.

If you think your child's depression is so deep that he or she is considering suicide, treat the situation seriously but calmly. Do not just dump your child in a therapist's office. Find someone, who may or may not know your child, with whom you can talk about your child's problems and what kind of program might be appropriate.

Crisis intervention may be necessary to weather an immediate storm; there are different types of assistance available, including individual, family, or group therapy with a psychiatrist, psychologist, licensed family or child counselor or therapist, psychiatric nurse, or medical or psychiatric social worker. These professionals may work in private practice, a private clinic, or a community clinic. Seeking professional help can be a sign of strength rather than weakness, for it means that an individual admits there is a problem and is willing to learn how to solve it.

When Your Child No Longer Lives at Home

The time may come when it is no longer possible or best for your child to live with you. If your child has a normal life expectancy, there is every reason to believe that he or she will outlive you. And although most younger children do better at home, the time may come when you can no longer care for your child at home. But much before that time, your child may want to live alone or with people of the same age or to get married. Choosing the best living situation for a child you can no longer care for is difficult, but if you keep in mind the best interests of your child as a member of your family, learn from other parents, teachers, and members of local or national organizations that help children like yours, and utilize the services of a social worker or other health-care professional involved in your child's care, you can make the best choice.

The establishment of their own home is the choice of most young adults. You may think you can provide the best physical and emotional care, but a maturing teenager may prefer to live alone or with people of the same age in an independent-living situation. Independent living for the disabled means being independent enough to make one's own choices about how one lives, even if one needs the help of friends or attendants.

Respite care (also called short-term foster care) is necessary if you or your family need an emotional or physical rest from the responsibilities of caring for your child, or if you have problems that preclude your being able to give your child the necessary care. There is nothing wrong with admitting that you need help, and it is better to ask for it when you need it than to collapse while trying to appear stalwart and brave. Check with the various service organizations in your community to see what possibilities for respite care exist. Respite care is sometimes available even as a child reaches adulthood, particularly if the program is run by an organization involved with developmental disabilities.

Long-term out-of-home placement may be necessary if you realize, after weighing the respective needs of all the members of your family, that respite care is not enough. This is often a very difficult decision to make, for you may not only have conflicting feelings but you may well receive unsolicited opinions from all sides, ranging from "How could you do that to your child?" to "You wouldn't want to care for him at home, would you?" But whereas others can offer suggestions, ultimately you have to decide. Possible alternatives include foster care, placement in a group home, placement in a private residential facility, or placement in a state hospital or institution.

Foster care is provided by most county welfare departments for children who can no longer be cared for by their parents. Whereas foster-care placement is often available only for short periods, it can continue until the parents decide to give their child up for adoption to a family willing to provide the necessary ongoing care the child needs. Most counties do not provide foster care after a child is considered an adult (either 18 or 21, depending upon state law). Therefore, this may no longer be an alternative for your child.

Group homes and family-care facilities provide the alternative closest to living at home. Usually, a small number of children (between 6 and 12) live together in a home that provides 24-hour-a-day nonmedical care, often in a residential neighborhood. Family-care facilities, as the name implies, are usually run by members of a family, such as a husband-and-wife team, while group homes are run by a hired staff. When more nursing care is needed, your child may go to a home called an intermediate-care facility. In most areas, there are more children who would like to live in group homes than can be placed. If you are serious about placing your child in a group home, you may have to become actively involved in starting one or helping with the ongoing needs of one. Although many homes receive some financial assistance from government agencies, often this does not cover all operating costs. So unless the home has a large endowment, parents often become involved in fund-raising activities.

Group homes are often the choice of parents who know their children will never be able to live alone, particularly if they have developmental disabilities. Since such children may well outlive their parents, the latter often work to establish a group home run as a nonprofit foundation so the home continues to exist after their death.

Private residential facilities are larger than group homes and, therefore, also more institutionalized. Since most disabled or ill children require much care, such facilities need large staffs, which makes the cost of running them very high. You, of course, help pay for this through your child's fees. Professionals in your community may be able to offer the names of reputable facilities and help you make up a list of questions to ask the director of the place you visit. You will probably get the most objective statements about a specific facility from a professional who has visited there but is not affiliated with it. If you cannot find anyone locally to help, call the national headquarters of organizations serving children such as yours and ask for recommendations. When you visit a facility, allow enough time to see how the place is actually run. When you ask questions, remember that most administrators are more apt to tell you of the strengths than of the weaknesses of the facility.

State hospitals or institutions provide less expensive care, but in many states parents must contribute toward their child's care, often on a sliding scale. Due to the sheer size of the institution and the need to keep operating costs as low as possible, state care is also the least personalized of the four alternatives.

Vocational Planning

While it is not easy to decide which vocation would be best for your child before he or she has any experience, and while final choices should not be made prematurely, advance planning is important. A disabled child who is old enough or ready to join the work force may have less part-time work experience than his or her able-bodied contemporaries. In spite of the equal employment opportunities ensured by Section 504 (see page 204) the child may have difficulty finding appropriate employment. Hence career planning can aid your child in reaching a vocation sooner, and by choice, rather than later and by chance.

Your teenaged child must take an active part in any such planning. Carolyn Vash, who is disabled herself, has tried to help others consider viable vocational alternatives. Here is her ad-

vice. Help your child make a list of the following:*

1. Interests: Things I like and dislike.
2. Abilities: Things I do well.
3. Aptitudes: Things I can do easily with little or no training.
4. Values: Things I feel are important for self-satisfaction.

These four factors can then be related to the following six "worker resource" areas:

1. Brawn—the ability to use one's body as a "power machine" or a mover of material. This includes such components as strength, endurance, and agility (coordination plus speed).
2. Brain—the ability to use one's intellect to perform operations on information and ideas. This includes such components as intelligence, creativity, special aptitudes, and knowledge.
3. Hands—the ability to use one's hands to create or manipulate objects. This includes such components as dexterity, special talents, and learned skills.
4. Personality—the ability to use one's personality to influence the attitudes and behavior of others. This includes such components as dominance, energy level, and learned interpersonal skills. (It should be stressed that this dimension is limited to that aspect of personality used as a work tool, much as we use our bodies, brains, and hands. Some jobs demand high levels of it—psychotherapist, teacher, trial attorney, receptionist, manager—and some require little or none—statistical clerk, laborer, bench assembler. It does not include aspects of personality that relate to getting or keeping jobs in general, such as poise, adaptability, and grooming habits.)
5. Communication—the ability to receive and transmit information accurately and efficiently. This breaks down into the components of visual/auditory reception and vocal/written transmission. Comprehension and other "data processing" abilities are considered brain resources. Persuasive effect of communications is considered a personality resource. This variable is defined solely in terms of receiving/transmitting abilities.

*Carolyn Vash, *A Predictive Model for Vocational Rehabilitation*, position paper prepared for the California State Department for Vocational Rehabilitation at Sacramento, CA, 1973, as quoted in Vash, *The Psychology of Disability* (New York: Springer Publishing Co., 1981), pp. 170–171.

6. Emotional stability—the ability to perform a job adequately in the face of stress and to behave appropriately on the job.

These variables will help you define how any disability your child has relates to potential vocations. For example, a quadriplegic might rate low on "brawn" and "hands," and high on "brain" and "personality," and a retarded person might rate low on "brains" but have other important areas in which he or she rates high. The important thing is to be realistic about the variables in which your child ranks low. Then remain optimistic about the areas in which your child either already does well or could learn to do well. Creative thinking, in terms of these six variables, about vocations in which your child might have an interest will help you to be more imaginative in considering future vocations and get you away from such stereotypes as that the blind only tune pianos or sell pencils—today there are blind doctors, lawyers, and so on. Simplistic statements like "You are going to have to use your head rather than your hands" can be less than helpful, particularly to a formerly active child who became disabled in a diving or motorcycle accident. There is no reason to think that a child who was not intellectually oriented before an accident or illness will necessarily be so afterward. It is far better to encourage your child to pursue an existing vocational interest rather than one in which he or she has no interest at all.

Of course, not even careful vocational planning and education will ensure financial independence for every child. Some children are not able to work in the competitive job market because of their handicaps, be they mental, emotional, or physical. And others, particularly the severely physically disabled, cannot afford to work, because if their incomes rise above a certain amount they are no longer eligible for Supplemental Security Income payments and the accompanying medical benefits (discussed more fully in Chapter 17). But for all these individuals, it is almost always better to do something than to sit at home. Seriously consider sheltered workshops or volunteer work if your child cannot find employment in the competitive job market.

Vocational planning begins in high school. When your child leaves school, you have to assume much more responsibility to make sure he or she receives appropriate vocational counseling and training. Many states provide vocational rehabilitation programs as well as vocational counseling at state institutions of higher learning such as community colleges and universities. But these counselors are usually quite busy and won't go looking for you. Your child, with as much assistance from you as necessary, has to learn to seek needed help. Career education may be a matter of systematically coordinating all school, community, and family components to aid your child's search for economic, social, and personal fulfillment. Providing this guidance is well worth the effort in terms of your child's human dignity and self-esteem.

PART 4

MEETING THE NEEDS
OF THE WHOLE FAMILY

16
Organizing Your Household

In order to care for a disabled or gravely ill child, your household must be organized. Caring for such a child takes more time than caring for a "normal" child, and there is no time for "seek and find." Also, people helping you will have to know how to do what is necessary. There are two issues to consider in keeping your home running smoothly: how most efficiently to organize your house, and how to find and work with any household help you may need.

HOUSEHOLD ORGANIZATION

Setting Priorities

Since you probably have more tasks you would like to accomplish than you have time for, you must establish priorities. Keeping your place spotless may make you a grouchy nervous wreck who never has time to take the family on a picnic, to spend an afternoon with the children baking cookies or reading stories, or to worship in the place of your choice. You may be providing for your family's physical needs, but you are ignoring their emotional, mental, and spiritual ones.

Moreover, finding time for your ill or disabled child, but not for your spouse or other children, is also to ignore your duties and the needs of your whole family. In such a case your disabled child may become a wedge separating you from your family rather than a bridge uniting you. Consider the basic needs of your whole family and what work needs to be done. Then set priorities,

try to organize your household, and figure out who can best help you keep it all running smoothly.

Organizing Your Living Space

Organize your living space for your own convenience and your child's safety. Although your house may not make the pages of a decorators' magazine, it will serve your family's needs, which is what a house is for. For example, if your child uses an electric wheelchair, you might take up the living-room carpets and move all the furniture against the walls so there is more room for your child to drive around. If your child spends a good part of every day having some kind of therapy, you might arrange a room that is a center of family activity around your child's therapy. This might result in a dining room that looks like a respiratory-intensive-care unit, but if your child needs help for hours every day it should be given where it is possible to participate in the life of the family.

If you have bathrooms upstairs but none downstairs, the kitchen may have to double as a children's bathroom. In addition to normal kitchen furnishings, you can keep a potty, hair brushes, and toothbrushes there.

Architectural elements such as stairs and narrow doorways may become barriers preventing full utilization of the space in your house. For example, while stairs may be merely an inconvenience with a small disabled child, they can be an intolerable obstacle with an older, heavier child. At that point, you need to consider moving, installing an elevator, or remodeling your home. Weigh the alternatives carefully. If you decide to remodel, look for an architect who is not only an expert in this field but who is also interested in your needs in caring for your child.

Sound barriers that prevent you from hearing your child can be overcome with intercom and alarm systems.

An intercom system may enable your child to spend some time alone. Also, with an intercom your child can learn to let others listen for any calls for help rather than insist that one specific person always sleep in the same room and care for him or her. In the long run, you will sleep better in a room separate from your child; you will hear your child even if you are a heavy sleeper. If your child has a large lung capacity, strong vocal cords, and a lusty cry, almost any intercom system will work. But if your child has a weak cry and you have to monitor breathing, you need the system that best amplifies those sounds you must hear clearly without interference or static. Many electronic-supply stores and telephone-supply stores carry room-to-room intercom systems. These consist of two or more units that plug into the electrical outlets in different rooms. The sounds are transmitted from room to room over radio frequencies; FM is less vulnerable to interference than AM. While most such units effectively convey sounds within the range of normal speech, some (particularly cheaper) models may have interference and may not satisfactorily transmit sounds in the lower-frequency range such as breathing and choking. Before you purchase an intercom unit, ask to try it out in your own home to be sure it adequately amplifies the sounds you need to hear.

If no commercial intercom is adequate, you may have to construct your own unit with the help of a friend or shop owner who knows about electronics and stereo components. Your intercom will consist of a microphone, connected to a preamplifier, connected to an amplifier, connected to a loudspeaker. It is best to buy a unidirectional microphone that can be placed or hung as close to your child's head as is safe and convenient so the pickup of ambient noise will be reduced. The lines connecting the microphone to the preamplifier should be short (less than 15 feet, if possible) to reduce electronic interference. The lines between the preamplifier and the amplifier can be as long as 40 feet. Lines between the amplifier and the loudspeaker, using ordinary lamp cord, can extend up to 100 feet. Special techniques (such as using 70-volt lines) may be required to span longer distances. Such a system should give clear amplification of any sounds your child makes. While you will not be able to talk back through the system to your child, if he or she calls you will probably have to go there to help anyway. If you are using an ultrasonic nebulizer in your child's room, be sure to wrap any of the components located in that room in plastic bags containing silica gel so they don't get wet or salty.

A call switch is nothing more than a switch connected to an alarm. If you do not have an intercom system in all rooms, you can place a battery-powered alarm near an immobile child (on a wheelchair tray or bed) so when the child touches the switch the alarm signals you to come. You may need an ultrasensitive touch plate such as the one made by Med-Labs (7036 Madera Drive, Goleta, CA 93117). If your child cannot operate this, Med-Labs will try to custom-make one your child can use.

A pressure-sensitive mat will alert you if your child gets out of bed. Just place such a mat where your child's feet would touch the floor when getting out of bed and wire this to a buzzer in your bedroom. This can be helpful, for example, if your child is mentally confused, cannot care for himself or herself, would not call you, or might try to go to the bathroom or elsewhere alone during the night. You can get the mat, buzzer, and items you need to connect them from an electronics-supply store.

A warning system in case of electric-power outage is crucial if your child depends on an electric life-support system. After your doctor verifies your child's medical need with your local electric-utility company, the company will record your child as a critical priority patient and make special note of your home on its district records and circuit maps. You will then be given advance notice in case of a planned outage and will be contacted as soon as possible in case of an unplanned power failure. In either case you will be given an estimated time for restoration of power, but you should understand that this is difficult for your utility company to predict with accuracy. If your child cannot survive long without electricity, discuss with your doctor what you should do in case of an outage. Since most hospitals have backup gas generators, your doctor may want you to take your child to the nearest hospital. Most large communities are on more than one circuit, so a friend in another part of town may have power when you don't.

You can attach a battery-powered alarm to your electric system to alert you immediately of any power failure. Such an alarm is not difficult for a person with some knowledge of electronics to construct.

Beepers, such as those used by doctors, may be worth considering if you feel you must always be in contact with whoever is caring for your child. If you feel you need a beeper, your doctor will be able to tell you which company he uses, and perhaps something about other companies. You will have to consider what services they offer and how much they charge.

Safety factors also demand your careful consideration. If you can't watch your toddler at all times, be sure that knives, cleaning solutions, medications, and other dangerous items have permanent homes up high so your child can't reach them. You may need gates with locks separating parts of the house or separating the yard from the street. Be sure all your friends close these when they come to visit. A sight-impaired child will fall over shoes in the middle of the floor. But you should keep the floors clear for yourself as well. If you spend time carrying a child or dashing to the rescue when your child rings an alarm, be sure everyone knows that the stairs are to be left clear at all times. Keep the pathway between your bedroom and your child's clear, especially for midnight dashes. There should be nothing to impede your way to your child. This is especially important when you are tired and not as light-footed or alert as usual.

Storage is the next item to consider. Now that you can fully utilize your space, having overcome architectural and sound barriers as well as having attended to safety factors, you must get the objects in that space organized so you and your helpers know where things are. Since you may have to give instructions verbally, you must be organized so people can help you readily. For example, if you need someone to fix a sandwich, it is not good enough to say the bread is in the kitchen somewhere. You must be able to say that it is in the cupboard above the toaster, bottom shelf, right-hand side, and that the butter is in the refrigerator, middle shelf, right, and so on.

Especially your medical equipment must be meticulously organized at all times. You (and everyone else in the house) must know where things are (and how they work) in case of emergency. Store your medical equipment where it is most likely to be needed. For example, the suction machine your child might need in an emergency must be stored in a permanent, readily accessible place. Although you may have more available storage space in an upstairs linen closet, a suction machine might live in a kitchen cupboard, since if your child aspirates while eating that is where he or she will most likely be.

Medicines also have to be well organized. Depending on storage requirements, this may be in the refrigerator or in a high cupboard out of reach of young exploring hands. Anything poisonous must be so hard to get at that even you should need a chair to reach it. If your medicines are well organized, you can see what you have on hand at a glance and can reorder before you run out of essentials in the middle of the night.

Getting the Jobs Done

Since you will not have time to do everything you would like to do, you must establish priorities in your daily life so things get done in order of importance. "Doing" doesn't just mean cleaning the house, it means living as a family. You can muddle through a few days or even weeks when your child needs intensive care with the Band-Aid approach to living, but if you anticipate weeks, months, or years of life with your disabled child you must decide what must be done daily (like cleaning the medical equipment, medical treatment, feeding people, getting enough sleep), weekly (food shopping, vacuuming), monthly (paying bills), and yearly (income tax). Consider what needs doing in basic areas such as:

- Earning a living
- Medical care
- Child care
- Spouse care
- Cleaning
- Food preparation
- Household repairs
- Yard work
- Errands
- Accounting
- Education
- Recreation
- Spiritual growth

Think about how you can streamline your household to eliminate certain jobs. If knick-knacks and figurines need dusting and you barely have time to vacuum the floor, you may decide that these treasures might be happier in the dustfree environment of a box in the attic for a few years. Other jobs may get done less frequently. Clean windows are nice, but you can still see through dirty ones. Cleaning medical equipment daily takes priority over mopping the kitchen floor.

Job allocation is important. After you have eliminated the unnecessary jobs, you must allocate the others. Your family will develop an allocation of jobs to suit your needs. For example, if one parent is often up for hours at night with a sick child, this parent might sleep for as long as the child does the next morning while the other fixes breakfast and gets any other children off to school. Obviously, if one parent enjoys a job in which the other has no interest, the interested parent should do that job. However, you must be flexible. One of you may be marvelously handy and the other may hardly ever try to fix things. But if you start having chronic mechanical problems with a piece of equipment your child needs, the unmechanical parent may find it worthwhile to learn how to make minor repairs.

Lists help organize yourself, your time, and consequently your household. While your own list of chores may be short and lacking in details, your family, friends, and paid help may require their instructions fully spelled out. You may think you don't have time to make a detailed list, but doing so will actually save time, since complete and concise instructions make time-consuming explanations unnecessary. Besides, if you must constantly correct the help because your verbal instructions were unclear, or if some of your needs are unusual, you may appear to be overly demanding. With a detailed list, you merely indicate that in your house things are to be done a certain way, and your help will not get in the habit of doing something *their* way because they don't know yours.

Your list of how to clean your living room will probably be quite different from anyone else's; it will also reveal a few idiosyncrasies about your family. For example, a living-room list might read as follows:

1. *Daily:*
   a. Put yesterday's newspapers in the brown paper bag on top of the refrigerator.
   b. Pick up all books and papers from the floor and couches and place them in a neat pile on desk chair. Do not touch desk.
   c. Put all toys neatly on the toy shelf.
   d. Straighten pillows and furniture.
   e. Sweep floor.
2. *Monday, Wednesday, Friday:*
   a. Vacuum floor.
3. *As needed:*
   a. Vacuum furniture and cobwebs.

Note that some chores, like window-washing, aren't even mentioned, because they are probably too far down on the priority list.

It is important to go through the list verbally with the person using it at least once and then post the list where it will be available for easy reference and won't get lost. The inside of the kitchen-cabinet doors serve this purpose well. This way you can also suggest that the help periodically check their work, or you can call their attention to parts of jobs you would like done differently.

It may also be helpful to suggest how long a job should take. A helper may be so meticulous that he or she becomes overwhelmed by the amount of work. You can show how work can be done more efficiently, corners cut, and jobs even eliminated if necessary.

Cleaning is important, especially if germs are a serious health hazard for your child. There are four major ways to create a less-germ-infested environment. (Making lists of these cleaning procedures gives an air of impersonality to what might otherwise be considered ridiculous requests.)

Prevent germs from even entering the house. Have everyone (family, friends, teachers, nurses, doctors, *everyone*) wash their hands when coming into the house. Don't worry about your doing things differently, but take the time to explain why hands must be washed. No one with a cold or other contagious illness should be allowed in the house except family members, and even they should expect a certain amount of isolation. Try to keep any sick siblings as far from your chronically ill child as possible and try to arrange bedrest for sick adults. Since illness is most contagious before the person even feels symptoms and since the sick person will keep breathing and filling the air with germs, isolation is not foolproof. But if colds are a critical problem, isolation may be appropriate.

Clean all washable surfaces with solutions containing germicides. Door and faucet handles need regular washing, for many germs come to rest there.

Sweep or vacuum surface dirt on nonwashable surfaces. If your child has respiratory or allergy problems, you may have to evaluate the efficiency of the suctioning and filtering system of any vacuum cleaner you use. The suctioning action of a good upright is usually better than that of a cannister. If you have carpeting and prefer cannisters, it may be wise to get one with a power nozzle that has a revolving brush and beating action to help get dirt out of the carpet. The filtering system includes what the dirt goes into (water or bags made of cloth or paper) and through what the exhaust air is filtered before leaving the vacuum cleaner.

If you think you need a new vacuum cleaner, talk with dealers who sell several brands and also have repair services, for they can not only tell you the comparative virtues of different machines but also how well the machines hold up over time. A good dealer will also have different types of carpeting (and free dirt) available so you can try out their machines on a flooring that approximates what you have at home.

Deal with airborne germs, pollen, and dirt if necessary. Your child's medical needs will determine the method most applicable to your situation.

Air-filtering machines of adequate size can filter the air in a room many times per hour, trapping dirt, pollen, and even airborne bacteria and viruses. There are electrostatic precipitators and high-efficiency purified-air (HEPA) filters, the latter probably being the style of the future. If you are thinking of purchasing a machine, be sure that you can easily replace the filters yourself (without sending the machine back to the factory) and that servicing is readily available.

Room sprays kill only those germs they actually contact. Hence there is no guarantee they will make an area germfree. Breathing aerosol sprays may be contraindicated for children with respiratory or allergy problems.

When you have determined what you would like done, you have to weigh this against how much time and help you actually have. Make up your cleaning lists accordingly.

Errands can be circumvented if it is difficult for you to get out of the house. First consider what stores in your community will deliver at little or no cost. Then consider what can be ordered by mail. If someone actually has to run an errand for you, you can make much more efficient use of his or her time (and your money, if you are paying) if you phone ahead to make sure the store has the item you want. Occasionally you can even request the item to be held at the cashier in your name. If you establish a good working relationship with the public library, the librarian may be willing to take a phone request and have the books waiting for you at the circulation desk.

Be polite and thank people for going out of their way to help you. Even if someone tells you gruffly that his establishment couldn't possibly help you in the manner you suggested, you can still politely thank the person for his consideration. In doing so, you may plant a seed for helpfulness to another person in the future.

Food shopping is another job that can easily be done for you. If someone shops for you regularly, it helps to have a master list, organized to follow the layout of the neighborhood supermarket. While the list may also include sections for items from the health-food store and the local deli, it is not economical to pay someone to go to more stores than that. (It is also more difficult for a helper to learn the layout of many stores.) Make a master list of everything you want to have in your house. Keep this list as simple but complete as possible, organized into logical sections that might include dairy, canned fruit, canned vegetables, paper and staples, fresh vegetables, fresh fruit, frozen items, meat and fish, condiments, and anything else you need.

Next to each item indicate how much you want to have on hand. In this way anyone can go through your cupboards and refrigerator to see what you need and then go shopping. If you are really organized and indicate on your list every time you use up or have almost used up an item, your shopping list will always be ready. After you have written out a master list, make a few photocopies so you can use it for a while and make any changes. Then you can photocopy enough to last for a few months.

Keep an ample stock of food, finding extra storage space in a closet or the garage if necessary. A second refrigerator helps if you have room.

Dinner time must be organized. Family members can prepare their own breakfasts and lunches, but try to arrange it so the family sits down together for dinner.

If your child eats very slowly, dinner is a good time to have friends over to visit, especially if it is difficult for you to go visiting or to stay up late. In this way you can have companionship and contact with the outside world. You might even have an "open door" policy, encouraging friends to drop in and join you for dinner. If you know friends are coming, you can ask them to come a bit early and help or even bring some of the food.

The dinner hour should be pleasantly calm. You may need to institute a nap or at least an afternoon quiet time for everyone.

If your child is very ill, it may be difficult to ensure ample time for meal preparation every day. Simplifying your meals or cooking ahead will help avoid rushing. Double your recipes and freeze half for another meal. Keep a list of what

is in the freezer so you can find something to eat on days when you don't have time to cook a complete meal. During a particularly rough time you can even ask friends to bring dinner; most people are delighted to help.

Getting sufficient rest is important for every family member to help maintain the whole family's health and good cheer. It is amazing how quickly fatigue can cause a person to become grouchy and lose perspective on things.

It is best to get uninterrupted periods of sleep at approximately the same time every day. Avoid using sleeping pills. While a sleeping pill may help you fall asleep, you may not feel very refreshed when you wake up.

It may be difficult to get enough of such regular uninterrupted sleep, especially when your child is sick, but since sufficient rest is so important for everyone in the family, consider the following:

When and for how long will your child sleep? While this varies greatly among individuals and can be influenced by illness, you will see patterns in your child. For example, you may find that your child needs about 12 hours of sleep a day, and may sleep from 7:00 P.M. to 7:00 A.M., from 9:00 P.M. to 9:00 A.M., or from 9:00 P.M. to 7:00 A.M. with a two-hour nap in the middle of the day.

You may find that naps are beneficial for you and your child. If you never get enough sleep at night because your child calls and needs help, a nap can give both of you essential sleeping time. It will also give you a break from constantly being together; both of you need time away from each other. And a nap provides an opportunity to take off any equipment your child may be wearing and give him or her a chance to change positions, lie down, and relax. Naps are easiest to establish and maintain if your child has always had them. However, if you have to reinstitute naps or quiet times, it is most effective if you also rest. If you are banging around the house, your child may just listen to the noises and feel that he or she is missing out on the fun. However, remember that children will sleep only so many hours per day, so if the naps are too long your child may be up late at night or be unable to sleep if you put him or her to bed too early.

Where should your child sleep? It is best if your child can learn to sleep in his or her own room, for if you are together all day long you both need a breather from each other, and parents need some time alone. If you get an intercom system you will be able to hear your child should he or she need help during the night.

What can you do to help your child call as infrequently as possible during the night? First, make sure all essential needs are met before your child goes to bed: make sure your child is tired, has been toileted, has had a drink, is correctly positioned and adequately covered. If you think you have satisfied all reasonable needs and you are still being called, try to make your child understand it is time to go to sleep. But if your child cannot move unassisted and is dependent upon an intercom system, do not ignore the calling; your child may panic, thinking that the intercom is not working. It is far better to yell down the hall or up the stairs, "Go to sleep!"

If in spite of all this your child still calls often during the night, you and your spouse might consider taking shifts during the night (one goes to bed early, the other is on duty, etc.). Or if one adult works outside the home and needs more sleep during the week, this parent could take call on Friday and Saturday nights. If you both wake up every time your child calls and consequently neither of you gets sufficient sleep, you may want to consider at least sometimes sleeping in separate rooms so one person can spend the night undisturbed.

HOUSEHOLD HELP

Finding the best help for your needs can be difficult, and it may sometimes seem that a good helper leaves as soon as you get him or her trained. This can cause, to say the least, mild exasperation, but you can use it as an opportunity to learn gratitude for every bit of help you can find.

What Kind of Help Do You Need?

The search for help is on when you realize that, in spite of organization and efficiency, you cannot manage alone. First you have to consider exactly what kind of help you require. Do you need assistance with medical care, help to keep the household functioning, or both? Do you need this help weekly or daily? Are there certain times of day when help is especially necessary— mornings, afternoons, dinner time, evenings, nights?

If your child's condition is progressive, the medical care you give may become more and more time-consuming, in which case you will need more and more help with the daily household chores of dinner preparation, laundry, cleaning, etc. If it becomes increasingly difficult for you to leave the house, you will need someone to do the marketing and run errands too. In this case, while helpers should be trained to care for your child, their primary job is to help in the house. You must decide which jobs you would rather do yourself and which you need to have done for you. You might favor help in the mornings and again in the evenings at dinner time over a straight eight-hour shift.

Who Can Help You?

Once you decide upon your needs, you must consider who can best help you meet them.

Friends who offer to help are genuinely interested in doing so. Often you have to make specific requests, at the same time insisting that you want an honest answer of yes or no. Friends are usually happy to help with child care, errands, cooking an occasional meal, and even cleaning in case of dire need. Don't worry about paying them back. You may not be able to do so for years, and even then your help may go to another person in need. This is what real friendship is about.

Service groups in your community are sometimes willing to help. Although "nonprofessionals" may not be able to give sophisticated medical assistance, they can often help with ongoing household chores, errands, and even child care. A local high-school service club may arrange for some of its members to come and play with your child, taking turns visiting every Saturday for an hour. Having someone there will not only give you a free hour but will provide your child with friendship and stimulation from the outside world.

If your needs are greater than the occasional help your friends and volunteers can provide, you must consider other types of help.

Registered nurses (RNs) have extensive medical training. Therefore, they are usually the most expensive source of help. Private-duty registered nurses usually want to work only for whole eight-hour shifts. Since they generally want to provide only nursing care, they are probably not interested in helping around the house. So ask yourself whether you really need someone who is willing to provide only medical care and whether you can really use that person for a whole shift. Your child may have very specific medical needs; in such a case you may need to teach anyone who comes to help, even a nurse.

Visiting nurses and public-health nurses are trained to come into the home for short periods of time, say an hour, and perform certain functions or assess your child's condition and needs. Their fee is often determined by your ability to pay. It might even be a good idea to spend an hour every week training one nurse from the local Visiting Nurses Association so one more person will be able to help you if you are "between" helpers or have a medical emergency. Although it may take as long to train this person as it does your other helpers, you may need the expertise from time to time. Visiting nurses can be very helpful if you occasionally need specific medical help, but you should learn to do anything that your child needs regularly, such as injections or the changing of dressings, yourself.

Licensed vocational nurses and paramedical assistants have less training than nurses and therefore charge less for their services. You may well have to teach them how to help your child.

Homemaker services are available in some communities, either through the Visiting Nurses Association or through commercial employment agencies. Hiring help through an agency does not guarantee competence. Also, the cost of employee benefits is unfortunately passed on to you. Persons hired under such a contractual

agreement may be limited in what they are allowed to do or by what they consider to be their job.

People you find and train yourself make up the last and, perhaps, the most important category. If what you need is a bright, level-headed, and responsible individual who is willing to learn how you need things done and is willing to pitch in when needed, there is no guarantee that formal training will provide it. You might do better training students, young people, housewives, or grandmother types.

College students, having made one commitment (schooling), will often be good at carrying through on another commitment (helping you), particularly if your pay makes it possible for them to stay in school. They are often bright, quick learners, and they may have some flexibility in arranging their class schedules to accommodate your needs. They are often more willing to help where needed with housework, child care, errands, and so on than someone with professional training and expertise—for example, a nurse. Students usually have their own interests and circle of friends, which means they have lives of their own to live and are not too dependent upon you. Of course, the student may want to go home for vacations, in which case you'll need alternative help or will just have to muddle through alone.

Nonstudent younger persons may have more time, but they sometimes don't show the commitment of a student intent upon completing his or her education. Young persons working full-time don't have the time to help you much. Those who work part-time may lack real commitment to their jobs and have no compelling reason to stay in your area. They may therefore be less committed to staying with you for a good while.

"Au pair" girls from foreign countries are sometimes willing to come and live with a family for a year. Usually you have to pay their transportation and a limited salary. The hitch is that you usually have to keep them for a year, which is marvelous if things go well but difficult if they are unable to learn what they need to learn to help you. Of course, before you commit yourself to an "au pair" girl you should make the nature

of the job as clear to her as possible.

Housewives working for you part-time may know more than younger helpers, yet they may be more set in their ways. They may also be less willing to take instructions from you, especially if you are younger than they are. If they have children of their own they will be experienced with children, but they may be unable to come to help if their own children fall ill.

Grandmother types are often very reliable and experienced but may be set in their ways and less willing or able to help as needed, especially with heavy housework and lifting.

The sex of the helper you choose may be influenced by the age and sex of your child (and any other children) as well as the type of help you need. Interview both men and women rather than remain bound by stereotypes; many men are great cooks, and many women are very handy with repairs and such.

How Can You Pay the Help?

The help you can use and the help you can afford are often two different things. While you may buy any equipment you need in the hope that you can find financial assistance, you will quickly learn that it is very difficult to get financial aid for household help. If you have very little money, the amount of help you have may be limited to the help you can barter and pay for with the financial assistance you can obtain from government agencies and service organizations.

Bartering room and board in exchange for help is the cheapest in dollars and cents since, if you have the room in your home, the only cash outlay is for feeding the additional mouth. This type of exchange can be very attractive to a student with no local home. Such live-in help will be available to help here and there as needed rather than only at set hours. However, you have to be careful not to "use" the person.

Since live-in help is part of the family, eating meals with you and being around much of the time, it is important that you get along well.

You may decide to hire a part-time helper to supplement the live-in helper. The live-in helper might cook dinner, do the marketing, and baby-sit in exchange for room and board. The second helper might be paid hourly to come in and help with the usual morning tasks of breakfast, packing lunches, the laundry, the cleaning, and errands. By having two helpers, not too much responsibility falls upon one individual, and if one helper quits you still have the other to tide you over until you find a replacement.

Insurance usually covers only registered nurses, and your share of the cost is usually 20 percent. A private nurse willing to work only a complete eight-hour shift may not only be expensive but also inappropriate if what you really need is daily paramedical or homemaking assistance for shorter periods of time. Visiting nurses usually come in to do specific treatments. Since community Visiting Nurses Associations are usually nonprofit organizations and often base their fees on your ability to pay, an insurance payment may sometimes be accepted as sufficient payment. Paramedical and homemaking assistance is usually not covered by insurance, but check your policy to be sure.

Government programs vary from state to state. Medicaid will usually pay for nursing care only in a facility. However, some states have special programs to provide specific services, which may include homemaker or paramedical assistance. As discussed fully on pages 228–232, begin by making phone calls to anyone you think might be able to help you, such as your doctor, social worker, county welfare department, Crippled-Children's Services, developmental disability programs, and the Supplemental Security Income office. If they can't offer assistance, maybe they know of someone who can. Since programs and their eligibility requirements frequently change, you must periodically check what is available in your area. If you are told that your child does not qualify for assistance, check again in six months, for the requirements may have changed and your child could be eligible.

Voluntary health agencies ("charities") usually have their funds earmarked for research and specific types of services such as summer camps, wheelchairs, orthopedic devices, etc. They are rarely interested in paying for the daily help you need to keep things running. There is no reason why you shouldn't present your case as forcefully as possible, but probably the most help you can expect is a special fund in your child's name, and that amount will usually be much too small to pay for ongoing household help.

How Can You Find Help?

Once you have determined what kind of help you need and how much you can afford, you need to learn how to find the help.

Your doctor may be the first person to whom you should turn. Your doctor knows both your child's medical needs and the needs of your family. You should feel free to talk to him or her about anything concerning your child, which of course includes the daily household routine. While your doctor may be able to tell you about available sources of help within your community and which funding sources might help pay their wages, he or she probably won't have the time to do the actual searching for you.

Social workers, whether they are connected with a hospital, government agency, or voluntary health agency, may be of assistance in finding help. But as in the case of your doctor, you must indicate the type of assistance you need. Social workers are usually busy with many clients and often need specific requests from you to initiate action.

If you are extremely lucky, an efficient, determined social worker with good connections will find you helpers.

Often any helper paid for with government or voluntary-health-agency funds has to be hired through an approved agency. Even if this is the case, be sure to have a say in who is hired. Sometimes you can convince the agency or social worker that you want to find your own helper. The agency can then officially hire that person to work for you. This technique is the least work for the social worker, although the private-hire system probably complicates someone's paperwork. Occasionally you can get the money paid directly to you, to be spent on employing the person of your choice.

You may have to find your own help if you are the one who has to pay or if the agency helping you is unable to find an appropriate helper quickly. You know what you need and want. If you feel comfortable doing so, you might begin by trying to find a friend willing to come and be your paid help. Next ask your friends if they have any friends, so the new helper won't be a total stranger. Then call any community college or university nearby, leaving specific job descriptions with their housing and part-time-employment agencies. Your ads, which you can run in the college and local newspaper concurrently, might be worded something like this:

Responsible student to help part-time with housework and child care (bright, cheerful, physically handicapped 8-year-old girl and 5-year-old boy) in exchange for room and board. 364-9752

When the phone starts ringing, give as much information as possible. If the person is interested, jot down name, phone number, and any other relevant information on a list. Then arrange interviews with the most likely applicants. Talking to someone is one thing, seeing how a person works is another. You might ask a serious applicant for a live-in position to help fix dinner and eat with you, for this will give you the opportunity to assess each other.

Deciding whom to hire is always difficult. Ideally the person should be efficient, willing to learn, and cheerful. You don't want someone who will burden you with personal problems or try to solve yours. And it is best if your values and life styles are compatible. You should therefore tell any prospective helper about the way your family lives. If, for example, you do not allow smoking in your house, you should tell this to your applicants. Especially if a child is terminally ill, conflicting religious beliefs can cause problems; it may, therefore, be appropriate to discuss these too.

After interviewing a few people, make an offer to the best applicant. Give the person 24 hours to decide. This will give the applicant time to reflect upon what the decision implies. It is important to give a realistic picture of the advantages and disadvantages of working for you. After all, it is to everyone's benefit if your helper likes to work for you and will stay for some time.

Work to Establish a Good Relationship with Your Helper

It takes time and effort to establish good rapport with your helpers if you want them to interact effectively with your family and be more than just "the hired help."

Take time to explain how your household is run and how the person can best help. It is futile to try to tell helpers everything they will need to know on the first day; no one could retain it all and anyone would feel overwhelmed. Teach your helper a few things at a time, feeling free to point out specific responsibilities. For example, a college student working for you might not have to bring in the food or clear the table at home, but it may be very helpful if this were done for you if you are busy with your children during meals.

Stress the necessity of asking questions, for some people are shy or feel stupid if they don't understand or remember what you told them. This also means that if they ask you to do something, try to do it, and emphasize that if you forget they should remind you again and again.

Work for open communication. In every family problems can develop because of lack of communication. You might assume that if you asked a helper if he or she would like to do a special job the helper would answer truthfully yes or no. Yet many helpers will feel that they have to say yes to every request and consequently may feel overworked and annoyed. So explain in advance that an honest answer to such a question is important, and that a no will not jeopardize the helper's position. Also stress that your helpers should tell you anything that disturbs them, for otherwise tensions can arise.

Expend the time and effort to establish a good relationship between your child and the helper. Your child may dislike having new helpers learn how to care for him or her. Try to help your child to understand the importance of patience and the ability to teach. And try to stress to your child and the helper that it may take a helper time to learn what is needed.

Teach the helper about your child's condition. When you teach helpers any special procedures make sure they understand the purpose of the task. Also indicate potential difficulties while at the same time emphasizing your faith in their ability to learn. Never leave a helper with a child until both he or she and you are confident that the helper can manage emergencies.

Express thanks to your helpers for their assistance. Especially if you are overworked, it is easy just to tell someone the next job to do, as you would mentally tell yourself if you were going to do it. However, helpers are not workhorses but humans, helping you in what is often a somewhat stressful situation. They need positive reinforcement for their efforts.

Problems

Don't despair if you choose the wrong helper. We all misjudge character sometimes. If you think the help really cannot learn to do the job well, politely ask him or her to leave. You needn't list all your grievances: simply say you don't think things will work out.

Neither should you despair if your help doesn't stay with you forever. Particularly if your child has severe problems, working for you may entail a lot of responsibility and commitment, more than most people are willing to carry for a long time. It is a genuine nuisance to have to look for help, and you may panic when your first help leaves. But you will survive the transition periods, and you will come to be grateful for all the help you receive.

17
Paying for the
Medical Help You Need

Your child should have all his or her medical needs taken care of, including all the *functionally* best medical equipment. So, for example, no child needs a gold-plated wheelchair, but he or she may have an electric outdoor and indoor wheelchair, especially modified to meet his or her needs. To pay for your child's medical expenses you will probably need the financial assistance of public and private agencies. You may need help not just for tens or hundreds but for thousands of dollars year after year. And if your child's medical expenses rise, the search for funds has to expand. Although you will surely be grateful for the generosity of others, the efforts to find funds can become so difficult that you may begin to feel that you are scrounging for money. But if you need financial assistance, you have to find out how to get it. Think of your search as a treasure hunt. This attitude will help you keep your perspective on the matter.

YOUR FINANCIAL NEEDS
AND RESOURCES

First you must consider not only your child's medical needs but also how your family spends its money. If you are frugal and try to save, yet still need more money for medical expenses than you have available, you have to consider outside sources of help, which in our society are of three basic kinds: tax-supported government programs at the local, state, and national levels; insurance; and voluntary health agencies.

Various individuals can help you search for

funds. Doctors can often direct you to sources of financial assistance in your community. Social workers working for hospitals, government agencies, and sometimes voluntary health agencies can also help. These are people to work *with* you, not for you, meaning that you must do your part, indicating your needs and providing any necessary information. Parents of other special children can also be helpful regarding support and information, especially if they have been successful in obtaining money.

When you look for help in finding financial assistance, remember that you are most familiar with your financial needs and medical problems and that you can be your child's best advocate. You must be able to provide all pertinent information to anyone helping you in your search for assistance.

THE REQUEST FOR ASSISTANCE

Regardless of which agency you contact for assistance, the appropriate approach is important.

Telephone Inquiries

Telephone inquiries are the first step in your search for financial assistance. There is a technique to making an effective phone call:

* *Consider what points you want to cover before placing your call.* It may be helpful to write these down.

- *Introduce yourself in a friendly voice:* "Hello, this is Judith Smith" (or "Judith Smith, the mother of Belinda Elizabeth Smith," if such identification is appropriate). People like to know who is calling, and a friendly tone gets things off to a good start.
- *State with whom you wish to speak and why.*
- *Write down the name of the person with whom you speak.* If someone gives you information, you may want to call him or her back for more later. Furthermore, if someone gives you a commitment of some kind, you need to remember who that person was.
- *Be well organized and concise.* Refer to any notes you have made before calling if this will help.
- *Take notes* during the phone call. Do not assume you will remember everything you are told.
- *Be friendly and polite.* Since people have good and bad days, don't take a grouchy or curt response personally. Even if you get no for an answer, watch your manners. You may be able to get the party to change his or her mind or at least to help you or someone else in the future.

Interviews

If an agency is interested in more information about your request, its representative may wish to see you in person and an interview should be arranged. Make an appointment for a time when you know you will be punctual and calm and when you will have the attention and interest of the agency (which excludes appointments on Friday at 4:45 P.M.). Your general appearance is important. If you come bedecked with diamonds, people may wonder if you are really a needy case. But if you arrive looking bedraggled and worn you won't create a positive impression either.

Again, be organized and write down notes in advance, for you must be able to convince people that yours is, indeed, a worthy cause. Since many professional people are very busy, don't take up more of their time than necessary.

You can sometimes arrange interviews at home. Not only may this be more convenient for you, but it will enable the social worker or other agency official actually to see your child in the home environment and thus better appraise your child's needs. Also, someone who has been to your home is more likely to remember you when you contact him or her again.

Written Requests

You will probably need to put your request for assistance in writing. Written requests may take time to formulate, but they ensure that an agency has all the relevant information. A written request makes the best impression if it is neatly typed on standard 8½ × 11″ white paper. You can give a person your written request at the time of an interview or mail it following a phone call. A written reply to your letter will then give you verification of the agency's general policy or a specific response to your request.

Refusals

Do not take any refusal personally. People are not saying they don't like you or your child. They are saying that, as they perceive the situation, they can't help you.

Be sure you know why a request is refused. In some cases, a refusal is due to an inflexible policy. But in other cases policy is open to interpretation. Check with the agency to make sure you have given all the information they need.

Don't be afraid to ask again. Assistance programs exist to assist people. If you think you have a reasonable request, keep making it. People must perceive your need before they can help you. Also, some programs change. While you may not be eligible for something now, you may well be later.

GOVERNMENT PROGRAMS

Although government programs and regulations are constantly changing, there are various major sources of government assistance for your child: the federal Medicaid program (and its equivalent on the state level), the federal program assisting the disabled (Supplemental Security Income), state programs for disabled children (often called the Crippled Children's Services or simply Children's Services), and state programs aiding the developmentally disabled. Other programs provide assistance to specific groups of individuals, such as children of veterans or of Social Security recipients. Aid from these programs varies from state to state; some parents facing huge and ongoing medical expenses have actually moved to another state in order to get more comprehensive government assistance. But some aid is available in all states. Unless you can easily pay for your child's expenses, you should find out what assistance is available.

Medicaid

Medicaid is the federal program assisting the medically needy. Some states have supplemental programs providing additional benefits. But wherever you live, there are certain factors to consider.

Apply immediately for these programs at your county or city welfare or Social Security office. While sometimes payments are retroactive and may be made as long as three months after an expense has been incurred, often you have to apply *before* expenses are incurred. So, for example, if you think your child may be disabled, apply before any testing is done. If you think your child needs hospitalization, apply. If an emergency such as an accident or sudden severe illness arises, apply. You can get preliminary information by phone. Often a friend or relative can do initial legwork for you.

Eligibility requirements not only vary from state to state but are constantly being updated. If you are considering applying for assistance, call your local welfare office to find out what the general requirements are. Although you may not qualify to go on welfare, you may well qualify for a program for the "medically needy only." Such a program may provide free medical assistance or a "share of cost" (see pages 230–231).

Residency is usually a requirement for eligibility. You are usually eligible only for a program within the state in which you reside. Therefore you are not eligible when traveling in another state or abroad. Likewise, foreigners are not eligible for U.S. programs unless they are here not as visitors but as resident aliens.

Property is usually the primary determinant of eligibility. Call your local welfare office for the exact information. Do this *before* you see an agency worker, so you will know what information to bring to your first meeting. A phone call can not only save you a trip if you are ineligible but may also inform you how you could become eligible. Medicaid determines eligibility on the basis of cash and savings, but it does not take into account your outstanding bills, loans, mortgages, etc. As an example, assume the Medicaid limit of cash on hand is $1,500. If you have $3,000, you might consider paying off bills, loans, or part of your mortgage to qualify. If it is also legal in your state to purchase a "paid in full" life insurance policy of $1,500, you might consider that.

This is by no means a suggestion that you be dishonest. Rather it is a realistic picture of how you will have to work within the system and will have to understand the rules and requirements of that system. There are requirements you will not be able to work around, however. For example, a requirement may be that you not own more than one home. If you own two and sell one, the money is then part of your financial worth, probably making you too rich to qualify. You may not give property away to become eligible.

Income may or may not determine eligibility. Free medical assistance will be given if necessary. However, assistance is often granted only on a cost-sharing basis. Based upon your income and the government's cost-of-living calculations, the government determines an amount that you must pay every month for medical expenses. The government pays the rest. The amount you pay refers to your out-of-pocket expenses: if you have insurance, you pay that amount *after* the insurance has paid its portion. If you are eligible, your eligibility is from the first of the month in which you apply, and your expenses are reviewed on a monthly basis. If in any one month your expenses are high enough, you will receive assistance. So, for example, if your share of cost is $400 and your out-of-pocket expenses are $650, the government will pay $250. Since the government's calculations of monthly living expenses are very low, you may find your share of cost is very high. Your income may be high enough that you will qualify only when your child has especially high expenses, as during hospitalization. In that case you may have to reserve this program for what the medical world calls "catastrophic illnesses" and use medical insurance and private agencies to help you with regular expenses.

You are legally liable if you lie about your finances. There are occasional audits of state and county records, as well as of individual files.

The referral service provided by the welfare department's social services division can be invaluable, for that department has much information that can help you find assistance with either another government agency or a private one. This referral service is provided even if you don't qualify for Medicaid.

Crippled Children's Services

All states have programs assisting children with disabling conditions (including birth defects, accidental disabilities, and chronic diseases). Whereas the title of the program may vary from state to state, it is often called either Crippled Children's Services or simply Children's Services. Since the funding is provided by both state and local governments, the benefits can vary not only from state to state but also from county to county. The programs are usually run by the department of health or welfare.

Assistance usually provided without proof of financial eligibility includes physical and occupational therapy, which are often administered through the schools free of charge. Diagnostic testing is usually paid for only if a doctor's authorization is received *before* testing is done. This is why you should apply for assistance as soon as you think there may be a problem and not wait until one is diagnosed. Often in an emergency, coverage can begin from the time phone authorization is given by your doctor, with the understanding that you will complete any necessary paperwork as soon as possible.

Assistance based upon eligibility is often available to middle-income families who do not qualify for Medicaid. Depending upon your financial status, either your child qualifies for free services or you must assume a share of cost. Often many

of the treatments prescribed by a physician are covered, including doctors' visits, testing, hospitalization, and orthopedic equipment.

Some states provide this assistance only on a loan basis, which means that you will have to repay the money over time.

Programs for the Developmentally Disabled

Most states provide assistance for the developmentally disabled, aiding children with neurological problems (mental and motor) caused by birth defects, illness, or accidents. Although these programs can be run by the departments of health, welfare, or social services, there also are private, nonprofit agencies contracting with the state for funds to provide such services. Your county health or welfare department should be able to tell you if any such agencies exist in your state. Such an agency will often first help you determine if your child is eligible for other public funding. If not, it may help you purchase services such as diagnostic testing, appropriate schooling, day care, and sometimes even homemaker services (such as cleaning and cooking). Such assistance is provided particularly if it will help maintain the child at home or in the community rather than in an institutional setting.

Since an individual agency may have some freedom in deciding how to allocate its funds, it may be up to you to indicate your need and to convince people that your child indeed represents a worthy cause. Such pleading cannot be based just upon feelings but must be substantiated by facts. For example, if you can find out how much it would cost the state to institutionalize a child in a state facility for one year and then estimate how much you would need to get enough help to allow your child to remain at home, you could show that it would be far cheaper for the state (and ultimately the taxpayer) to assist with home care than to institutionalize your child.

Supplemental Security Income

Disabled individuals with little or no income of their own may qualify for Supplemental Security Income. However, unless your child is over 18 or does not live at home, your whole family income is considered. So whereas this program may well aid your child when he or she gets older, it may not do so now. But check on present eligibility requirements, because these are constantly changing.

Social Security

When a parent on Social Security dies or retires, his or her severely disabled child will receive Social Security payments until the age of 18. The amount is determined by how much the parent(s) paid in. After age 18 the monthly payments continue if the child's condition prevents "substantial gainful work."

Benefits to Children of Veterans

There are programs aiding children of veterans who are at least 50 percent disabled or who have died as a result of military service. Call your nearest Veterans Administration office for details.

Title 19 Federal Deeming Waiver (Model Waiver for Disabled Children) enables a disabled child to receive assistance from Medicaid and Supplemental Security Income even though he or she would not qualify under the regular federal regulations. The first child to receive such a waiver was Katie Becket, a ventilator-dependent child who was hospitalized since birth. Her parents, appealing first to elected state officials and later to President Reagan, were finally granted a waiver of regulations so that their child would get the necessary financial assistance for home care from Medicaid and Supplemental Security Income. Do check to see if your state government has passed legislation permitting Title 19 Federal Deeming Waivers. If it has not, encourage your elected state representative to do so, for even if you don't need such assistance, some other family might.

MEDICAL INSURANCE

If you cannot find enough government assistance to pay for medical care, middle-income families in particular should next consider medical insurance.

This is another complicated matter for the lay person, for a variety of plans are available from many different insurance companies. Basically, medical insurance operates on the principle of "spread the risk," meaning that if everyone pays in a small amount to a central fund, the few who need a large amount of assistance can be aided.

Benefits vary greatly. Generally the more you pay in, the greater the coverage. Most plans cover two major areas.

The basic plan covers the smaller medical expenses, such as diagnostic testing, X rays, lab work, and medication. However, there is usually an upper limit per illness or per year.

Major-medical covers most costs not covered by a basic plan. Major-medical often requires you to pay a "deductible," like the first $100 of medical expenses per individual per calendar year, after which the insurance company usually pays 80 percent of the expenses. Sometimes there is a "stop-loss clause": after a large amount, let us say $2,000 of expenses incurred in a calendar year, the company will pay 100 percent of all subsequent claims in that year. Usually there is a lifetime maximum of benefits to be paid to one individual of about $250,000. If your child is about to reach his or her lifetime maximum, there may be other ways to get financing (see pages 239–241).

Exclusions are those items that the plan will not cover, such as preventive medicine, annual physicals, outpatient care, rehabilitation, maternity benefits, hearing aids, glasses, and sometimes preexisting conditions, which are medical conditions existing *before* the policyholder took out the insurance. So be sure you read the small print of every plan and go over it with the person enrolling you in the insurance program. If your child has a medical problem, *be sure that the plan includes preexisting conditions for all family members* from the day the policy is taken out, for otherwise the child will not be covered. All additional children should be covered from the moment of birth with no 30-day waiting period. (A newborn infant needing surgery or other expensive medical care in the first month can run up a very high bill.) Although the exclusions provide general guidelines, you may try to get the medical review board of the company to consider special needs once you are insured.

Group Insurance

Group insurance is almost always a better buy than private insurance because lower premiums can be offered to a group of individuals, such as the employees of a firm or a college or members of a professional association.

Some employers offer a choice of programs. If you have a choice, the person enrolling employees for insurance should be knowledgeable and able to advise you as to the comparative virtues of the plans. If your child has problems, you are almost always better off taking the highest amount of coverage possible. The two most common options are a basic plan with major-medical and a health maintenance organization (HMO).

The basic plan and major-medical have just been discussed. If you have a choice of insurance companies, check the benefits to see which plan will give the best coverage for the types of expenses your child usually incurs.

A health maintenance organization is made up of a group of doctors, usually in one clinic, who emphasize preventive care and early detection and treatment of problems for the employees of one company. You are limited to the doctors at the clinic unless you have to be referred to an outside specialist.

Since the emphasis is on preventive medicine, coverage is available for items often not covered by regular insurance plans such as well-baby care, immunizations, periodic checkups, and sight and hearing examinations. While some expenses are covered 100 percent with no deductible, you often have copayment (a portion you must pay) on various things such as office visits, prescriptions, elective procedures (such as family planning), or treatment of mental or nervous conditions.

Most HMOs request that you pay the copayment before receiving services, which simplifies your paperwork. Such a plan may cost 20–30 percent more than a regular policy, but if your child has high medical expenses the additional coverage will probably offset this cost.

The main disadvantage of a health maintenance organization is that you are limited to the doctors in the program. If you have a choice of health maintenance organizations, check which doctors are involved in which program. If your child is already being seen by a nonaffiliated doctor with whom you have a good working relationship, you may have to consider whether improved coverage is worth changing doctors.

Preexisting conditions are often covered in group insurance. If your child has a preexisting condition so you cannot insure him or her privately, or only at very high premiums, you might consider changing employers to find a group plan that would give you the insurance coverage you need. This may sound extreme, but if your child has extensive needs you may find that where you live, where you work, and what hours you work will all be influenced by your child.

If your insurance covers preexisting conditions, never take a leave of absence or quit that job until you have another policy that will cover your child.

If your employer offers a variety of programs, preexisting conditions will usually be covered only if you take out the insurance at the time of your initial enrollment or if you change policies during the annual "open enrollment period," which is usually one month of the year. If you change plans at any other time, the company can demand a physical and thus exclude persons with preexisting conditions. The only time you can add a person with preexisting conditions to your policy during the rest of the year is if that person loses coverage from another company. For example, if parents get divorced and the employer of the parent with custody offers a group insurance policy that covers preexisting conditions at the time of enrollment, that parent can enroll the child at any time and get the benefits.

Private Insurance

The cost of private insurance is high. If you are specifically trying to insure a child with preexisting conditions, it is often astronomically high. If you cannot get group coverage and think you need insurance, make sure you have all the relevant information before taking out a policy.

Find a reputable, experienced agent who sells medical insurance and has access to a variety of plans. Again, recommendations from friends or other persons knowledgeable about the field are helpful. If you are forced to turn to the yellow pages, try to find a firm that advertises that it has been active locally for many years. Then call and ask to speak to the owner, the manager, or the head salesperson for medical insurance. Do not settle for less. You want an experienced agent so when you describe your situation he or she will be able to ask you additional questions to determine your needs. It helps if you ask the agent specific questions about whether the insurance plan covers medical expenses you think your child might incur. (The preceding pages on medical insurance should give you ideas about questions to raise.) If the agent seems unable to answer your questions readily with detailed knowledge of the actual coverage of the plan, he or she may sell you an inappropriate policy. If in doubt, call another agent to discuss your situation. If your child has unusual needs and no agent can satisfactorily answer your questions, call (collect) the national offices of a few insurance companies and discuss your problem with people well versed in medical insurance. Make sure you receive any policy explanations in writing.

Mail-order firms with whom you have no personal contact have limitations precisely because it is difficult for you to know what you need without talking to an informed agent. Also, your local agent is your advocate in case there is a claim problem. The exception here may be plans with limited coverage, such as those offering, say, a limited amount for every week you are hospitalized. If you know that your child will be hospitalized for several weeks every year, you might want to take out such a policy in addition to your regular one for extra protection.

Consider the cost. If your medical expenses are going to be very high, if the cost of private insurance is also going to be very high, and if your income is only moderate, you have three choices. Consider carefully the financial virtues of each.

1. Buy the insurance.
2. Change jobs so you can get a policy that will cover the preexisting conditions of your dependents.
3. Don't buy insurance and simply rely on government programs, such as Medicaid and your state's Children's Services, augmented by the help you can get from private agencies.

Getting the Most out of Your Insurance Policy

Simply being insured is not enough. You have to learn how to use the policy. Since you may have many and frequent claims, sometimes for extraordinary items, consider the following.

Withhold payment of the medical bill until you receive insurance payment if you are on a tight budget. If you explain your financial situation to your doctor, he or she may let you withhold all or part of your payment until you are reimbursed by the insurance company. The monthly statements from the physician's office will remind you to file your claims regularly and will draw your attention to any slow processing of your claims. Legally, you have to make only a small payment every month (as little as $1) to keep the bill collector at bay.

Work directly with one particular claims examiner. If you have many claims, you should deal with a person who knows your child's problems and who has the authority to help you. If your claims are not processed locally, you can try to find the appropriate person by mail, but it is usually faster and easier to call the supervisor of claims for your area and discuss your situation. (Place a collect call to the insurance company, stating that you are a customer. Your call will either be accepted or you will be asked for your number for a return call on their line. If this fails, dial direct, since that is cheapest.)

When you reach a knowledgeable person, explain your problem and ask if in the future you may send your claims directly to him or her. If so, the examiner will get to know the special problems of your child and be able to write instructions on your child's chart and enter the relevant information into the computer, thus greatly facilitating the processing of your claims.

If the company is slow in paying or rejects a claim, you can then call this individual and ask for help. Be sure to keep notes on telephone conversations about your child's claims, including the date, agents, and decisions reached.

Submit claim forms methodically. It saves time and effort if you ask all vendors of medical services to submit bills directly to the insurance company for you. However, many will ask you to pay and then submit your claim form to the insurance company for reimbursement. Have a separate "Claims Submitted" folder for each member of the family.

Fill out claim forms carefully. It is better to spend a few extra minutes to do so than to have the insurance company withhold payment because it needs additional information.

- Make sure you fill in every blank in the form.
- Make sure the form is submitted in the claimant's full name. For example, if your child's name is Belinda Elizabeth, she may be known in your community as Betsy, but the insurance company's computer will probably recognize claims only for Belinda Elizabeth Smith.
- Do not abbreviate anything. You may, for example, be tempted to write MS for muscular dystrophy or CP for cerebral palsy. If the same claims examiner does not always process your claims, the form may be returned to you for further information.

Make a copy of every claim form and bill you submit. If your forms are numbered and you are using carbon paper on an extra form for your own copy, be sure to write in the number of the original claim on your copy. However, some computers now assign a new number to a claim form when it is processed, rendering that original number useless to you and them. Your copy is important protection against loss of the original in the mail or by the insurance company; you will need it for your own reference when you receive claim payments.

Mark the upper corner of your copy with the initial of the given family member, numbering

that person's claims consecutively. Your daughter Belinda Elizabeth's eleventh claim for the year would be numbered B-11. In this way you can easily keep track of any bills that are being held up. When your folders fill, these numbers are easier to refer to than the dates of the bills' submission. If, for example, you note that B-3 has not been paid but all others through B-10 have been, call your insurance supervisor collect and inquire about B-3. Sometimes claims get lost, in which case you will have to resubmit. Since you have a copy of the claim and the bills, this will not be difficult. Remember, you must always retain a copy so you can refer to or resubmit the information if necessary.

Keep a list of prescription numbers with names of the drugs in your folder. Often your receipts will list only the number of the prescription; however, the insurance company wants the drug's name. If you buy at only one pharmacy and have a charge account there, your complete monthly statement should include all prescriptions filled. If the statement lists only the prescription number, phone the pharmacist and add any new drugs with their numbers to your master list. This record will greatly assist your record keeping.

Don't claim too many different kinds of items on one form. If one item is rejected, usually the processing of the whole form is delayed. Even though the form is divided into two parts, such as health-care services and prescriptions, fill in only one part. Although you will end up with more pieces of paper this way, by limiting how much you submit on each form you will ultimately simplify and expedite the processing of your claims.

Recording Claims Payments

Submitting a claim is only part of the task. Keeping track of the payments is equally important.

Start a "Claims Paid" folder for each family member. When you receive a payment, you will also receive information on how the claim was handled, often called the "Report to the Subscriber."

Be sure the claim number corresponds to the number on your original claim. If it does not, the computer may be assigning its own numbers, so check vendor, date, and cost.

Mark the report form with your code, say, B-11, and staple the report form to your copy of the original claim.

Indicate on the report form exactly what you did and when. For example, if you sent the insurance check directly to the physician, laboratory, or other vendor, note this, including the amount of the check, the vendor, and the date on which you sent it. If your insurance covers, say, 80 percent of the cost and a voluntary health agency has agreed to pay the outstanding 20 percent, send the agency a copy of the "Report to the Subscriber" with a letter reiterating the payment agreement previously reached and thanking them in advance for their assistance. This letter should then be placed in a special file for that specific agency.

Place the original claim, bill, and "Report to Subscriber," all stapled together, in your "Claims Paid" folder.

If you get a check that does not correspond to the total of any single submitted claim, the insurance company may have lumped items of different claims together. So try to add some items from another unpaid claim to the one indicated by the payment number. You may need to add up several different items to unravel the mystery. Also, some items will be paid 100 percent, while others will be covered only 80 percent, so you may have to try to figure out which items are fully covered and which only partially (and maybe even which were refused). If you are still baffled and can't solve the mystery, call your claims examiner.

Questionable and Rejected Claims

Learn what to do with rejected claims. The principle is never to take no for an answer if you think your claim is valid. Even if your child needs some unusual items, you should try to get the insurance company to pay for them. If you know when you originally submit the claim that an item may not be covered, attach a letter from your physician indicating why the item is vital for your child's medical care. If you neglect to send this cover letter and payment for the item is rejected, ask your doctor to write a support letter and send it to the supervisor, requesting that your claim be forwarded with this letter to the company's medical review board, which considers unusual claims. Since it is always difficult to get people to change their minds once they have said no, it is best to supply all convincing information when any extraordinary claim is first submitted.

Letters must be as forceful as possible. Since doctors are busy people, they do not always write long, informative letters. Therefore you may be able to work out an arrangement with your doctor whereby you provide a list of salient points, or you may even draft a letter that your doctor can then edit and have retyped on his or her letterhead. This is not being devious. Rather you are saving your doctor time and ensuring that the request has the best possible chance of being honored the first time you make it.

A questionable item is something not commonly used for medical purposes, such as a whirlpool bath, or something not purchased from a regular medical vendor, such as cleaning solution for medical equipment. If you can prove that you need the item for medical purposes, or that you can get it cheaper from a nonmedical source, the insurance company may pay for it.

VOLUNTARY HEALTH AGENCIES

After you have discovered which expenses can be defrayed by government agencies and medical insurance, if you still have more medical expenses than you can pay yourself, consider voluntary health agencies. These are established to help individuals with special needs; they vary greatly in what they can and what they are willing to provide. Since their help can be invaluable, we should indeed be grateful to them. But in case you have the impression that they simply give away money, you should be aware of how they function.

Although people working for voluntary health agencies usually genuinely desire to help, they may not understand your economic straits. Also, since these agencies work very hard to raise their money, they are usually very cautious about how it is spent. Persons in charge of fund allocation are held accountable for how they spend that money. They have budgets and bookkeeping procedures to follow that do not allow for maximum flexibility. Also, sometimes an agency will want to show the public that it is indeed helping needy individuals, so it will stress public-service projects, such as supplying a taxi van for the disabled, because this generates much more publicity and community support than providing orthopedic shoes. This is not to say that one item is more important than another but to indicate that it is sometimes difficult to get help for direct services (assistance given directly to specific persons for their individual medical needs).

Some agencies are a joy to work with; others can be extremely difficult. However, an agency is established to aid needy individuals, and you can provide it with the opportunity to assist.

Discovering which agencies can help you is not always easy. Begin by contacting all agencies that might be even remotely interested in your child's problem. All agencies provide a variety of information services, including advice about other groups that may be able to help you. While some agencies provide direct financial assistance, it is usually only for certain items or services. Therefore you may come to rely on a number of organizations for different services and funding.

Contacting the agency is the first step toward receiving assistance. Sometimes a doctor or social worker will refer you to an agency. Ordinarily you have to make contact yourself. Usually it is best to telephone the agency first to see if it can indeed help with your child's needs. At some point, personal contact must be established. Sometimes its social worker will make a home visit, in which case it is much easier for you to show him or her your living situation, your child, and your child's medical needs. If no one from an agency wants to come to you, try to take your child to the agency at least once so the personnel will know you both and have a better understanding of why you are making your request.

Financial need is usually the criterion for assistance. While a few agencies will pay for any "standard" item for someone with the designated disability or illness, regardless of your financial need (for example, the Muscular Dystrophy Association of America will buy wheelchairs), most agencies will want to assess your financial situation. If you think you have a legitimate need, it is your responsibility to prove it. Often you will have to fill out a standard form that may not clearly depict your financial situation. So feel free to add any information you think is relevant.

The actual request is your opportunity to convince an agency that your need is reasonable. Since agencies must respond to written correspondence, even if you discuss the matter by phone, make every request in writing (typed if possible), clearly and concisely stating your child's medical need and backing up your request with a written prescription or a letter from your doctor. Again, since not every doctor has the time or interest to write as complete a letter as you might desire, you will be doing both yourself and the doctor a favor by writing down all the relevant details and conveying them to your doctor in person or by mail, or at least dictating the information to his or her secretary over the phone. As mentioned before, your doctor may not mind if you draft a letter for editing. Remember, a good letter may convince the agency to help you.

Unusual requests will arise if your child has extraordinary needs. Examples of such requests, which must be convincingly made if payment is to follow, fall into three main categories:

1. *Items routinely or frequently rejected by insurance companies,* such as hearing aids or orthopedic shoes, are readily paid for if you can find an agency addressing itself to persons with that particular disability and need. However, there are other items, such as a whirlpool bath, which are requested infrequently and for which the medical

need could be considered questionable. In this case, if you can convince the insurance company to pay 80 percent (see page 236), a local agency may agree to pay the remaining 20 percent.

2. *Items no one ever paid for before* can be submitted. If your child needs unique items, perhaps made especially for you by a nonmedical person, you may be able to convince a local agency to pay for these.

3. *Costs of maintenance and repair of equipment* may be covered by whoever paid for it originally. So if the insurance company paid 80 percent of the purchase price of a piece of equipment and an agency paid 20 percent, you can try to get the same split for maintenance and repair. You can probably convince the insurance company and the local agency that the maintenance and repair of equipment your child uses regularly are ongoing costs and it is cheaper to help with this than to replace the equipment.

Retroactive requests are disliked by most agencies because they cannot carefully analyze whether the request is justified. In addition, an agency may feel pressured to provide financial assistance for an item a family has already purchased and doesn't feel it can pay for itself. An agency greatly prefers that you have prior medical authorization for all expenditures and that the requests proceed (often at a snail's pace) through the appropriate channels. Unfortunately, you are not always able to perceive needs in advance. For example, in an emergency, you need additional equipment immediately, not three weeks later after the appropriate committee has met and the board has given approval. Sometimes equipment can be rented, with the first month's rent deducted from the purchase price. This gives you 30 days to find the money. In other cases, you may have to buy the item and then start the laborious process of finding someone to pay for it.

Special funds may be established by an agency if you are constantly coming up with unusual requests, often of a retroactive nature. With strong support from your physician, you may be able to work out an agreement with an agency to set up a special fund allowing a certain amount of money per year for your child's care. This way you will not have to send in a physi-

cian's support letter for every request. Such a fund could cover any amount not covered by your insurance (while it is, of course, understood that only a certain sum is available). Payment will probably be made by the charity directly to the vendor upon receipt of the bill from you, without your needing to establish the legitimacy of each item. This arrangement saves time and effort for your doctor, the agency, and you.

Refusals are not uncommon. Despite all your carefully planned efforts, you may find that getting an agency to part with its money is very, very difficult.

If you get annoyed about the refusals you are sure to encounter, it is hard on you and your family and this won't help establish a good working relationship with the agencies whose assistance you really need. Keep smiling, and remain determined and persuasive. Polite insistence can work wonders.

Keeping records is vital when you are successful in getting assistance from agencies. Begin by starting a folder for each agency and keeping in it a carbon or photocopy of any correspondence or bills submitted to that agency, using a numbering system as with insurance, where B-1-CP would indicate the first claim to the United Cerebral Palsy Association for your daughter Belinda Elizabeth for that year. Also add to your folder any notes of telephone conversations. Keep careful track of bills submitted and bills paid, especially if the agency pays a vendor directly for services for which you have been billed. Computers often get very confused when an agency, rather than the individual, sends money and doesn't clearly indicate whose account should be credited.

Give thanks for any help received from an agency. It's a good idea to write thank-you letters (keeping copies in the agency's folder), since correspondence is often read at board meetings. A carefully drafted letter will help board members better understand the needs of individuals such as your child. Even if you have had extreme difficulty in getting help from a particular agency, you should still be polite to have the strongest effect. Factual information such as the date of the request and the final date of assistance received will indicate an excessively slow pace without your pointing this out specifically.

Official complaints are sometimes necessary. If you think that an agency is running a particularly abysmal show and that the needs of other children are not being met either, complain. If only your requests are being turned down, try to figure out why.

Complaints can be lodged with whoever is next up the line in the agency from the person with whom you are experiencing difficulty. If a committee reviewing your request moves very slowly, contact the director. If the director is incompetent, contact the chairman of the board. However, since incompetence is a serious accusation, be sure that it is not just a personality conflict but that the director's brusque and rude manner, tardiness in returning phone calls, etc., make it difficult for many members of the community to work with this individual and that the agency's image is being tarnished. Since you are trying to help people understand and empathize with the needy, have factual information to support any complaint, and proceed with tact. If you think insufficient monies are being spent on direct services, substantiate your claims with a review of the actual expenditures of other non-profit organizations, which must be open to the public.

You can follow up a series of telephone complaints with a carefully drafted letter if you really feel the agency is not serving the needs of the community. If you proceed tactfully, your action should not adversely affect your future requests for assistance. Any responsible board will want to know of any serious, unwarranted difficulties a client encounters.

Becoming a board member has pros and cons. Through board or committee membership you can express gratitude, help others, and learn how such organizations function. But active participation takes time and energy—sometimes nervous energy if the agency is poorly run. You will have to decide if you can learn enough and be effective enough to make being a board member worthwhile at this time, particularly if caring for your child is very demanding.

Interagency meetings can be arranged if your child has high medical expenses and receives support from different agencies. Your social worker may coordinate work among agencies, but you know your child's needs best and are therefore often his or her best advocate. If you think a meeting including you, your physician, and representatives of the agencies that are (or that you would like to have) involved in your child's care may be helpful, discuss it with your doctor. If he or she thinks it is appropriate, let your doctor choose the meeting date and then arrange the meeting yourself, unless you have a competent social worker to do it for you. You might try to have such meetings at your house so the people can meet your child and see how he or she lives and what he or she needs. Since the main purpose of such a meeting is to establish one's financial need, and a parent can often do this best, always prepare a comprehensive financial statement (with copies for everyone) so each participant can see how much financial assistance you need and who is contributing in which areas. A sample statement is shown in figure 17-1.

Creative Financing Through Friendly yet Forceful Persuasion

Sometimes, in spite of your best efforts, you may see your child's medical bills mounting, with no way to pay them. At that point, you may need help from someone in your community or at the state level who has learned how to develop and present a comprehensive plan of an individual's financial needs to insurance and/or governmental agencies in such a way that the package is irresistible. For example, say a ventilator-dependent child who is hospitalized for $40,000 a month could be cared for at home for about $12,000 a month. And if it placed these funds into an interest-earning account, within three years the interest would pay for any continuing home care for the child. Who could resist that? And if there is no way to show irresistible savings, then one can still appeal to the finer humanitarian qualities in people. If, for example, your child has almost reached his or her lifetime insurance limit, the directors of the insurance

MEDICAL EXPENSES FOR BELINDA ELIZABETH SMITH, 1985*

	EASTER SEAL	MUSCULAR DYSTROPHY	REGIONAL CENTER	VISITING NURSES	SMITH FAMILY
Physicians:					
Pediatrician					
Chiropractor					
Orthopedist					
Radiologist					
Respiratory diseases specialist					
Rehabilitation medicine specialist					
Pediatric dentist					
Laboratory work:					
Prescriptions:					
Food supplements:					
Vitamins, protein powder, etc.					
Equipment:					
IPPB machine					
Emergency bed alarm					
Wheelchair repair					
Orthopedic equipment:					
Leg splints					
Body jacket					
Registered nurses:					
Paramedical assistance:†					
TOTALS:					

*Another sheet could read "Projected Expenses, 1986."
†Item not covered by insurance. All other amounts listed are the 20% not covered by insurance.

Figure 17-1   Sample financial statement.

company certainly wouldn't want you child to go without the health care he or she needs, would they? If carefully presented proposals fall on deaf ears, it is always possible to appeal to the public by getting the media to present your case to the people after you have told officials involved in providing financing for your child's care that unless some progress can be made by a certain date you do think the individuals in your community should be made aware of the problem. After all, the media are always looking for human interest stories and are happy to help individuals get the services that they truly need.

Some creative doctors and directors of state children's services have always managed to get their children the services they need; you can too.

PLANNING FOR THE FUTURE

Life Insurance

Unless you have a large extended family or group of friends who can financially help you in case of need, consider life insurance, if the premiums are not too high.

You may want to buy life insurance for both parents, for if your child requires a great deal of nursing care and one parent dies, the other parent will either have to stay home or hire someone to do so while he or she goes out to work.

There are both private and group life-insurance plans. Group plans are cheaper and less likely to have preexisting-conditions clauses that exclude anyone with a known medical problem of a serious nature. Sometimes there are modified preexisting-conditions clauses indicating that the policy will pay after a person has been enrolled for a certain length of time, such as two years. Preexisting-conditions clauses are meant to prevent terminally ill persons from taking out large policies right before their deaths.

Carefully consider if you want to insure the father, mother, or both and whether you can insure dependents. Since many family plans do not have preexisting-conditions clauses for children, such insurance could be valuable. If your child has a progressive illness and you buy life insurance for him or her, you may pay premiums for years. But if your child does die, any life-insurance payments could help offset medical expenses you incurred.

Wills and Trusts

Every parent should have a will. This is especially true for parents of an ill or disabled child. Two important factors in your will will be who will be your child(ren)'s legal guardian and what will happen to your estate.

Any will should be drafted by a competent attorney who has experience in this specific type of estate planning.

A legal guardian is necessary for any minor. If your son or daughter is now unable to care for himself or herself and will probably continue to be unable to care do so as an adult, it is vital to make provision for your child's care should both parents die. To ensure that your child remains in a family and is not institutionalized, see if a close friend will agree to be designated as legal guardian of your children and estate. (Usually both of these responsibilities are delegated to one party unless you have a very large estate.) If you don't ask your friends if they would be willing to be legal guardians, your child could become a ward of the state after your death.

If your child is living at home, you might want to make an agreement with another family, recorded in the wills of both, that if the parents in one family die the other family will become the legal guardians of any surviving children and take them into its home. If your child is not living at home, he or she will still need a legal guardian until he or she comes of age.

The inheritance of your assets is the other factor to consider. If you do not have a will, any family assets will be divided equally among the surviving children. However, if your disabled child, either intentionally through your will or unintentionally through your failure to make a will, inherits assets having a value in excess of an amount specified by the government (presently $1,500), he or she will no longer be eligible for Supplemental Security Income. This can be very important if your child is very ill or severely disabled. In the absence of SSI qualification, it is often extremely difficult to qualify for any of the other state and federal benefit programs. The money provided in your bequest or gift to your disabled child may be totally insufficient to meet his or her needs, but those funds will have to be exhausted to the dollar limit before eligibility can be reobtained. This means that if you leave your child assets, either through a poorly planned will or through lack of planning, your child may be denied services to which he or she would otherwise be eligible if only the disability were considered. Therefore carefully draft your will so some portion of your estate can supplement the government benefits without disqualifying your child for those benefits. The key to financial eligibility for government benefits is the "availability" of the funds to your child. If the assets are put in a properly worded trust for your child, he or she is not considered to *own* them; rather, the assets in the trust are used to supplement other assets owned by the beneficiary or in which the beneficiary may have some interest. In other words, it should be clear that the trust is not intended to provide primary support for the ill or disabled person. The trustee (the person who manages the assets) should have complete discretion to determine when and if the beneficiary needs any supplemental services or programs. Payments that are made from the trust go directly to the persons who supply goods or services to the beneficiary. A "spendthrift" program should be included in the trust, indicating that the beneficiary has no ownership interest whatsoever in the assets placed in the trust. You can also name someone to receive the funds when your disabled child no longer needs them. A provision can even be included that would require a distribution of the remaining assets in the trust to a nondisabled family member in the event that the state brought litigation against the trust or refused to provide benefits to the disabled beneficiary because of the existence of the trust. You might contact your local association for mentally retarded persons to get the names of reputable lawyers who are well versed in the pertinent state and federal laws and who have experience in setting up such trusts and wills.

Even if your child is not so disabled as to require careful estate planning to ensure any needed government services, remember that if you do not set up a trust your child will receive his or her total inheritance upon coming of age. A trust may be appropriate if you want to give guidance for the allocation and use of funds after your child comes of age.

PART 5

IF YOUR CHILD
IS DYING

18

How to Care for
Your Dying Child at Home

Long ago in India there lived a woman named Kisa Gotami. When her only child died, in her overwhelming grief she visited all the homes in the village, asking for a curative medicine. Though the neighbors sympathized, they could provide none and felt she had lost her senses, for the boy was indeed dead. Finally she met a man who said, "I cannot give thee medicine for thy child, but I know one who can."

And the woman pleaded, "Pray, tell me, who?"

The man replied, "Go to the Buddha."

So Kisa Gotami went to the Buddha and cried, "Lord and Master, give me medicine that will cure my boy."

The Buddha answered, "I need but a single mustard seed, but it must come from a house where no one has lost a child, a husband, a wife, a parent, or a friend."

Kisa Gotami again went from house to house, asking for mustard seed. Even the poorest were willing to give her some, but when she then asked if anyone had died there, she found that in every house some beloved person had died. Finally she came to understand that death is common to us all, that there are no means by which those who have been born can avoid dying, for death is as much a part of life as creation. Her mind at peace, she calmly buried her child and returned to the Buddha, thanking him for sharing his wisdom with her.

People who have cared for the dying will tell you that although there are some "difficult" deaths,

just as there are "difficult" births, the actual moment of death is, from all outward appearances, peaceful. And although no one who has died has come back to tell us what it was like, people who have been declared clinically dead but who were later revived give similar accounts of the death experience, reporting it as an overwhelmingly calm and positive event and saying that they will never fear death again. Nevertheless, most of us are not prepared for death as an event and have difficulty finding meaning in it. This is especially so for the death of a child, which you can only accept according to your own set of beliefs. Whether you turn to religion, friends and family, or professional counseling, you must come to terms with the death of your child so you can be grateful for what he or she contributed to your life and remember your child in a positive, enriching way.

If your child is terminally ill, you will have to consider the following:

- How do you talk to your child about death?
- How do you decide to stop treatment and provide only comfort care?
- How do you care for your dying child?
- How do you keep your household running in the last stages?
- What are common signs of impending death?

Talking to Your Child About Death

If your child has a life-threatening illness and is getting worse, honest communication about death is vital. It may be extremely difficult to bring yourself to discuss death and dying with your child, but a child who is sick enough to die knows it and has a right to the information he or she wants or needs. And as difficult as it may be for you to initiate a conversation or to answer your child's questions about death, you too need the opportunity to share your feelings with your child through honest communication. In all this it cannot be overemphasized that there is no one right way to think and talk about death, just as there is no one right way to live life. What is true is that it is much easier to live with things you can talk about, and this includes death.

If you are reluctant to speak to your child about death, your child will sense this and his or her very real need to talk about it will be unmet. Moreover, a child who feels that you must be protected from the discomfort or pain of discussing death carries an unnecessary burden at a time when he or she already has enough to cope with.

If your child is not afraid that you are reluctant to discuss death, he or she will probably ask you questions about it. These questions may be oblique: "What will happen if I'm inside my oxygen tent and a fire breaks out?" or "What happens to the mouse when Pussy catches and eats it?" When your child asks such questions, try to pick up on what is really being asked. At other times, your child's questions may be more specific and direct, such as "What is heaven like?" It is perfectly fair to return the question and ask what your child thinks so as to gain your child's perspective before sharing your own.

Never give your child a dishonest answer to the most important questions he or she has ever asked—"What is it like to die?" or "Am I dying?" A lie at this point can break the communication between you and your child, whereas the truth may provide great relief to your child, who will be grateful that you told the truth (and told it yourself) and will realize that it is possible to communicate honestly with you. Your child will know if your answer is dishonest or evasive and will look elsewhere or turn inward for answers that a child is poorly equipped to provide.

Being truthful to your child involves learning to say the right thing in the right way at the right time. The day your child is diagnosed with a fatal illness is probably not the time to give him or her all the details of the illness and the projected treatment, but eventually your child will need to be given this information. In like fashion, your child will need to know that he or she is going to die, including the fact that no one can say exactly how (although an older child should know what the possible alternatives are) or exactly when.

Since the unknown is much harder to deal with than the known, your child's questions about dying and being dead may center on those six questions a newspaper reporter asks to get the whole story: who? why? what? where? how? and when? Obviously, one difficulty in answering these questions is that we do not know the exact answers. Nevertheless, you should share what you do know with your child and listen to what he or she thinks.

"*Who* is going to die?" might be phrased "Am I dying?" This is a vital question that must be answered honestly to keep communication open. A child can become afraid of dying if he or she thinks death is imminent but no one will admit it.

"*Why* am I going to die?" is a question you probably cannot answer with certainty. It is all right to say you don't know—better to be honest than to try to simplify your beliefs in a way that distorts them but still offers no great solace. Most children would rather be with their mothers and fathers than anyone else, even God. So to say your child is dying because God wants him or her may not make your child feel better at all and may actually confuse your child. If you tell your child that God loves him or her so much that God wants your child in heaven, your child may believe, for example, that by being naughty he or she will live. And make sure your child doesn't have the common misconception that he or she is dying because he or she was bad. The simple fact that sometimes our bodies become so ill that they cannot function anymore and they die tells why physical death occurs.

"*What* is it like to die?" Judging from interviews with people who have been pronounced dead but revived, death is a peaceful event, whether the person is an atheist or a devout believer in God.

"*Where* do people go after they die?" Often what children fear most is loneliness—that regardless of where they go, Mother and Father will not be there with them. If your child has such a fear, you have to try to explain, within the context of your child's beliefs, that he or she will not be alone. You might say something like: "My love will be with you. Since you will be in a different state, this will be as strong as my physical presence now." Others may believe they will be with God. Do not tell your child that he or she will be alone in a grave.

"*How* am I going to die?" At one level, it is perfectly true to say that no one knows how a person will die. But doctors can predict the course of the last stages of many illnesses and should be willing to share this information. Children who have been hospitalized may have an idea of what will happen, but if they want more information they should be given it. Some children, especially after long and painful treatment, come to fear pain. These children need to be assured that good pain control can usually be obtained as death approaches and that dying is seldom painful; rather it is a release from pain.

"*When* am I going to die?" This is a question no one can answer in advance. However, if a family has consciously decided to stop treatment, they may be told approximately how long their child will live and should be willing to share this with the child in a loving way that always leaves room for some hope. "You'll die before June 1" is different from saying, "You'll probably die in the next few weeks, but we'll make you as comfortable as we can, and we look forward to the joy each day will bring us." A child who says, "I hope it won't be long. Will it be long?" may not need your opinion in the matter as much as he or she needs to know that it is all right to die and that you will be there until the end. Since the most fearful aspect of death for some children is their separation anxiety, children need to know that their parents will be emotionally and physically close to them while they are dying. Exactly what is said is less important than keeping open communication.

Some parents whose child could never or can no longer speak wonder whether they should tell their child that he or she is dying. Even if a two-way conversation is not possible, it is important that you share what you know with your child. Take as an example a boy with a brain tumor who has had CAT scans in the course of his treatment. His condition deteriorates, he can no longer speak, and the latest scan indicates that, indeed, the tumor is growing. Now even if the child can no longer verbally ask the results of the test, he may still wonder what the results were. Not to tell him can begin that conspiracy of silence when the parent knows the result and the boy probably intuitively knows it too and knows that his parents are not being honest and open. It is as unfair to place the burden of silence on this child as on a speaking one. In a very real sense you show your respect for your child by sharing what he or she is entitled to know about the future. Information about his or her condition can help a child prepare for death in his or her own way. A major, ground-breaking book on the subject of death is Elizabeth Kübler-Ross's *On Death and Dying*, which is important reading for the families of terminally ill patients as well as for the patients themselves, if they are old enough to understand it. See Appendix 3, "Suggested Reading," for this book and others that can help you if your child is dying.

How Do You Decide to Stop Treatment and Provide Only Comfort Care?

While modern medicine can cure some diseases and arrest the progression of others, a point may come when you must ask yourself whether using drugs with only the remotest hope of a remission or cure, or prolonging life through use of medical technology, is worthwhile. In other words, a time may come when medical care may prolong your child's life but neither cure the condition nor improve the quality of life, when extending the dying process may not extend the meaningfulness of life. If you come to such a point, you have to make an extremely difficult decision on the basis of the information you have, and you may never know what would have happened had you chosen otherwise. The only certain thing is that a decision must be made.

Discuss these matters periodically with your doctor; if a crisis arises, you might have to make a decision immediately and you should have seriously considered in advance what you truly feel should be done. It is no easier to unplug life-support systems once they have been connected than it is not to start them; perhaps it is more difficult.

And while there are some illnesses in which a crisis may precipitate the need for a quick decision, there are also chronic illnesses in which the time may come when the treatment becomes worse than the disease, and you will have to decide whether or not to continue treatment. If your child is not an infant, he or she should probably be involved in this decision. An article in the *Journal of Pediatrics* (vol. 101, no. 3, September 1982) called "Therapeutic Choices Made by Patients with End-Stage Cancer," by Ruprecht Nitschke, M.D., et al., deals with the role of children in deciding on treatment. The article reports on a program in a children's hospital in which, with parental consent, all cancer patients older than three are informed that they have cancer that will result in death if not treated. While details given vary according to the child's age and intellectual capacity, the therapy and side effects are discussed. When children over five no longer respond to standard therapy, the nature of the disease, its recent progression, and the unavailability of any other drugs known to be effective are discussed. The remaining therapeutic choices are then considered as objectively as possible: supportive care with the imminence of death or the use of experimental "phase II" drugs. Of the 44 families included in the study, all but one felt that their child should be included in the final-stage conference and help make the decision about further therapy.

This pioneering study is very important because it shows that medical professionals, parents, and children can all work together to answer an extremely important question: Should I stop trying to treat my child's disease and concentrate on supportive care? Be sure that not only your child but also the doctors know how you feel, so if they need to make a decision based upon their medical expertise it will be in accordance with what you would wish for your child.

Each case is different and each family must make its own decision as to when person-oriented comfort care is more appropriate than disease-oriented treatment.

Comfort care means exactly what the words imply—making the child as comfortable as possible, which is usually at home. It means eliminating drugs and procedures not needed to relieve symptoms. Emergency measures to avoid death (often called heroic measures) such as cardiopulmonary resuscitation or the use of life-support systems may also no longer be appropriate. The active care is in providing the food and liquids your child wants (if any), relieving as much discomfort as you can, letting your child rest, and providing the love, understanding, and support he or she needs for peace of mind and the knowledge that you will be with him or her to the end. With the help of health-care professionals and your own child, you can learn how to care for your dying child.

How Do You Care for Your Dying Child?

Most children would rather die at home, and most parents can learn to care for a dying child at home. If you have been caring for your severely ill child at home for some time, the knowledge that he or she will soon die may not greatly alter the routine you have established. If you have not, you should discuss with your physician what would be involved in home care and then decide what you think would be best. Most parents who decide on home care are happy that they do and find that they can manage. Some parents decide to take a child back to the hospital if they are exhausted themselves or if they can no longer handle their child's medical problems. But even families who take their child back to the hospital are usually happy to have had some time at home together.

If you decide that disease-oriented treatment is no longer appropriate, you can learn, with the assistance of health-care professionals, how to provide person-oriented comfort care for your child at home. Considering the following factors may help you get the information and organize the resources you will need.

How will your child die? It is most helpful if you have some idea what will happen in the last stages of your child's illness. Ignorance may be easier as long as there are no major changes in your child's condition, but ignorance can also cause fear, because either you worry about what might happen or you panic when changes in your child's condition do occur.

If you ask your doctor how your child will die and he or she doesn't know, this not knowing is very different from your not knowing. Your doctor may not know exactly what is going to happen but he or she probably thinks one of a number of alternatives will occur. Try to learn what these alternatives might be, and the possible signs of approaching death, so you can act with knowledge rather than out of ignorance. If you are prepared for changes you can, step-by-step along the way, talk with your doctor and together intelligently decide what to do next on the basis of answers to questions such as:

- What is happening now?
- What would be the best thing to do from now on?
- Will this make my child more comfortable or prolong my child's life?

Whom should you contact if you need help during the day, at night, or on weekends? It is very important to plan with your doctor what you should do in case of need. Some doctors will always want to be contacted directly even if they are not on call; others will ask you to contact the physician with whom they share call. If your doctor's partners may be responding to your call, request that your doctor keep them informed as to your child's condition from day to day.

Can you manage alone or will you need any health-care professionals to help? Frequently a doctor who agrees that you should care for your child at home will also be willing to make house calls as needed. If for some reason he or she cannot, the doctor may want a visiting nurse to come by periodically. It is important to have some health-care professional see your child regularly, since such a professional has the knowledge and training to appraise your child's condition and help decide if any changes in treatment are indicated. Even if the visiting health-care professional only tells you to do more of the same, this information can be very reassuring. You may of course need a professional to help you every day if your child needs specialized care.

Is there a local hospice organization that can help you make arrangements and offer support?

How can your family best provide the necessary nursing care? If you decide to manage without professional help, try to arrange for your family to work in shifts, so someone is always with your child but everyone has some hours off to sleep or just get out of the house. However you arrange things, it is very important to remember to take care of yourself. If you get totally exhausted, you will not be able to provide the help your child needs—neither the physical care nor the compassion and loving support.

How can you best provide for your child's daily nurturing care? Detailed instructions on this are given in Chapters 7 through 12. However, there are certain points worth mentioning in regard to the dying child.

Equipment (including wheel chairs) can sometimes be borrowed from the Visiting Nurses, the Cancer Society, or whatever organization in your community has a loan closet.

Bedding. If your child will spend much time lying down and you have not modified his or her bed, consider getting a foam pad to put under the sheet or a synthetic sheepskin to place on top of the sheet, since these can make lying more comfortable and help prevent bedsores. Consult a rehabilitation specialist or other health-care professional involved with your child as to the best device. A wedge-shaped pillow or a hospital bed may provide more comfort for the back than propping your child up on pillows, which do not support the spine. However, if your child doesn't want anything that brings hospitals to mind, don't push it.

Toileting. If your child can no longer use the regular toilet, read pages 141–145 on toileting.

Constipation can be a side effect of some pain medication, so check that your child is having regular bowel movements. If he or she is not, discuss with your doctor if you should do anything about it. However, shortly before death bodily functions often start to shut down, so your child may urinate and defecate less frequently than before, if at all.

Your child may get concerned when he or she can't control bodily functions; you have to be loving, supportive, and tactful, explaining that it's fine to do things differently than before if this is easier and more comfortable.

Bathing. If showers or tub baths are no longer practical, you can just give your child a sponge bath. Although we may feel more comfortable if we bathe every day, you shouldn't feel you must give your child a complete daily bath unless he or she wants it or needs one for medical reasons.

Hair care. Here again comfort is more important than looks or what you have done in the past. Wash your child's hair only if he or she really wants it done. Also use your discretion about brushing hair.

Mouth care. Most people feel more comfortable if their mouths are clean. If using a soft tooth-brush and toothpaste becomes difficult, you can use a lemon-glycerine swab or a Q-tip dipped in Gly-Oxide (a special type of pleasant-tasting peroxide). A child who is eating very little and becoming comatose would probably be just as happy if you didn't bother brushing his or her teeth. If you see that your child's lips are becoming chapped and dry, apply some lip ointment.

Eye care. A child who becomes comatose may not blink very much anymore and the eyes will become dry. Ask your doctor if eye drops might make your child more comfortable.

Massage. Sometimes gentle massage can make your child more comfortable, especially if he or she is stiff and sore. Let your child tell you what feels good, trust your hands, and soon you will find what works best. Using a body lotion or powder may feel good.

Food and liquid. While diet may have been very important before, now that you have decided upon comfort care, give your child what he or she says tastes good, even if it seems peculiar to you. If your child decides not to eat or drink much of anything, that is fine too. Giving intravenous feeding at this point may prolong your child's life but won't make him or her more comfortable, for dehydration may actually decrease the pain your child feels. A child who feels thirsty but can't keep liquid down might like to suck on ice chips.

If your child does want to eat, don't let him or her become a tyrant. Give your child a choice, prepare the food, and serve it. Overindulgence doesn't do anyone any good, not even a dying child, who still needs to feel that there is some structure in his or her life.

In all these aspects of nurturing care, let instinct be your guide, for you know best what your child has preferred in the past and what might feel most comfortable now. However, don't hesitate to call your doctor if you are not sure what you should do.

What medical care does your child need? Once you have decided on comfort care, the only appropriate medical care is that which will make your child more comfortable, and this you will have to discuss with your doctor. Providing medical care at home is discussed in Chapters 4 through 6, but there are certain factors worth mentioning about terminal care.

Set up an account with a pharmacy. For more information about pharmacies, see pages 45–46. If you have not already been going to a local pharmacy, ask your doctor for recommendations, especially if your child will need infrequently used medications, for some pharmacies have larger stocks of these than others.

Strong pain-relieving drugs (analgesics) contain narcotics. Some states have special dispensing regulations; for example, the pharmacist may have to receive a nonrefillable written prescription from the doctor and also make a written report to the state. Many pharmacists do not carry such medications in stock for fear of being robbed; rather, they quickly special-order them from their wholesalers. Others may carry limited amounts in stock but certainly would not tell you if you phoned and asked unless you were a known customer. Therefore, if your child will need strong pain-relieving drugs, make sure you know the procedure for getting the prescriptions filled and plan ahead. Don't wait until you have only one pill left on a Friday afternoon before contacting your doctor.

In an emergency most hospitals will fill a prescription, especially if no pharmacy in town carries what you need or if you suddenly need something in the middle of the night. However, it is best to plan ahead and give your pharmacy the time to fill your prescriptions.

Make sure you understand what medication your child should take and why, as is more fully explained in Chapter 5. When a child is terminally ill, you no longer worry about addiction and it may be appropriate to use medications differently than before. Your doctor may also decide to discontinue medications that no longer serve a useful purpose. (He or she may decide that you should slowly taper off, for your child may have a reaction if you stop a medication suddenly.) The goal now in giving medication is to comfort your child. Your doctor may request that you increase or decrease dosages as your child's condition changes. If your child suddenly gets worse after taking medication, you should never blame yourself for causing the change. If a child dies shortly after receiving medication, never feel that giving the medication caused the death. Changes are bound to occur, and what you have tried to do is make your child as comfortable as possible.

Some dying children experience pain, particularly those with cancer. These children may need analgesics (pain-relieving drugs), which, as just mentioned, often contain narcotics. While narcotics may depress respiration, the positive effect of reducing pain usually outweighs the potential negative effect. The goal is to have your child as painfree yet as conscious as possible.

Your doctor will value your impressions as he or she works to determine which drugs in which amounts are best for your child. Usually one tries to give pain medication *before* the pain recurs. Since fear of pain can aggravate the experience of pain tremendously, your child should know that he or she will get the needed medication regularly as needed to prevent the pain from recurring, or at least to keep it to a minimum.

Nausea and breathlessness can also cause discomfort. Nausea can often be relieved with medication. While breathlessness can sometimes be relieved by providing a slow steady stream of oxygen, being short of oxygen is in itself an analgesic and a sedative. It is therefore not necessarily all bad and can even be advantageous to the dying. Your doctor will have to decide whether or not your child should use a small oxygen mask or a nasal cannula. You should understand that this doesn't really prolong life, but it may make your child more comfortable. (If you have not used oxygen or nasal cannulas before, see pages 68–71. Note that you will have to monitor how much oxygen the cylinder contains so you don't run out.)

Learn when you should contact your doctor. Discuss with your doctor not only what you should do now but what changes in your child's condition warrant contacting the doctor. He or she may want to leave certain decisions to your good judgment. At critical times you might check with your doctor every day to report on how things are going and to ask what you should do if things get worse—that is, what you should try to handle and when you should call for help. While this can prevent unnecessary calls in the middle of the night, if you really don't know what to do, call your doctor.

How Do You Keep the Household Running in the Last Stages?

A calm, quiet atmosphere is undoubtedly best. Exactly what that means to you will, of course, be determined by your life style.

Decide who should help with your child. A child who is approaching the end may slowly withdraw and want only those very close to him or her about. This doesn't mean your child no longer loves friends and relatives; it may just be that social contact is a strain when he or she is preparing to let go.

It is often a good idea always to have with your child a parent and a helper-friend who will fetch items, make phone calls, fix snacks, or get the other parent. Try to be calm, warm, and loving, with your emotions under control. This doesn't mean you have to be so brave as to never shed a tear. A good cry alone can be cathartic. Such signs of grief are important and, since honesty has been your goal, your child should know you are sad. But at some level you can only convey to your child that it is all right to die if you act that way in his or her presence as much as possible.

Remember and include the other children in your family. When your child is dying, try to be very factual with any siblings, telling them that their brother or sister is very ill and might die. As your child's condition gets worse, tell any siblings that their brother or sister will probably die. Healthy children cannot be expected to be quiet for long periods of time and need to continue their normal daily routines as much as possible. Although your dying child will require much care, try to spend time with your other children, not just explaining what is happening but also playing with them. Also try to keep your other children on their regular sleeping and mealtime schedule at home. They might spend part of their days with friends who live nearby so they can come back regularly to see their brother or sister. Or you might find it more practical to have a relative or friend come and live in the house to care for the children and run the household. It is important that your healthy children be able to interact with your dying child if they so desire. However, some dying children may want to be only with their parents. This is more apt to occur if the siblings are younger and may seem too noisy or active. If your dying child starts to withdraw, respect his or her wishes while also explaining to any siblings that their brother or sister loves them but no longer has the energy to interact with them.

Call on friends for help. If your child has been chronically ill for some time, your relatives and friends may not even know that he or she is dying. And even if they do know, they often don't know what to do to help. Therefore you help them and yourself most if you make specific requests for help. Make sure to indicate that you understand if they are unable to help at this time. Friends can help with child care, running errands, or doing the wash. You may just want to let the dirt pile up, but if it is getting to you, ask a friend to come in and do a bit of cleaning. Or you might ask friends to bring meals. If your stomach starts to feel weak, don't hesitate to give menu suggestions.

Take care of yourself. It is most important that everyone in the family gets the love and nurturing care they need, including, of course, the parents. You will be of more help to everyone if you get some sleep (even if only in four-hour shifts) and if you occasionally get out of the house (even if just to sit in the sun for ten minutes or to walk around the block). You can't run full-steam forever; you have to pace yourself, for you don't know how many days your child will need inten-

sive care. Your friends want to help you, so let them do the things you don't have to do yourself. You may not feel much like eating at all, but it's important to keep eating a relatively balanced diet. Since it's important for parents to keep their own brains as sharp as possible, drinking alcohol or taking drugs at this difficult time is probably not helpful to either the parents or the child.

What Are Common Signs of Impending Death?

When death is imminent, there may be times when you or your spouse want to leave the room for a while. If neither of you feels comfortable with your dying child and you don't think you can care for your home any longer, call your doctor to discuss the matter. It is important to remain flexible and to do what you feel is best for you and your child. Parents should never feel that they must force themselves to stay with their dying child; neither should one parent blame the other for being unwilling to do so. And it is all right if you decide you'd rather take your child to the hospital.

If you decide to keep your child at home, you will be better off if you have an idea of some common signs of impending death. Talk with your doctor so you will be prepared calmly to give your child the care he or she needs.

Certain things are more apt to occur with some illnesses than with others. The following are possibilities, which can happen in any order and may occur in conjunction with each other. Some are easier to observe than others.

Fading of consciousness. "Fading" is a very descriptive term, for losing consciousness can take several days. Your child may at first become confused, perhaps perceiving a few minutes as a few hours, or seeing things where or as they are not. For example, a child may ask you to move a table that isn't there. If this happens, there is no need to argue about reality. Just calmly pretend to carry out the request and assure your child that it has been done. A child may also cry out in sleep or half-consciousness. If this happens, it is usually better not to wake your child; let him or her have the needed rest. If pain or discomfort is really severe, the child will awaken and ask for help. A child may tell you about events that happened when he or she was very young, or even see a kind of review of his or her whole life. If any of these things occur, it is best to be calm and supportive, for what a child is experiencing is important to him or her in some way, even though you may not comprehend the meaning. Your child will probably lose the ability to speak. Many people feel that a child's sense of smell, touch, and hearing remain long after the ability to speak fades.

Try to have someone in the room with your child, for the physical presence of someone the child loves is very important. While you might sometimes want to sit by your child and hold his or her hand, you don't need to focus on your child every moment. There may be times when it is appropriate for you to do other quiet activities in the room, such as reading silently or out loud, writing letters, or doing paperwork. The word "quiet" is important because the atmosphere should be calm. As adults we all know that if we are very sick we don't want the television, radio, or stereo blaring, although we may find quiet music soothing. Do what feels right, but remember that even if your child can no longer talk with you, he or she may in some way be aware of what is going on. Discussions in the room should be honest, even if the doctor comes and you discuss what is happening to your child. Since honest communication has been your goal, this is not the time to become secretive. Whispering may actually be very annoying to a dying child. If you really don't want to discuss something in front of your child, go into another room to talk.

Difficult or irregular breathing. When your child is near the end, breathing may become difficult or irregular. It may even make a rattly sound as saliva trickles into the windpipe. Watching your child breathe toward the end, you may feel that dying seems to be hard work. If your child is conscious, it may help if he or she can be encouraged to breathe deeply in a relaxed way. But the main thing is not to panic at what you see. It is normal and will pass, even if this means your child dies. While labored breathing may not look pleasant, while it may

even look painful, it should be seen as part of the dying process and is probably not as painful to the dying person as it appears to us to be. As mentioned before, a lack of oxygen in a way anesthetizes a person.

In rare instances, as with certain brain tumors, a child may stop breathing and after a few minutes suddenly start to breathe again briefly. Even with other conditions, as long as 15 minutes after a child has stopped breathing and you no longer feel a pulse the child may suddenly inhale or exhale one more time. Muscle twitching may also occur for several minutes after death. While all this is quite rare, it is worth mentioning, for it could be quite shocking if one did not know it could occur.

Irregular pulse. It may happen that your child's pulse begins to beat so fast you cannot even count it. The pulse may even out again for a day or so and then become irregular before death. While this may be a sign that death is near, when you have decided against heroic measures there is nothing you should do for an irregular pulse. However, knowing that an irregular pulse can occur may keep you from panicking.

Change in color and temperature of the body. As a child gets less and less oxygen, the skin may fade from the pinker glow to a more grayish or mottled color. The hands and feet may become cool.

Specific illnesses have their own indices. For example, a leukemic child may have fading of consciousness or seizures, gastrointestinal bleeding evidenced by bloody stools or vomit, or a very severe nosebleed. If you know that these can occur, you will be prepared. As parents it may be difficult to watch something like this happen, but the realization that it is not that painful and that your child's suffering will soon be over can make it seem all right.

"No Code" for the Hospitalized Child

"No Code" in hospital terminology means specifically that there should be no efforts at cardiopulmonary resuscitation if a person stops breathing or if the heart stops beating. More broadly, "No Code" in many hospitals means no heroic measures should be taken to continue life. If your child is dying in the hospital and you have decided against heroic measures, it is very important that the hospital staff know of your decision. Make sure the doctor has written those instructions on your child's chart. If your child suddenly stops breathing when you are with him or her and you do not want attempts at revival, you may have kindly but firmly to tell anyone who is not aware of your "No Code" decision and, if necessary, ask them to verify this on your child's chart.

19

Looking to the Future

Although as a parent of a terminally ill child you may have difficulty admitting that your child will die, looking thoughtfully to the future and thinking about what kinds of details will have to be taken care of is not a macabre way of hastening destiny. Rather, looking to the future can not only help you become aware of what to expect but can also give you the opportunity to think about decisions you may have to make. While all this may not be easy to do before your child dies, it certainly won't be any easier afterward. It is not just the physical details that need attention. You also have to reflect upon how your life will be changed and how the love and happiness your child brought into your life can be a positive force in the days, weeks, and years to come.

Arrangements That Can Be Made Before Death

Who should be notified? Make a list of family and friends to be notified and decide who should do so. If all your relatives live far away, you may feel that it would be better not to phone them in advance of your child's death, since they will probably not be able to come to help and would probably only worry. However, if you wait until the day after the death of your child to notify loved ones, you may sound so upset that you will shock them more than necessary. It will be easier for you and for those you notify if you inform family and very close friends when your child approaches death rather than after death. This doesn't mean they have to rush to the bedside. If you do not think this would be appropriate, you

can always have someone tactfully request that they don't. But at least people will have time to prepare themselves mentally for the eventuality and won't be so shocked when the death occurs. If you do not feel up to phoning perhaps the most composed member of your family or a good friend can call close relatives and friends.

Which persons living at a distance will have to be notified by letter or printed notice? Again, make a list of names, and decide what should be sent to whom.

Should you join a memorial society or just contact a local funeral home? Memorial societies are designed to offer inexpensive arrangements while allowing you to add any extras you want. If you deal with a mortician after your child dies, you may spend more money on funeral arrangements than is appropriate for your family. Membership in a memorial society is inexpensive and usually transferable between societies should you move to another community. Usually you have to join *before* a person dies. Most memorial societies contract to work with one mortician in a community.

Funeral homes are run by professional morticians. While all in your community may offer approximately the same services, you may be able to work better with one than another. You can ask friends, doctors, or nurses whom they recommend. Feel free to call a number of morticians to discuss your concerns with them. Look for a kind, compassionate mortician who will respect your views, have reasonable prices, and not demand payment in advance.

When should the medical examiner or coroner be notified? Your doctor will report the death of your child to the coroner's office. A death is a "coroner's case" if the child was not regularly attended by a physician or died due to an accident, an unknown cause, or suspected violence. However, in some communities the police have to make a report on any home death unless the medical examiner has been contacted *before* the death and been told of the impending event and its causes. Therefore, check with your mortician and your doctor about your local law so they can make any necessary arrangements before your child dies. You may not want to deal with such a detail before a death, but it is better to do so than to have a policeman at the door with a list of questions when you really don't feel like talking.

Decisions That Can Be Made Before Death

Many decisions about how you will want to proceed with what needs to be done after death can be made in advance.

Is an autopsy necessary? In most states, an autopsy is not required if a doctor has seen the child within the last 20 days and if the cause of death is known. The coroner has the authority to do an autopsy in any coroner's case. Even if your doctor has seen your child regularly, he or she may suggest an autopsy for the sake of increasing medical knowledge of your child's disease, for this may benefit another child in the future. Your physician may discuss the question of an autopsy before your child's death to give you time to think about the request. If you decide upon an autopsy and your child dies at home, part of the mortician's role is to transport the body to the hospital for the autopsy and then on to the funeral home. In case of a sudden unexpected death of a chronically ill child, a doctor may suggest an autopsy so the parents will know the cause of death, for some may feel that certainty, however harsh, is better than lingering uncertainty. If you are against autopsies for religious reasons, tell your doctor.

When should the mortician pick up the body? Many people have the idea that if someone dies the mortician should be called immediately to come and get the body. But if you want to spend some time with your child after death this is perfectly all right and your desires should be respected.

If your child dies in the hospital, it is reasonable to request that your family have some quiet time alone with the body before it is removed from the room. If your child dies at home, you may not want the mortician to come until your family and any close friends have spent some time with the body. If your child dies in the middle of the night and you have other children, even if you wake them after the death, it may be important to let them see their brother or sister when they are really awake in the morning and talk about the death with you in the privacy of your own home. The main thing is that you can decide what timing is best for your family.

Although most of us will not be interested in this option, it is legal in some states to bury the body yourself on private property without even calling a mortician.

Who arranges for the completion of the death certificate? Unless you bury your child yourself, the mortician will arrange that the death certificate be completed and will order any certified copies you need, such as for a life insurance company. Do not be surprised if the cause of death is not written out as you expected, for the doctor must express it in medical terms.

Should the body be embalmed? Embalming is the replacement of a person's body fluid with a preservative fluid. This is *not* required by law in most states unless the body will be transported across state lines by a public carrier such as a plane or train. If you plan to have the burial or cremation within about 24 hours, it is not necessary to embalm the body, for it can be refrigerated. However, if the viewing, burial, or cremation won't take place for three or four days, embalming will be needed.

Should you have a viewing? Some parents may want the family and maybe even close friends to view the body at home. After the body is taken to the mortuary, some families do not want to see it again. Others want a private family viewing or a public viewing for family and friends. The casket can be present at the funeral, open as guests arrive and then closed, or left open throughout the service. Some people feel a viewing can help them accept that the death has occurred and is final, especially a sudden or accidental death. Others do not want to see the body again.

If you think you will want a viewing, it is important to know that morticians may use cosmetics. If your child never used makeup and you'd prefer to see him or her once more as a remembrance, discuss with the mortician whether cosmetics should be used at all and in what way. If the mortician tells you he or she always uses makeup and that the results are lovely, you may be inclined to seek another one who doesn't use makeup so your child will look more as he or she did in real life. You can provide clothing for your child to wear.

Viewings are a personal matter. Do what you feel is most appropriate for your family.

Do you need to buy a casket? If your child is to be buried, you do. The cost can range from a few hundred to thousands of dollars. Buy what you think is appropriate, but don't feel that the only way of showing love and respect is by spending lots of money. For cremation without a viewing, a very inexpensive casket may be needed to transport the body to a crematorium. If your child is to be cremated but you are having a viewing, ask your mortician if he or she can provide alternatives like laying the body out on a table or renting a casket for the viewing.

Should you have a funeral or a memorial service? The difference between a funeral and a memorial service is that at a funeral the body is present, at a memorial service it is not. If the family decides on burial, a brief graveside service may be held either before or after the memorial service or funeral. You have the option of being present at the actual interment (burial). Whatever type of service is chosen, it provides family and friends an opportunity to express their love for the person who has died and for

each other in a fitting closing to that person's life. You must decide what would be most meaningful and in accord with your beliefs. It is important to include any surviving children in the service, even if their ages and attention spans must influence what you plan.

Services for the dead can range from traditional church services, to memorial services in parks where friends of the deceased tell what the person meant to them, to home memorial services with only a few friends present. While you, as a parent, may wonder if you have the strength to go through *any* service, you will. Having no service leaves things hanging, whereas a service, planned to be meaningful for your family, will provide an appropriate ending to your child's life.

If you have a religious affiliation and worship with others regularly, you may want to plan the service with the head of your congregation. If you have not, the mortician can contact either the head of the congregation of your choice or an interdenominational chaplain, should your local hospital or college have one. The clergy have shared their knowledge and compassion often with families such as yours. If you do not have strong affiliations of some kind, you may want to arrange a service that would be meaningful to your family and friends, perhaps including eulogies, music, readings, prayers, or recollections of your son or daughter, all done by people who knew your child. Again there is no right or wrong way, only what is right for you.

Should your child be buried or cremated? This is a matter of your preference. Burial of the body is more expensive since you have to pay for a plot, a marker, and the opening and closing of the grave. With cremation, you can have the ashes stored in a niche in the cemetery or in a columbarium (crypt for ashes) or have the remains strewn in a meaningful place by an employee of the crematorium or by yourself. If you decide to scatter the ashes yourself, you should realize that these may contain bits of bone.

Do you want to bequeath organs or the whole body to science? All states allow people to donate all or parts of their bodies to hospitals and research or educational institutions. If you think this would be appropriate, discuss it with your doctor. Organ donation is more common in cases of sudden death than after lingering illness. Some people have very strong feelings as to whether or not this is right; you must decide.

What do you do if you have no money at all? Nearly all communities provide for the burial or cremation of individuals whose families cannot afford to do so. There are usually certain regulations regarding use of such public assistance. For example, you may not have a choice as to whether cremation or burial will occur and funds may not be provided for a service. If you can't afford a memorial society, or you don't feel that it is appropriate to pay for a burial or cremation, what is legally called "abandonment" is an alternative.

Would you prefer flowers or donations to a worthy cause? Often friends like to express their love in some way. Some families prefer receiving flowers for the funeral or memorial service. These can then be given to the church, to rest homes, or to hospitals after the service. If the flowers are taken to the cemetery, they will be removed after three or four days. Others prefer monetary donations to an organization that helped with their child's medical care, such as a hospital, a Visiting Nurses Association, a hospice, or a foundation working to help children with their child's specific medical disorder. Donations may also be given to a youth group, the public library, a museum, a school, or a religious organization. State your preference in the newspaper obituary notice.

What should be included in a newspaper obituary notice? Note that the question is not "Should you put an obituary notice in the newspaper?" This is because you should. If you have no notice, or an announcement so small that many people may not see it, you will frequently talk to people who call for your child or who ask how your child is for quite a while after the death. Dealing with those well-meant inquiries is much more difficult than getting the news through a well-planned newspaper obituary to those who will not be contacted directly after the death. Some suggestions for an obituary notice are:

- Include a picture. People tend to notice pictures of children and read on.
- Request that your child's first and last names be used, even if you have already held or plan to hold private services. This is particularly important if you have a common name. For example, "Sarah White" will attract the attention of some who might not read an article entitled "White Services."
- State your preference for flowers or donations.

Obituaries normally include only name, age, surviving family, and whether the person died of a sudden or lingering illness. If you would like other details included, feel free to furnish the newspaper with the relevant information. In smaller communities, newspapers will probably print whatever information you submit, although they will sometimes edit it to fit the available newspaper space for that day. Larger metropolitan newspapers may have only paid announcements, in which case you will have to decide how much information you want to include.

Arrangements to Be Made After the Death of a Child

Everything we have talked about so far can be considered *before* your child dies. While any decisions you make in advance will give you fewer to confront after your child's death, certain details can be taken care of only after the death of your child.

Phone your doctor. It is a legal requirement that a patient be "pronounced dead" by a doctor or the coroner before the latter can sign a death certificate. Your doctor will probably come to your home, even if it is in the middle of the night.

Notify your mortician of the death and state when you would like him or her to come to your home. If your child dies during the night and you do not want the mortician to come until morning, it is not necessary to call and wake him or her up. You may prefer to leave the room when the mortician picks up the body, if you will find it hard to watch your child's face being covered by a sheet. These are the only two things that have to be taken care of right away. You don't have to do anything else immediately. It may be more important to get some food, rest, or spend time with other members of your family, especially any surviving children. When you are ready to attend to the remaining details, you can ask someone to help you. But don't let well-meaning friends act without specifically delegating responsibility to them, for otherwise you may later regret that things were not arranged as you really would have wished.

Decide on the time and place of the funeral or memorial service.

Notify family and friends. Whereas you may want to make some calls yourself, others can be made by another family member or by friends. If the services will take place very soon, friends and relatives should also be informed of the time and place of the services. Notify people very soon by phone or letter to avoid the difficult situation of friends dropping by to say hello to your child.

Arrange for the obituary notice in the newspaper, as discussed in the previous section.

Consider asking friends or relatives for assistance with child care, meal preparation, cleaning the house, and so on. People are very willing to help; they only need to be told how. You can ask a friend to coordinate any assistance you need.

Make any necessary hotel or motel reservations for family or friends coming from out of town.

Notify life and medical insurance companies.

Notify persons living at a distance by letter or printed notice.

Send notes of gratitude to persons who have been particularly helpful. These might include your child's doctors, helpers, the visiting nurses, school class and youth groups, the school board (if the district provided special services), and other organizations that helped your child.

While it takes time to compose the right letter, such a message can not only be an expression of thanks but can also give the recipient more than just a phone call, which could leave a person somewhat taken aback, especially if the death was unexpected. A letter can indicate the calm of the passing and the fact that, although your life will be different now, you are grateful that your child was a part of your family and for the way in which the recipient enhanced your child's life. Once you have carefully composed the core of your letter, it can be modified for each person. For example, to a former helper one could write:

Dear Kim,

As your mother may have written you, Maria died peacefully here at home on Friday, March 25. You were one of her favorite helpers, and after you left she often talked happily of the things you had done together. Thus we want to thank you not only for your assistance but also for your friendship.

Maria believed that everyone's life is an opportunity to learn special things. Thus she didn't view herself as handicapped. Rather she felt that, although she lived with definite physical limitations, there was much to learn, and she looked forward to what each new day would bring and lived it to the fullest. And indeed she learned much of courage, friendship, patience, and cheerfulness.

Maria wanted people to be happy when she died, for she had learned that in the East people celebrate an individual's death, as people only die when they have learned that which they were to learn in that lifetime.

Thus we are sure she would want to be remembered in this way—and it is now perhaps our turn to learn from her example.

Thank you again for your friendship!

How Can You Pass Through Mourning and Move Ahead with Life?

It will take time to accept the fact that your child has died and to make the necessary adjustments, especially if the child required intensive care for an extended period of time. If you have been a full-time mother and nurse for a long time, you may suddenly feel unemployed. You might consider what you will do with your life after your child dies. When he or she does die, not only will you have to restructure your own life but everyone in the family will have to move on and find new and appropriate ways of doing things. Grief and mourning are common to all of us, but each of us expresses it individually.

Don't rely on alcohol or drugs. Alcohol and drugs may help you view the world through rose-colored glasses, but they also veil reality, which must be accepted. At some point you have to face things as they are. To help you get a move on through grief, consider the following.

What is grief? Grief is the suffering or pain we feel after an acute loss, often the death of someone we love. In a sense we grieve not for the person who has died, for that person's suffering is over. Rather we grieve for ourselves and our own sense of loss. We have to come to separate ourselves from our sorrow, to regain our sense of humor, and to look ahead to what each new day brings.

It can take months or even years to overcome grief completely. The important thing to remember is that with time the good days will outnumber the bad, not because you no longer love your child but because you have accepted your child's death.

Grief can manifest itself not only emotionally but physically and mentally as well. Physically, you may feel exhausted, have trouble sleeping, lose your appetite, and have indigestion, diarrhea, or constipation. You may feel hot or cold, may feel your heart rate and breathing are too fast or too slow, and so on. While they are different for different people, a variety of physical symptoms may occur. When grief affects you mentally, it may be difficult to concentrate or to remember things. You may even "see" your dead child or "hear" your child talking to you. This is part of grieving; do not feel that you have gone insane. However, if you have concerns about this phenomenon and it persists, feel free to discuss your symptoms openly with your doctor.

Some people don't express their emotions much. While self-control is a virtue, keeping things bottled up inside can cause problems. Parents, both fathers and mothers, need to realize that it is all right to feel and express emotions, even to cry. If a surviving child sees you crying and asks why, answer truthfully. Some parents find it helpful to agree to wake each other up in case one cannot sleep and discuss their thoughts. A surviving child may also need to be assured that he or she can come and talk with parents in the middle of the night.

Guilt can be very strong during mourning, especially in cases of accidental death or suicide. But you cared for, taught, and loved your child as best you could, and you must hold to this knowledge. You were responsible for your child's life, not his or her death.

Anger, frustration, or guilt may take the form of blame, directed at others—the doctor who cared for your child, the person who might have prevented an accidental death, the family member who didn't react as you would deem right. If in your discontent hatred starts to fester, it is destructive for everyone involved. You must realize that everyone else was and is trying just as hard as you to do their best.

A large part of grief is a sense of powerlessness, the feeling that you couldn't control the course of events. It takes courage and wisdom to accept what can't be undone by yourself or others, to know that you cannot reverse time and go back to live in the past but that you can utilize what you have learned as you live each day to the fullest from now on.

Do all adults grieve in the same way? It is important to realize that your spouse and any other adult relatives and friends close to you may work through their grief in different ways and at different rates than you do. Marital conflict and crises can arise if you don't respect the way and the pace at which your spouse grieves. While each family has its way of doing things, basic to every family is the realization that every family member is an individual and that you can't turn your back on the needs of another.

How do children grieve? Children differ from us not in kind but in age. So they too feel grief. In a family with several children, each child may respond to the death in an individual way. As a parent, you have to try to be aware of the particular needs of each of your children at this time. They may need your help in understanding why the death occurred and in overcoming any negative emotions they feel. Guilt can arise in a living child who feels that he or she caused the death by wishing one day that the sibling would drop dead. In such a case, the child needs to be assured that such wishes are natural and that bad wishes don't come true. Guilt can occur if a surviving child doesn't think he or she was kind and loving enough, or if he or she felt annoyed that the deceased sibling got so much attention. Some children may even think that such unkind thoughts can precipitate death. Or a child may become angry that a sibling died and is no longer with him or her. A young child may even tell you that the dead brother or sister will come back, which may be denial or simply an age-appropriate notion that death is reversible. Whereas you probably prepared your surviving children just as you prepared your dying child for death, your surviving children need you now to help them understand and accept what has occurred. While you provided the best physical care and attention for your deceased child that you could, you now have the opportunity to help your surviving children through any emotional or spiritual turmoil they are experiencing.

Surviving children should understand why their sibling died and that other members in the family will not die now too. (Of course, if the cause was an accident or a contagious or hereditary disorder that has also placed the lives of other family members in danger, an honest discussion of the situation is important.) Listening and clarifying may be more helpful than just telling. A surviving child may develop fears. For example, a child who has heard that dead people "go to sleep" may fear going to bed. Such a child may also fear being alone or may have nightmares.

Children sometimes don't verbalize their fears and grief the way adults do. Therefore you may have to be alert and sensitive to any significant changes in the behavior of your remaining children, such as an unwillingness to eat, the inability to sleep, regression in toilet training or other skills, acting up, stealing, and so on.

Clarifying any religious misconceptions your surviving children have is important. If after the death your surviving children heard that "It was God's will" or "Now the child belongs to God" and they do not understand the philosophical basis for such statements, they may become confused. They may even develop an awesome fear of God, who appears to be an all-powerful being from whom even parents cannot protect them. Furthermore, if some members of the family become very religious, and others do not, friction may develop. While religion can be a solace and guide in one's own life, there is danger in indicating to another that one's own belief is the only true one, especially at a time such as this.

A child may seem either to withdraw or constantly want to go out with others. Either behavior may be a sign that the child needs your help and an indication to you not to get too wrapped up in your own sorrow. Home has to be a happy place for children, and when you reach out with good cheer to help your children overcome their grief you will find it also helps you overcome your own.

Finally, some surviving children act quite normally with very few outward expressions of grief. This should not be taken as a sign that the child didn't love the deceased sibling. As one child so aptly put it, "Thinking about my brother is like looking at the sun. You know the sun is there, you glance at it every once in a while, but you can't stare at it all the time or you'll go blind."

What should you do with your child's belongings? It may take a while to give up the physical ties with your child, so give yourself time to change your child's room and to make decisions about what to do with clothes, toys, and other possessions. Trust your own feelings about when is the right time for you to do it. Well-meaning relatives and friends should understand that it is important that you do this yourself unless you specifically ask for their help. Consider whether your surviving children would like any of their brother's or sister's things. It may be good to let them have now any objects they would like. You may also want to pack some things away until a surviving child is old enough to use them. And you may want to choose mementos to give to your child's special friends.

By deliberately sorting each item—some for removal, some for gifts, and others for saving—you go through a personal separation process. This can be done alone or with members of your family, at your own pace and in a manner unique to the lost relationship. If you can't decide what to do with an item, save it for another day. While such decision-making is sometimes painful and brings tears, it is a necessary part of letting go. After all, the only alternative would be to leave your child's room unchanged, rather like a museum. This will not aid you in moving ahead to realize that true memories of your child are held in the heart, will always be there, and can help you as you try to do your best each day.

Will you need to restructure your family? Just as during the illness of your deceased child he or she and the rest of the family were aided by maintaining some structure and order, the same applies to the surviving members of the family. While in the beginning of your mourning it may be helpful to ask a friend to lend a helping hand, with time you have to reassume the normal daily chores of cooking, cleaning, shopping, gardening, and so on. Although you may not feel like resuming the family routine, inactivity may be harder on you, for it can emphasize your loneliness and grief. Inactivity may also be hard on the rest of your family, because when you can't provide the nurturing care they have realistically come to expect from you, you aren't helping them cope either.

Helping others in your family regain a sense of proportion is important but difficult. You don't want to let others wallow in their misery; neither do you want to order others to pull themselves together and get back to the business of daily life. It is often difficult to say the right thing in the right way to people we love. But saying nothing can be just as bad, and communication is extremely important in times of crisis.

While talking with another is helpful, constantly pouring out your grief and leaning on another family member as a crutch can cause friction. Finding a friend with a good ear or joining a group of bereaved parents may give you the opportunity to verbalize your thoughts and feelings without unduly leaning upon another family member during his or her own grief. At other times, if grief seems truly overwhelming, it may be a sign of strength, rather than of weakness, to seek professional help.

You and your spouse have been through a lot together: the illness of your child, special arrangements that may have entailed, and now

death. Especially if the illness was a long one, it may take time to focus again on each other, reestablish your relationship, and find what is now the most appropriate way of living together. If you haven't had much time alone together, if you shared your child's care, sleeping different hours or even in different bedrooms, you may simply have to begin by reestablishing intimacy and modes of expressing your love. Sex may be a problem. While one partner may feel sex is a good way of expressing love, the other may feel sex at this time is disrespectful. Or sex may remind one partner of how your child was conceived and overwhelm the person with sorrow. A partner who feels much more reticent than the other should try to express love or at least accept love; this may help renew feelings of love and the ability to express them.

Whether or not to have more children is a question sometimes related to sex. If the mother has been acting as a full-time nurse, she may suddenly feel unemployed. If she liked her job, she may want to get back to work by having more children.

The father, on the other hand, may feel that they have spent enough years on intensive child care and should move on to something else. Or the roles can be reversed, and the mother may have had enough of being at home while the father feels that home is not a home without children. Whenever you are not agreed on whether or not to have more children, it is best to wait. After all, a child is not a passing fancy but a long-term commitment. If your child had a genetic disorder, genetic counseling is important to help you decide if you want more biological children or if you'd rather adopt.

While the number of living children you now have may not lessen your sense of loss, it may influence whether you want to have more children, particularly if you had only one or two children. If you had two children in part out of the conviction that you didn't want to have an only child, you may now envision all those disadvantages you thought only children had. But as families with only one child will tell you, there are advantages too. If your only child dies, the problem of whether to have more children is different, for then you have to ask whether you want to have a family with children again or not.

It is important to remember that you can never replace a child you have lost, so don't attempt to do so by having another child, whether it is by being a foster parent, adopting, or having a baby. When parents add another child to their family while still grieving, the unresolved grief can influence their attachment to the new child in a way that is not to the child's advantage.

You may also want to consider how adding another child would affect any surviving children, who may have strong preferences for or against it. While these shouldn't determine your decision, they may influence it. However, knowing your other children's attitudes may help you explain any decision you make to them.

You and your surviving children. While your children may need assistance with the mourning process, they also need the continuity and security that a daily routine provides. Small changes such as rearranging the seating at the dinner table or redistributing chores may be helpful, but holding to your established expectations in terms of behavior, responsibilities at home and in school, and use of free time is important. Of course, in expecting your children to assume responsibility for reasonable behavior it is only fair that you try to follow suit.

Keeping established patterns from the past in mind as guidelines can help, for as a parent you can err either on the side of being too lenient because your child is sad or you don't have the strength to supervise, or on the side of being too strict because you fear something might happen to your remaining children. Neither extreme is good.

How can you best express the memory of your child? Honor your dead child by remembering your child as he or she was, neither better nor worse. To say that your son or daughter was always good and fair, especially to hold your child up as a paragon of virtue to any surviving children, is not helpful to anyone. While dwelling on the memory of your child can increase your sorrow, sharing the things you did together is an acknowledgement that he or she was part of your family and that what you learned from your child will always be with you. If you speak of your child, in both weakness and strength, you will show friends that you talk of your child and that they are welcome to do so too. When people don't know what to say, they often say nothing.

How can you reestablish friendships and activities outside the home? Shortly after the death of your child, you may wonder if you will ever be happy again. You may not want to go out to friends for dinner, go to a movie, go on a vacation, or celebrate the holidays. But if you think of what your child would have wanted to do when he or she was alive and what he or she would want you to do now, you will see that you better honor the memory of your child with laughter and joy than by holing up in despair at home. It is hard to move out into the world again, but in doing so you move ahead.

Of course you should not run about so hard and fast that you're never at home; but there are activities that are good for your whole family, and it is good to do things together. Some may like quietly to take up activities as a family, others may also want to take an adult-education class or become involved in some community activity.

A support group including other bereaved parents not only provides a setting in which to share any and all experiences and feelings but also helps to see that others have not only survived the death of their child but look forward to the future.

The good things in life will live on. Although your child is gone, you can still be grateful that your child shared his or her life, however brief, with you.

Stephen Crane once wrote,

A man said to the universe:
"Sir, I exist!"
"However," replied the universe,
"The fact has not created in me
A sense of obligation."

Certain things are as they are, and that includes the fact that your child is dead. How you continue your life, how you honor your child's memory, is up to you.

APPENDIXES

Appendix 1

Oxygen Cylinder Capacity and Flow Chart

GAUGE PRESSURE IN CYLINDER	CYLINDER SIZE	LITER FLOW PER HOURS AND MINUTES				
		1	2	3	4	5
2200	H or K	115:08	57:34	38:22	28:47	23:01
	D-122	57:34	28:47	19:11	14:23	11:30
	E	10:16	5:08	3:25	2:34	2:03
	D	5:52	2:56	1:57	1:28	1:10
2000	H or K	104:40	52:20	34:53	26:10	20:56
	D-122	52:20	26:10	17:26	13:05	10:28
	E	9:20	4:40	3:06	2:20	1:52
	D	5:20	2:40	1:46	1:20	1:04
1800	H or K	94:12	47:06	31:24	23:33	18:50
	D-122	47:06	23:33	15:42	11:46	9:25
	E	8:24	4:12	2:48	2:06	1:40
	D	4:48	2:24	1:36	1:12	:57
1600	H or K	83:44	41:52	77:54	20:56	16:44
	D-122	41:52	20:56	13:57	10:28	8:22
	E	7:28	3:44	2:29	1:52	1:29
	D	4:16	2:08	1:25	1:04	:51
1400	H or K	73:16	36:38	24:25	18:19	14:39
	D-122	26:38	18:19	12:12	9:09	7:19
	E	6:32	3:16	2:10	1:38	1:18
	D	3:44	1:52	1:14	:56	:44
1200	H or K	62:48	31:24	20:56	15:42	12:33
	D-122	31:24	15:42	10:28	7:51	6:16
	E	5:36	2:48	1:52	1:24	1:07
	D	3:12	1:36	1:04	:48	:38
1000	H or K	50:20	26:00	17:26	13:05	10:28
	D-122	26:10	13:05	8:43	6:32	5:14
	E	4:40	2:20	1:33	1:10	:56
	D	2:40	1:20	:53	:40	:32
800	H or K	41:52	20:26	13:57	10:28	8:22
	D-122	20:56	10:28	6:58	5:14	4:11
	E	3:44	1:52	1:14	:56	:44
	D	2:08	1:04	:42	:32	:25

GAUGE PRESSURE IN CYLINDER	CYLINDER SIZE	LITER FLOW PER HOURS AND MINUTES				
		1	2	3	4	5
500	H or K	26:10	13:05	8:43	6:32	5:14
	D-122	13:05	6:32	4:21	3:16	2:37
	E	2:20	1:10	:46	:35	:28
	D	1:20	:40	:26	:20	:16
300	H or K	15:07	7:51	5:14	3:55	3:08
	D-122	7:51	3:55	2:37	1:57	1:34
	E	1:24	:42	:28	:21	:16
	D	:48	:24	:16	:12	:09

Appendix 2

Tube-Feeding

If you do decide to tube-feed your child at home, your doctor will instruct you on what and how to feed your child. If you have any questions, *ask them before proceeding.* If something doesn't seem quite right, call your doctor immediately. Your doctor may provide you with information that he or she has written, or may give you materials developed by companies that market tube-feeding formulas or supplies. Detailed information on tube-feeding is given here, but *this is not meant to replace instruction from your doctor.* Rather, it is meant to serve as an outline to which you should add any specific instructions your doctor gives you. Tube-feeding can be done at home if you proceed with caution.

The Tube-Feeding Formula

The formula will have to be determined by your doctor, sometimes with the help of a dietitian. Calories and fluid requirements are based upon age, weight, height, and the specific disease process. Since the small-bore silastic tubes are only about the width of a pencil lead, you will have to use a completely lumpfree liquid. Therefore it will be difficult to use home brews and you will most probably have to use a commercial preparation. Most of these contain a balance of protein, fats, carbohydrates, vitamins, and minerals, although special formulas are designed to meet individual dietary needs, particularly regarding protein, sodium, and potassium. Since lactose, the sugar found in milk, may cause diarrhea, few formulas contain any milk products. Formulas usually are constituted with 1 calorie per cubic centimeter or 30 calories per ounce of liquid.

Your doctor will determine not only how many calories but also how much fluid your child needs.

Your doctor will also tell you how frequently your child should be fed. Usually small tube-feedings are given every three to four hours throughout the day and evening. It is important not to have the feeding too concentrated in the beginning, for otherwise your child can get severe diarrhea. Therefore at first the formula is usually diluted to about half strength to see how well your child's digestive system can tolerate it.

If your child has been eating very little before you begin tube-feeding, be sure to give him or her very small amounts per feeding and build up to the desired amount slowly, for you may overload his or her system in your enthusiasm to nourish your child with what his or her little stomach may consider a huge feeding. Overfeeding can cause vomiting or diarrhea. Also, if your child is suddenly getting more nourishment, he or she will also need to eliminate more. So carefully monitor urination and bowel movements, being especially careful to watch for constipation.

It is important to weigh your child at regular intervals to see if the weight is stable. Weight loss can indicate dehydration, insufficient calories, or difficulties in assimilating the food. Gradual weight gain as an indication of improved nutrition is desirable, but weight gain can also be caused by the body retaining more liquid than it should.

The Equipment

The equipment will be selected by your doctor. Usually silicon-coated tubes, called silastic tubes, are used, since they slide in and out more easily than plain plastic and, therefore, cause less irritation. Tubes with weighted mercury tips are often prescribed, since a weighted tube is less apt to come up out of the stomach. Tube sizes are not in inches or centimeters but in "French," so your prescription may read "5 Fr. weighted mercury silastic." You will also need a feeding set, consisting of a long piece of tubing that connects the feeding tube to the formula bottle. The bottle itself can then be hung in a special plastic bag from an IV (intravenous-feeding) stand. A stand with telescoping legs of adjustable height on casters is the most versatile.

Inserting the Tube

This must be supervised by a doctor or nurse. Do not attempt this alone. As mentioned before, inserting the tube into the lungs by mistake and pouring in the formula could be fatal! This is not to say that you can't learn how to tube-feed your child at home. But you must learn under supervision. If eventually your doctor feels you are qualified, you can proceed as follows, but phone your doctor if you have any doubts.

The new silastic tubes can be left in for as long as six months, so you will not have to reinsert the tube daily unless it comes out by mistake, is pulled out by your child, or nasal irritation indicates that it should be placed into the other nostril. (Keep a few extra tubes on hand.) Since inserting the tube is the most complicated and tricky part of the procedure, your life will be simplified if you do not have to do this daily. Nevertheless, you should understand the whole process, start to finish.

1. Gather your supplies:
   —feeding tube
   —administration set and tubing
   —30–50 cc syringe
   —stethoscope
   —roll of 1″ silk tape
   —formula
   —feeding pump (optional)
2. Wash your hands.
3. Explain to your child, in a reassuring way he or she can understand, what you are going to do. Even if your child does not seem too alert, who knows how much he or she can hear and understand? Your child is a person, and talking to him or her cannot

hurt, whereas not explaining can. A soothing tone of voice helps even if your child can't understand the words.

4. Measure the length of tube needed to reach the stomach. Do this by using the tube to measure the distance from the tip of the nose to the tip of the ear and then from the tip of the ear to the end of the breastbone. Add two inches to this distance. This is the total length of the tube that should be inserted. Mark this spot with an indelible marker so you will know how far to insert the tube.
5. Prop up your child to at least a 30-degree angle during the tube-feeding and for at least 20–30 minutes afterward to prevent regurgitation and aspiration.
6. Lubricate the end of the tube with a water-base jelly such as K-Y Jelly. Be sure *not* to use an oil-base jelly. Insert the tube into the nose. If your child can swallow, the swallowing will aid in inserting the tube and guide it into the stomach rather than into the lung. If your child cannot swallow effectively enough to help pull the tube down, your doctor may during insertion want to stiffen this very flexible tube with a guidewire stylet. If you are to use a stylet, make sure it is locked in place behind the mercury-weighted tip before beginning to insert the tube. *Never reinsert the stylet when the tube is in the patient.*

   Never use force or attempt to advance the tube against resistance. Pull the tube up and try again. It may take some experimentation to find the best position for your child's head and body to insert the tube. If your child fights, you may need another adult to hold him or her.

If your child starts to turn blue, pull the tube out immediately, since you are blocking the airway. Usually a child with a gag reflex will choke like this if you start down the trachea. If the child starts fighting you, it may also be that the tube is caught and is just circling around in the mouth. In that case, pull it out and try again.

Always check that the tube is in the stomach and not clogged before beginning the feeding. This step is particularly important if your child has no gag reflex, for he or she will not choke and gag as the tube starts down the trachea. Check with your doctor as to how to verify tube placement. He or she may want you to use one or both of the following methods.

• Attach a syringe to the end of the tube and aspirate up stomach contents. Note odor and appearance to be sure the fluid is gastric juice.

- Use a syringe to inject quickly 5–10 cc of air (depending upon the size of your child) through the tube while listening over the stomach with a stethoscope. If the tube is in the stomach, a rush of air entering the stomach will be heard.

Secure the tube to the nose BEFORE *beginning the feeding.* One common method is to split a three-inch piece of hypoallergenic tape down the middle for one and a half inches. Wrap the two narrow ends securely around the tube, and then attach the wide end to the bridge of the nose. Make sure the tube is correctly and securely positioned between feedings. If it moves about, it will irritate the nasal passages, causing excess mucus production; worse, it may slip out of the stomach. Do not tape the tube up or across the nostrils, as this will eventually cause ulceration of the skin.

Feeding

1. Make sure the formula is at room temperature.
2. Start with 20cc of water to make sure the tube is correctly inserted. If the tube is in the lung, your child will start coughing, but the water can be absorbed by the lung—whereas if you get food into the lung, it can cause an inflammatory reaction.
3. Attach the feeding set and bottle.
4. Let the formula run down the tube slowly by gravity to force out the air.
5. Connect feeding set to tube.
6. Start feeding.
7. When the formula has been given, rinse the tube by quickly injecting 20cc of lukewarm water with a syringe. It is important to flush the tubes, for they plug up easily.
8. After feeding insert 5 cc of water into the tube and plug the feeding-tube set with its cap so the food won't drain out again.
9. Try to keep your child upright for at least 20 minutes after feeding.

Stop feeding immediately and call your doctor if: (a) your child starts vomiting; (b) your child says that he or she feels nauseated or that his or her stomach hurts; (c) your child starts choking.

Do not remove the tube after each meal unless your doctor has prescribed it, for putting the tube in and out is more irritating than leaving it in, especially if your child needs to be fed frequently throughout the day. Usually children are fed six times a day.

Some children just don't like being tube-fed. If this is the way your child will have to eat, try diversionary tactics. John howled when he was tube-fed until his parents realized that they could make his dinner time more enjoyable if they put on a Beatles record and one person pushed him around the room in his stroller while the other person fed. To one who has never had a severely disabled and retarded child, this procedure may seem a bit excessive, but if you have a child who hates to eat and you discover a way to make mealtime enjoyable, it seems perfectly sensible. You may also find that your child is much happier and more responsive when the tube is out. If he or she needs to be tube-fed, you will hope that with your support he or she will get used to the tube over time. However, if your child seems to become totally unresponsive and to "fade" when the tube is in, you may want to discuss with your doctor the advantages of taking it out overnight. John's parents finally decided to take the tube out every night. Having their child alert when the tube was out in the early morning and evening was worth the hassle of reinserting it every morning before daytime feedings.

If your child needs to be tube-fed over an extended period, your doctor may recommend that you use a feeding pump. This can deliver feeding at a constant rate and can be used so that feeding can be done during the night. In some communities there are home-care companies that can supply all the necessary equipment and formulas for tube-feeding. These companies may be able to answer many of your questions, and may even bill your insurance company for you. Although these companies may charge a little more, the convenience may make the additional cost worthwhile.

It is hoped that this information will be useful when you work with your doctor in learning how to tube-feed your child. But remember that your child may have special needs, so use this information to augment rather than to replace any instructions your doctor gives you. Remember, if you have any questions or problems, call your doctor immediately.

Appendix 3

Suggested Reading

The reading list below offers only a limited number of books relating to the material covered in this book. Those seeking more information should consider the following resources:

Bibliographic Guides

Azarnoff, Pat. *Health, Illness, and Disability: A Guide to Books for Children and Young Adults.* New York: R.R. Bowker, 1983.

Bibliography discusses books about a wide range of disabilities and the various experiences and feelings of children and their families.

Moore, Cory, Peg Gorham Morton, and Anne Southard. *Reader's Guide for Parents of Children with Mental, Physical or Emotional Disabilities.* Baltimore: Maryland State Planning Council on Developmental Disabilities, 1984.

Available through *The Exceptional Parent* magazine (see below).

Bibliographies Compiled by Family-Resource Libraries at Large Hospitals

These are usually very good, up-to-date, and well worth the small cost. The Association for the Care of Children's Health (see "humanizing health care" in "Helpful Organizations") can supply the names of family-resource libraries which have compiled bibliographies.

Bibliographies of Professional Literature

Sometimes books and articles written for professionals can be helpful, but make sure the information you read is current, for treatment for some disabilities and illnesses (such as cancer) is changing rapidly. Some health agencies compile bibliographies of professional books and articles, often centered on specific disabilities or more general problems. Organizations established to humanize health care often have bibliographies on a variety of subjects.

Your Local Public Library or Hospital Library

Your librarian will be happy to provide any help you may need in learning to use the subject index of the library catalog and to tell you if a book you would like can be obtained through interlibrary loan.

Service Organizations Focusing on Specific Disabilities or Illnesses

Read through the list of "Helpful Organizations," contact any you think might be helpful, and request literature about your child's condition or about any specific problem area. (Also check with organizations dedicated to humanizing health care.) Such literature might include:

- *Newsletters*, which often contain helpful articles and reviews

272

- *Bibliographies,* which give a more complete listing of written materials relating to the specific illness or disability
- *Publications focusing on a specific illness or disability,* published either by the organization or by a commercial publisher

Magazines Other Than Those Published by Service Organizations

The Exceptional Parent (605 Commonwealth Avenue, Boston, MA 02215) is the only magazine for parents of the ill or disabled child, and an excellent resource. It contains articles about the experiences of other families, how-to articles, information and advertising on new products, and a reader's forum in which you can request information from others with similar experiences.

Accent on Living (Cheever Publishing, Gillum Road and High Drive, P.O. Box 7000, Bloomington, IL 61701) is for disabled adults but contains the same range of articles as *The Exceptional Parent,* and its positive tone can help you and your child realize that the disabled adult can lead a full life.

Chapter 1   Learning to Accept Your Child's Condition

Ayrault, Evelyn West. *Growing Up Handicapped: A Guide for Parents and Professionals to Helping the Exceptional Child.* New York: Seabury Press, 1977.

Focuses on the psychological needs of the child and his or her family and giving suggestions on how and where to get assistance from health-care professionals.

Featherstone, Helen. *A Difference in the Family.* New York: Penguin, 1981.

A compassionate consideration of the pain and feelings experienced by the author (whose own child was severely handicapped) and by other families in the process of coming to accept a child as he or she is.

Frankl, Viktor. *Man's Search for Meaning.* New York: Pocket Books, 1963.

An autobiographical account of the author's experience in World War II concentration camps is used as the basis for developing the idea that every human being can find meaning in his or her life.

Jampolsky, Gerald, M.D., ed. *There Is a Rainbow Behind Every Dark Cloud.* Millbrae, CA: Celestial Arts, 1978.

Collections of writings and drawings by children with life-threatening illnesses; shows how they have overcome their fears and learned to live each day to the fullest.

Jampolsky, Gerald, M.D., and Gloria Murray, eds. *Another Look at the Rainbow: Straight from Siblings.* Millbrae, CA: Celestial Arts, 1983.

Stories, poems, and drawings by and for children who have brothers and sisters with life-threatening illnesses.

Kushner, Harold. *When Bad Things Happen to Good People.* New York: Schocken, 1983.

A rabbi's discussion of how those believing in God can find strength and hope when facing great difficulties.

McCollum, Audrey T. *The Chronically Ill Child: A Guide for Parents and Professionals.* New Haven: Yale University Press, 1981.

Practical advice and support for parents of chronically ill children, focusing on psychosocial needs of these children and the other members of the family.

Murray, J. B., and Emily Murray. *And Say What He Is: The Life of a Special Child.* Cambridge, MA: MIT Press, 1975.

The parents' sensitive and moving account of living with and caring for a severely handicapped boy; it charts the process of grief, acceptance, and restored satisfactions in life with a sick child in the family.

Perske, Robert. *Hope for the Families: New Directions for Parents of Persons with Retardation and Other Disabilities.* Nashville: Abingdon, 1981.

An optimistic book showing that your family can do more than just cope with your child.

Turnbull, H. Rutherford, III, and Ann Turnbull, eds. *Parents Speak Out: Views from the*

Other Side of the Two-Way Mirror. Columbus, OH: Charles E. Merrill, 1978.

Selections written by parents of children with a variety of disabilities; indicates not only problems families face, but also how they have overcome them.

PART 1   MEETING YOUR CHILD'S MEDICAL NEEDS

There are three major sources of information that may be helpful to you, as follows.

A basic reference book on child care such as:

Pantell, Robert, M.D., et al. *Taking Care of Your Child: A Parent's Guide to Medical Care.* Boston: Addison-Wesley, 1977.

Spock, Benjamin, M.D. *Baby and Child Care.* New York: Pocket Books, 1977.

A basic reference encyclopedia, giving more information than the above, such as:

Boston Children's Medical Center and Richard Feinbloom, M.D. *Child Health Encyclopedia.* New York: Delta, 1975.

Smith, Lendon, M.D. *The Encyclopedia of Baby and Child Care.* New York: Warner, 1980.

The Good Housekeeping Family Health and Medical Guide. New York: Hearst Corporation, 1979.

A medical dictionary (so you can look up terms you don't understand) such as:

The Bantam Medical Dictionary. New York: Bantam, 1982.

Dorland's Medical Dictionary, shorter edition. Philadelphia: W.B. Saunders Co., 1980.

Chapter 2   Finding and Utilizing the Medical Help You Need

Bursztajn, Harold, M.D., Richard I. Feinbloom, M.D., Robert M. Hamm, Ph.D., and Archie Brodsky. *Medical Choices, Medical Chances: How Patients, Families, and Physicians Can Cope with Uncertainty.* New York: Delta, 1983.

Shows how medical decision-making can become a shared responsibility between doctor and patient (and parent), aimed at helping the patient in the best way.

Cousins, Norman. *Anatomy of an Illness as Perceived by the Patient: Reflections on Healing and Regeneration.* New York: Bantam, 1981.

Discussion of how a patient's attitude and involvement in his or her medical care can influence the whole healing process.

Chapter 3   Hospitalization

Gots, Ronald, M.D., and Arthur Kaufman, M.D. *The People's Hospital Book.* New York: Avon, 1978.

A basic guide to how hospitals function and how to get the care a patient needs.

Harrison, Helen. *The Premature Baby Book: A Parent's Guide to Coping and Caring in the First Years.* New York: St. Martin's Press, 1983.

How to deal with the emotional, medical, and practical issues facing a family after the birth of a premature baby; provides more medical information than other books of this kind.

Howe, James. *The Hospital Book.* New York: Crown, 1981.

A book for children explaining what happens in the hospital, whom a child will meet, procedures and equipment, and how to cope with one's feelings.

Lund, Lois. *Eric.* New York: Dell, 1974.

A mother's account of her son's life, including much information about his extended hospitalization for cancer treatment as a teenager.

Rey, H. A., and Margaret Rey. *Curious George Goes to the Hospital.* Boston: Houghton Mifflin, 1966.

A delightful and instructive story for children (and adults) about a monkey who has been hospitalized after eating a piece of a puzzle.

Stein, Sara. *A Hospital Story: An Open Family Book for Parents and Children Together.* New York: Walker, 1984.

The illustrated story of a girl's tonsillectomy provides the background for clear and honest description of hospital procedures with one text for young children and a more complex one for adults.

Richter, Elizabeth. *The Teen-Age Hospital Experience: You Can Handle It.* New York: Coward, McCann and Goehegan, 1983.

A book for teenagers about hospitalization.

The Association for the Care of Children's Health (see "humanizing health care" in "Helpful Organizations") publishes many pamphlets about hospitalization. You may also order other publications about hospitalization through this organization. "The Hospital Game," a wonderful game developed by Elizabeth Crocker, a child-life professional, is also available through ACCH.

Chapter 4   Providing Medical Care at Home

Home care is a new field and it is often difficult to find the written information you need. Sometimes an organization aiding children such as yours may have materials. Hospitals, clinics, and research centers dealing with specific disabilities also sometimes develop materials on specific procedures for parents. Therefore, if the organization(s) you contact cannot provide the information you need, you might ask them or your doctor which clinics or research centers you can contact.

Any information on how to do specific procedures should be reviewed by your doctor and you should receive instruction from your doctor or the health-care professional he or she designates before providing medical care at home.

Montgomery, William H., M.D., and Thomas J. Herrin, M.D. *Student Manual for Basic Life Support: Cardiopulmonary Resuscitation.* Dallas: American Heart Association, 1981.

Basic information everyone should know on CPR.

Chapter 5   Medication

Books for the general public on drugs and medication:

Graedon, Joe. *The People's Pharmacy,* books 1 & 2. New York: Avon, 1981.

This and other books of its kind provide sound basic information, but may not include information about the drugs your child is taking.

Long, James W., M.D. *The Essential Guide to Prescription Drugs.* New York: Harper & Row, 1982.

Zimmerman, David R. *The Essential Guide to Nonprescription Drugs.* New York: Harper & Row, 1983.

Books for medical professionals on drugs and medication:

Huff, Barbara, ed. *The Physician's Desk Reference.* Oradell, NJ: Medical Economics Company (annual publication).

Quite a complete compendium, giving the manufacturer's opinion of its own products. Each manufacturer buys the space to include its drugs.

The United States Pharmacopeia: National Formulary. Easton, PA: Mack Publishing Co. (annual publication).

Giving Medications ("Nurses Photobook Series"). Edison, NJ: The Skill Book Co., n.d.

A book on how to give medication, written for nurses but clear and simple enough for parents. *Caution:* Never follow directions for any procedure unless your doctor has instructed you to care for your child in that way.

Chapter 6   Respiratory Therapy

A basic manual for patients with chronic lung diseases:

Moser, Kenneth M., M.D., Carol Archibald, R.N., Patsy Hansen, R.N., Birgitta Ellis, P.T., and Donna Whelan, R.R.T. *Better Living and*

Breathing: A Manual for Patients. St. Louis: C.V. Mosby Co, 1980.

A basic manual for nurses and respiratory therapists on respiratory care:

Respiratory Care ("Nurses Photobook Series"). Edison, NJ: The Skill Book Co., n.d.

Clear and simple enough to be used by parents. *Caution:* Never perform any of these procedures on your child unless your doctor has instructed you to care for your child in that way.

Your hospital should provide you with written instructions on tracheostomy care. If you also want to get these books, make sure your doctor reviews the material to be sure that it is appropriate for your child.

Alperin, Kenneth, M.D., and Howard Levine, M.D. *Tracheostomy Care Manual.* New York: Thieme-Stratton, 1982.

Tracheostomy Care (free manual by Shirley, Inc., 17600 Gillette Avenue, Irvine, CA 92714)

PART 2   MEETING YOUR CHILD'S DAILY PHYSICAL NEEDS

Source books which can give you an idea of available equipment:

Enders, Sandi, ed. *The Technology for Independent Living Resource Guide.* Bethesda, MD: Rehabilitation Engineering Society of North America, 1984.

Guide to equipment and technology, with practical application to the everyday life of a disabled person. Includes extensive references to useful publications, resource persons, and organizations that can provide assistance.

Hale, Glorya, ed. *The Source Book for the Disabled: An Illustrated Guide to Easier and More Independent Living for Physically Disabled.* New York: Bantam, 1981.

A well-illustrated text explaining the needs, equipment, and resources available to the ill or disabled person.

Kreisler, Jack, and Nancy Kreisler. *Catalog of Aids for the Disabled.* New York: McGraw-Hill, 1982.

Guide describing useful equipment and aids to enable more independent functioning for the disabled; appendix contains list of organizations, agencies, and suppliers of equipment described.

Lowman, Edward W., M.D., and Judith Lannefeld Klinger, O.R.T., M.A. *Aids to Independent Living: Self-Help for the Handicapped.* New York, McGraw-Hill, 1969.

Similar format to Kreisler, but much more extensive; no longer in print but may be available in your library.

Lunt, Suzanne. *A Handbook for the Disabled: Ideas and Inventions for Easier Living.* New York: Charles Scribner's Sons, 1982.

A practical guide to show you what is available, names and addresses of manufacturers and suppliers, as well as references to other sources of information. While this is written for the disabled adult, much of the information is applicable to children.

Directory of Living Aids for the Disabled. Washington, DC: U.S. Government Printing Office, #501-000-00158-3, 1984. Catalog of information on assistive devices to help disabled persons with daily living. Listings include brand name of product, description of function, name and address of manufacturer.

Catalogs of major suppliers of medical and therapy equipment are available free or at nominal cost. Ask your therapist or medical supplier which they recommend, considering your child's condition and who supplies your area. You might consider:

Abbey Medical
13782 Crenshaw Boulevard
Gardena, CA 90249

J.A. Preston Corporation
71 Fifth Avenue
New York, NY 10003

Fred Sammons, Inc: Be OK Self-Help Aids
Box 32
Brookfield, IL 60513-0032

How-to books:

Finnie, Nancie. *Handling the Young Cerebral Palsied Child at Home.* New York: E. P. Dutton, 1975.

A classic, comprehensive guide to caring for young children with cerebral palsy. Much of the material is relevant for children with other physical disabilities.

Chapter 7 Positioning Your Child: Beds, Wheelchairs, and Other Orthopedic Equipment

Caston, Don. *Easy-to-Make Aids for Your Handicapped Child: A Guide for Parents and Teachers.* Englewood Cliffs, NJ: Prentice-Hall, 1981.

A clear description of a variety of aids that parents can build for their child; aids can be made for the child's specific needs and are much cheaper and sometimes more appropriate than commercially produced aids.

Chapter 8 Exercises and Orthopedic Appliances

Froman, Katherine. *The Chance to Grow.* New York: Everest House, 1983.

A physical therapist's account of how parents can work with their disabled babies and young children at home.

Levy, Janine, M.D. *The Baby Exercise Book for the First Fifteen Months.* New York: Pantheon, 1975.

Exercises described are for the normal infant, but the material can be helpful for children with impaired motor development.

Chapter 9 Vision, Hearing, and Communication Problems

Vision (parents of blind children should check with organizations aiding the blind):

Nousanen, Diane, and Lee W. Robinson. *Take Charge! A Guide to Resources for Parents of the Visually Impaired.* Austin, TX: National Association for Parents of the Visually Impaired, 1980

A practical manual on how to find the medical care, special materials and equipment, and an appropriate education; excellent bibliography and source list.

Hearing:

Ogden, Paul W., and Suzanne Lipsett. *The Silent Garden: Understanding the Hearing Impaired Child.* Chicago: Contemporary Books, 1983.

A clear description of problems facing parents of a deaf child, of how to accept the disability and help the child learn to communicate with a discussion of the different approaches of oralism, signing, and total communication; resource list.

Speech:

Barach, Carol. *Help Me Say It: A Parent's Guide to Speech Problems.* New York: Harper & Row, 1983.

A helpful guide to how parents can help children overcome various communication problems or learn to cope with them; bibliography and list of resources.

Hagen, Dolores. *Microcomputer Resource Book for Special Education.* Reston, VA: Reston Publishing Company, Inc., 1984.

A book written specifically for parents and special education professionals on how microcomputers can be used to help disabled children and adults.

Closing the Gap. PO Box 68, Henderson, MN 56044.

A newsletter on computer technology for the handicapped with articles about new products helpful to disabled children. Also contains information on conferences and paid advertising.

Chapter 10 Bathing, Toileting, and Personal Hygiene

Chapman, Warren, M.D., Margaret Hill, R.N., and David B. Shurtleff, M.D. *Management of the Neurogenic Bowel and Bladder.* Oak Brook, IL: Eterna Press, 1979.

Handbook on how to meet the toileting needs of children with myolodysplasia or those who have had spinal cord tumors or trauma.

Geter, Katherine. *These Special Children.* Palo Alto, CA: Bull Publishing, 1982.

Handbook for parents of children with ostomies.

Mullen, Barbara Coor, and Kerry Anee McGinn. *The Ostomy Book.* Palo Alto, CA: Bull Publishing, 1980.

Handbook for adult ostomates, but much of the material is applicable to children.

Chapter 11   How and in What to Dress Your Child

Hotte, Eleanor Boettke. *Self-Help Clothing for Children Who Have Physical Disabilities.* Chicago: Easter Seal Society, 1979.

A well-illustrated pamphlet on choosing and making simple alterations on children's clothing, with a short section on teaching dressing skills; bibliography.

Kennedy, Evelyn S. *Dressing with Pride: Clothing Changes for Special Needs.* Groton, CT: Pride Foundation, 1981.

A manual written specifically for the person with limited knowledge of home sewing skills; shows how regular clothing can easily be modified or altered for ease in dressing and undressing, as well as for better fit.

Reich, Naomi, Patricia Otten, and Marie Negri Carver. *Clothing for Handicapped People: An Annotated Bibliography and Resource List.* Washington, DC: President's Committee on Employment of the Handicapped, 1979.

An excellent annotated bibliography and resource list covering all aspects of clothing for the ill and disabled.

Chapter 12   How and What to Feed Your Child

General nutrition:

Atwood, Stephen, M.D. *A Doctor's Guide to Feeding Your Child: Complete Nutrition for Healthy Growth.* New York: Macmillan, 1982.

Discussion of nutritional needs at various stages of normal development and of nutritional problems; although book does not focus on the needs of the ill or disabled child, much of the material is applicable.

Breast-feeding:

La Leche League International. *The Womanly Art of Breastfeeding.* New York: New American Library, 1981.

Basic manual on how to breast-feed a baby.

Brewester, Dorothy. *You Can Breastfeed Your Baby . . . Even in Special Situations.* Emmaus, PA: Rodale Press, 1979.

Gives practical suggestions on how most physically disabled, retarded, ill, and premature babies can be breast-fed.

Basic nutrition:

Robertson, Laurel, Carol Flinders, and Bronwen Godfrey. *Laurel's Kitchen: A Handbook for Vegetarian Cookery and Nutrition.* Berkeley: Nilgiri, 1976.

While part of the book is simply a vegetarian cookbook, the section on diet and the nutrients in foods (carbohydrates, fats, proteins, vitamins, and minerals) is excellent and is particularly helpful if you are trying to provide your child with specific nutrients.

Special diets: In addition to the following books, organizations assisting those with your child's disorder may have specific suggestions.

Diet and Nutrition: A Resource for Parents of Children with Cancer. Washington, DC: U.S. Department of Health and Human Services, 1982 (free publication).

Although there is one section on the side effects of cancer and cancer treatment, the helpful information on the importance of nutrition, ways to encourage your child to eat, and special dietary modifications is applicable to most children.

Feingold, Ben, M.D. *Why Your Child Is Hyperactive.* New York: Random House, 1974.

Discussion of how elimination of food additives (preservatives and coloring agents) can improve some children's behavior.

Gallender, Carolyn Newton, and Demos Gallender. *Dietary Problems and Diets for the Handicapped.* Springfield, IL: Charles Thomas, 1978.

Discussion of basic nutrition, eating handicaps and other dietary problems, and how an appropriate diet can be provided.

Smith, Lendon, M.D. *Improving Your Child's Behavior Chemistry.* Englewood Cliffs, NJ: Prentice-Hall, 1976.

Discussion of how some types of hyperactivity and behavioral problems can be lessened by controlling the intake of refined carbohydrates.

PART 3   MEETING YOUR CHILD'S EDUCATIONAL AND SOCIAL NEEDS

Clemes, Harris, and Reynold Bean. *Self-Esteem: The Key to Your Child's Well-Being.* New York: G.P. Putnam's Sons, 1981.

Perceptive book on how to help any child develop a good self-concept.

Mollan, Renee, M.A. *Yes They Can! A Handbook for Effectively Parenting the Handicapped.* Irvine, CA: Reality Productions, 1981.

Positive approach on how to help one's child reach his or her maximum potential.

Chapter 13   Play, Recreation, and Travel

Play:

Arnold, Arnold. *Your Child's Play: How to Help Your Child Reap the Full Benefits of Play.*

New York: Simon and Schuster, 1968.

A discussion of the importance of play as well as imaginative play ideas for children from infancy through adolescence.

Marzollo, Jean, and Janice Lloyd. *Learning Through Play.* New York: Harper & Row, 1972.

Discussion of the importance of play and how we can provide play opportunities for the young child.

Trelease, Jim. *The Read-Aloud Handbook.* New York: Penguin, 1982.

Why, when, and how to read aloud to children, followed by a listing of read-alouds for toddlers through teenagers.

Toys: It is often difficult to find appropriate toys for disabled children. *The Technology for Independent Living Resource Guide,* edited by Sandi Enders, is a good guide to sources of toys for your disabled child. See page 276 under "Meeting Your Child's Daily Physical Needs" for a full reference.

Recreation:

American Academy of Orthopaedic Surgeons, sponsor. *Sports and Recreational Programs for the Child and Young Adult with Physical Disability.* Proceedings of the Winter Park Seminar, April 11–13, 1983. Chicago, IL: American Academy of Orthopaedic Surgeons, 1983.

Excellent sourcebook on how to assess the orthopedically disabled child's ability, possible adaptations for various sports and recreational activities, available program resources, competition classifications, and bibliography.

Travel: Most books on travel for the handicapped are written for the adult traveler. While you might find that some of the ideas that are presented in such books are helpful, you should first check and see what you can borrow from your public library.

Access Amtrak
400 North Capitol Street NW
Washington, DC 20001

Airport Operators Council
Access Travel: Airports
International Consumer Information Center
Department 619f
Pueblo, CO 81009

Chapter 14   Teaching and Educating Your Child

Psychological testing:

Klein, Stanley D., Ph.D. *Psychological Testing of Children: A Consumer's Guide with Special Emphasis on the Psychological Assessment of Children with Disabilities.* Boston: The Exceptional Parent Magazine, 1979.

An introduction to the nature and use of psychological testing for individuals with little background information.

Wodrich, David, Ph.D. *Children's Psychological Testing: A Guide for Nonpsychologists.* Baltimore: Brookes, 1984.

A more complex discussion of the whole field of testing, including a consideration of the most frequently used children's psychological tests, when referral for testing is appropriate, and how to interpret and use test results.

Working with the schools:

Culter, Barbara Coyne. *Unraveling the Special Education Maze: An Action Guide for Parents.* Prairie Village, KS: Research Press, 1981.

A guide to help you understand how to get the educational services your child needs and how to advocate on his or her behalf.

Lillie, David L., and Patricia A. Place. *Partners: A Guide to Working with Schools for Parents of Children with Special Instructional Needs.* Glenview, IL: Scott, Foresman, 1982.

Information and strategies on how you can work with the schools to get your child the appropriate educational opportunities legally provided for under PL 94-142. Workbook form allows you to test your knowledge and evaluate whether you are being effective in getting your child the education he or she needs.

National Cancer Institute et al. *Students with Cancer: A Resource for the Educator.* Bethesda, MD: U.S. Department of Health, Education, and Welfare, 1980 (free publication).

While this is written specifically with the child with cancer in mind, it does offer sound general guidelines on how to reintegrate a child into the classroom after an illness or accident.

Learning disabilities:

Lerner, Janet W. *Learning Disabilities.* Boston: Houghton Mifflin, 1981.

Discussion of diverse approaches to learning disabilities and of assessment procedures, and a consideration of teaching techniques and materials. While this book is written for professionals, it provides valuable information for the parent of the learning-disabled child.

Chapter 15   Adolescence

Adolescence:

Lund, Lois. *Eric.* New York: Dell, 1974.

See Chapter 3.

Showalter, John, M.D., and Walter Anyan, M.D. *The Family Handbook of Adolescence.* New York: Knopf, 1981.

A comprehensive medically oriented reference book for parents and their adolescent.

Depression:

McCoy, Kathleen. *Coping with Teenage Depression: A Parent's Guide.* New York: New American Library, 1982.

How to recognize signs of depression, what you can do as a parent, and how, when, and why to seek professional help.

Sexuality:

Balis, Andrea. *What Are You Using: A Birth Control Guide for Teenagers.* New York: Dial Press, 1981.

Discussion of the need for and methods of birth control.

McKee, Lyn, and Virginia Blacklidge, M.D. *An Easy Guide for Caring Parents: Sexuality and Socialization.* Walnut Creek, CA: Planned Parenthood of Contra Costa County and the Association of Retarded Citizens of Alemeda County, 1981.

A discussion of sexuality and the social needs of children with mental handicaps and developmental disabilities.

Rabin, Barry, Ph.D. *The Sensuous Wheeler: Sexual Adjustment for the Spinal-Cord Injured.* San Francisco: Multi Media Resource Center, 1980.

Survey of current information on sexual functioning in general and especially in relation to spinal-cord injury as well as methods by which the disabled individual may achieve sexual adjustment.

The future of the ill or disabled teenager and young adult:

Feingold, S. Norman, and Norma R. Miller. *Your Future: A Guide for the Handicapped Teenager.* New York: Richards Rosen Press, 1981.

A practical guide to assist teenagers in choosing appropriate vocations, getting the necessary education, finding a job, choosing an appropriate life style that includes work, recreation, and the best possible living situation.

Laurie, Gini. *Housing and Home Services for the Disabled: Guidelines and Experiences in Independent Living.* New York: Harper & Row, 1977.

Practical discussion on helping the disabled live independently; excellent source materials included.

Lifchez, Raymond, and Barbara Winslow. *Design for Independent Living: The Environment and Physically Disabled People.* Berkeley: University of California Press, 1979.

Discussion of how environmental adaptations can make it possible for the disabled to live independently; biographical sketches of individuals.

Vash, Carolyn. *The Psychology of Disability.* New York: Springer, 1981.

Consideration of how the physically disabled can come to accept their disability and live full, productive lives.

PART 4   MEETING THE NEEDS OF THE WHOLE FAMILY

Napier, Augustus, Ph.D., and Carl Whitaker, M.D. *The Family Crucible.* New York: Harper & Row, 1978.

This book sheds light on how every individual's problems are rooted in the family. While this is not included to suggest that therapy is appropriate for all families or that family therapy is always better than individual therapy, the book does make clear the importance of family interrelationships.

Chapter 16   Organizing Your Household

While there are no books dealing exclusively with household organization for families with disabled or ill children, *The Exceptional Parent* magazine (see page 273) occasionally has articles on this subject. Books listed under Chapter 15, "Adolescence" and "The Future of the Ill or Disabled Teenager and Young Adult," give practical suggestions to promote independent living skills. Books for the general homemaker on how to run a household efficiently may occasionally also have helpful ideas.

Chapter 17   Paying for the Medical Help You Need

Apolloni, Tony, and Thomas Cooke. *A New Look at Guardianship: Protective Services That Support Personalized Living.* Baltimore: Brookes, 1984.

Exploration of the alternatives available to parents and other care providers considering not only relatives, friends, lawyers, and bankers, but also the emerging option of public and private group guardianship.

Russell, L. Mark. *Alternatives: A Family Guide to Legal and Financial Planning for the Disabled.* Evanston, IL: First Publications, 1983.

Discussion of factors the family of a disabled or ill child must consider, such as wills, guardianship, trusts, government benefits, taxes, insurance, and financial planning.

Swirnoff, Weinberg, and Daly. *Planning for the Disabled Child.* Minneapolis: Northwestern Mutual Life Insurance Company, n.d. (free publication).

Pamphlet discussing the advantages and disadvantages of various forms of estate planning for the disabled child.

PART 5   IF YOUR CHILD IS DYING

Understanding the dying child:

Kübler-Ross, Elisabeth, M.D. *On Death and Dying.* New York: Macmillan, 1969.

A classic book on the dying, their concerns, and how family can best help.

Kübler-Ross, Elisabeth, M.D. *On Children and Death.* New York: Macmillan, 1983.

Utilizing many letters from parents, the author confronts the difficulties faced by parents of dying children, such as talking about death with all family members, caring for the dying child at home with love, and overcoming grief in a positive way.

Sabom, Michael B., M.D. *Recollections of Death: A Medical Investigation.* New York: Harper & Row, 1981.

Interviews with people who have almost died and a review of literature in the field lead to the conclusion that most people do not feel anguish, pain, or despair at the moment of death, but rather tranquility and peace.

Personal accounts:

Lund, Lois. *Eric.* New York: Dell, 1974.

See Chapter 3.

Sharkey, Frances, M.D. *A Parting Gift.* New York: St. Martin's Press, 1982.

A doctor's moving account of how even she first feared caring for dying children but how she has now come to see the value of allowing and arranging for a terminally ill child to die at home.

Zorza, Victor, and Rosemary Zorza. *A Way to Die.* New York: Knopf, 1980.

Description of how the authors' daughter, who got cancer as a young adult, first lived independently with the help of her family, was then cared for at home, and finally spent her last days in a British hospice.

Chapter 18   How to Care for Your Dying Child at Home

Duda, Deborah. *A Guide to Dying at Home.* Santa Fe: John Muir Publications, 1982.

A manual on providing physical care as well as mental, emotional, and spiritual support for the adult dying at home; much of the material is applicable to children.

Martinson, Ida. *Home Care: A Manual for Parents; Home Care: A Manual for Implementation of Home Care for Children Dying with Cancer.* Alexandria, VA: Children's Hospice International, 1984.

Discussions of what is involved in caring for a child at home, including specific advice on providing medical and nurturing care, emotional concerns, community resources, payment for home care, necessary funeral arrangements, what will happen at death, and an annotated bibliography. While written with cancer in mind, much of the material is applicable to the family of any dying child. The implementation manual is written for health-care professionals, but if you are actively involved in your child's medical care, this can be very useful as a reference book.

Chapter 19   Looking to the Future

Conley, Bruce H. *Handling the Holidays.* Elburn, IL: Thum Printing, 1979.

Excellent short book on how to handle the holidays after a death in the family.

Church, Martha Jo, Helene Chazin, and Faith Ewald. *When a Baby Dies.* Oak Brook, IL: Compassionate Friends, 1981.

Short pamphlet provides insight into the grieving process, outlines options on leave-taking ceremonies, and considers how a family can come to cope with and look to the future, including a discussion about having another baby.

Duda, Deborah. *A Guide to Dying at Home.* Santa Fe: John Muir Publications, 1982.

See Chapter 18.

Grollman, Earl. *Living When a Loved One Has Died.* Boston: Beacon Press, 1977.

A compassionate discussion of how we can survive our grief and emotional turmoil in confronting the death of a loved one and in so doing come to affirm life.

Kushner, Harold. *When Bad Things Happen to Good People.* New York: Schocken, 1983.

See Chapter 1.

La Tour, Kathy. *For Those Who Live: Helping Children Cope with the Death of a Brother or Sister.* Oak Brook, IL: Compassionate Friends, 1983.

Designed especially to help siblings understand the death of another child in the family.

Lund, Lois. Eric. New York: Dell, 1974.

See Chapter 3.

Miles, Margaret. *The Grief of Parents . . . When a Child Dies.* Oak Brook, IL: Compassionate Friends, 1978.

Short, well-written pamphlet for parents on how parents and siblings can cope with their grief and loss.

Schatz, William H. *Healing a Father's Grief.* Redmond, WA: Medic Publishing, 1984.

A short booklet written specifically for fathers after the author's own son died; can be ordered through Compassionate Friends, listed under "death and bereavement" in Appendix 4, "Helpful Organizations."

Grieving, Healing, and Growing. Oak Brook, IL: Compassionate Friends, 1983.

A collection of some of the best articles from the Compassionate Friends newsletter from 1978 to 1982.

Appendix 4

Helpful Organizations

This list is alphabetized by condition or need and is cross-referenced for your convenience. However, since there may well be more than one type of organization that can assist you, it will be helpful to read through the entire list, and perhaps also show it to your doctor. The organizations listed here range from large, well-established ones that provide a variety of services, to small, informal parent groups that share information about specific disorders. Inclusion in this list should not be viewed as an endorsement by the author, but only as an indication of an available resource. You and the professionals working with your child have to consider whether information you receive from any given organization would be helpful in the care of your child.

If you cannot find an organization dealing with your child's disability in this list, specialized pediatric units treating similar children at large hospitals may know of regional support groups or any newly formed national organizations. The National Organization for Rare Disorders (listed under "rare disorders") and the National Maternal and Child Health Clearinghouse (listed under "government agencies") both keep excellent updated listings. If your child has a rare disorder and you want to find other parents in a similar situation, consider writing to *The Exceptional Parent* (see "Suggested Reading") and requesting that others write to you.

Information retrieval systems (often computerized) can assist professionals or patients locate helpful information. Since clearinghouses are continually being established, not all in the health field could be listed here. Ask any organizations you contact if they know of clearinghouses from which you might be able to get helpful information.

Data bases, which are computerized information banks, may also be of assistance. Some data bases are free, while others have a user's fee. Again, check with the professionals and organizations assisting your child to see if any relevant data bases exist for your needs.

While all the addresses and phone numbers in this list were correct at the time of publication, if you try to contact one of the organizations and your letter is returned, try to find it through telephone information in the same city. If you still have no luck, ask your local reference librarian to check in reference books of organizations for a current address or try contacting the resources mentioned above.

acidemia

See organic acidemias.

acoustic neuroma

Acoustic Neuroma Association
PO Box 398
Carlisle, PA 17013
717-249-3937

adrenoleukodystrophy

Adrenoleukodystrophy Project
JKF Institute for Handicapped Children
707 N. Broadway
Baltimore, MD 21205
301-955-4051

advocacy

American Coalition of Citizens with
Disabilities (ACCD)
1200 15th Street NW, #201
Washington, DC 20005

Center on Human Policy
Syracuse University
216 Ostrom Avenue
Syracuse, NY 13210

Disability Rights Center
1346 Connecticut Avenue NW
Washington, DC 20036
202-223-3304

albinism

NOAH: National Organization for
Albinism and Hypopigmentation
919 Walnut Street, #400
Philadelphia, PA 19107
214-627-3501

allergy

Allergy Foundation of America
118–35 Queens Boulevard
Forest Hills, NY 11375
718-261-3663
See also asthma.

amputation

National Amputation Foundation, Inc.
12–45 150th Street
Whitestone, NY 11357
212-767-8400

Parents of Amputee Children Together
West Kessler Rehabilition Institute
West Orange, NJ 07052
201-731-3600

anemia

See Cooley's anemia.

aniridia

Aniridia Information
1032 Croton Drive
Alexandria, VA 22308
703-780-8856

arson

See behavioral disorders.

arthogryposis multiplex congenita

AVENUES
5430 East Harbor Heights Drive
Port Orchard, WA 98366
206-871-5057

arthritis

Arthritis Foundation
1314 Spring Street NW
Atlanta, GA 30309
404-872-7100

asthma

National Foundation for Asthma, Inc.
PO Box 50304
Tuscon, AR 85703
602-624-7481

ataxia

Friedreich's Ataxia Group in America, Inc.
PO Box 11116
Oakland, CA 94611
415-658-7014

National Ataxia Foundation
600 Twelve Oaks Center
15500 Wayzata Boulevard
Wayzata, MN 55391
612-473-7666

See also muscular dystrophy.

autism

Autism Services Center
101 Richmond Street
Huntington, WV 25702
304-523-8269

National Society for Children and Adults
with Autism
1234 Massachusetts Avenue NW, #1017
Washington, DC 20005
202-783-0125

Batten-Vogt syndrome

See brain disorders.

behavioral disorders

Center for Hyperactive Child
Information, Inc.
PO Box 406, Murray Hill Station
New York, NY 10156
212-679-3959

Council for Children with Behavioral Disorders
1920 Association Drive
Reston, VA 22091
703-368-3293

National Firehawk Foundation (Arson)
PO Box 27488
San Francisco, CA 94127
415-922-3242

bereavement

See death and bereavement.

birth defects

See genetic disorders.

blindness

See eye and vision disorders.

bone disorders

See osteogenesis imperfecta.

brain disorders

Association for Brain Tumor Research
6232 North Pulaski Road, #200
Chicago, IL 60646
312-286-5571

National Head Injury Foundation
18A Vernon Street
Framingham, MA 01701
617-879-7473

brain injury

See brain disorders.

breast-feeding

La Leche League International
9616 Minneapolis Avenue
Franklin Park, IL 60103
312-455-7730

camping

The American Camping Association
Bradford Woods
5040 State Road 67 North
Martinsville, IN 46151

The Committee for the Promotion of Camping for the Handicapped
2056 South Bluff Road
Travers City, MI 49684

cancer

American Cancer Society
777 Third Avenue
New York, NY 10017
212-371-2900

Cancer Information Clearinghouse
Office of Cancer Communications
National Cancer Institute
9000 Rockville Pike, Building 31, Rm10A21
Bethesda, MD 20205
800-4-CANCER

Candlelighters Childhood Cancer Foundation
2025 Eye Street NW, #1011
Washington, DC 20006
202-659-5136

cataplexy

See narcolepsy; brain disorders.

celiac-sprue

Midwestern Celiac-Sprue Association
2313 Rocklyn Drive, #1
Des Moines, IA 50322
515-270-9689

cerebral palsy

United Cerebral Palsy Associations, Inc.
66 East 34th Street
New York, NY
212-481-6300

chromosome abnormalities

See Down's syndrome; trisomy 18/13.

cleft lip/palate

American Cleft Palate Educational Foundation
331 Salk Hall
University of Pittsburgh
Pittsburgh, PA 15261
412-681-9620

Prescription Parents, Inc.
PO Box 426
Quincy, MA 02269
617-479-2463

colitis

See ileitis.

colostomy

See ostomy.

Cooley's anemia

Cooley's Anemia Foundation, Inc.
105 East 22nd Street
New York, NY 10010
800-212-3571

Cornelia de Lange syndrome

Cornelia de Lange Syndrome Foundation
60 Dyer Avenue
Collinsville, CN 06022
203-693-0159

craniofacial deformities

Debbie Fox Foundation for Craniofacial
Deformaties
PO Box 11082
Chattanooga, TN 37401
615-266-1632

cri-du-chat syndrome

Cri-du-Chat Society
Department of Human Genetics
Medical College of Virginia
Box 33, MCV Station
Richmond, VA 23298
804-786-9632

cystic fibrosis

Cystic Fibrosis Foundation
6000 Executive Boulevard, #309
Rockville, MD 20852
301-881-9130

International Cystic Fibrosis Association
3567 East 49th Street
Cleveland, OH 44105

deafness

See ear and hearing disorders.

deaf-blind

Helen Keller National Center for
Deaf-Blind Youths and Adults
111 Middle Neck Road
Sands Point, NY 11050
516-944-8900

death and bereavement

AMEND: Aiding Mothers Experiencing
Perinatal Death
4324 Berrywick Terrace
Saint Louis, MO 63128

Children's Hospice International
501 Slaters Lane, #207
Alexandria, VA 22314
703-556-0421

Compassionate Friends, Inc.
PO Box 1347
Oak Brook, IL 60521
312-323-5010

dental problems

American Dental Association
211 East Chicago Avenue
Chicago, IL 60611
312-440-2500

National Foundation of Dentistry for the
Handicapped
1250 Fourteenth Street, #610
Denver, CO 80202
303-573-0264

diabetes

American Diabetes Association, Inc.
2 Park Avenue
New York, NY 10016
212-683-7444

Juvenile Diabetes Foundation
60 Madison Avenue
New York, NY 10010
212-889-7575

National Diabetes Information
Clearinghouse
Box NIDC
Bethesda, MD 20205
301-468-2162

disabilities

National Organization on Disability
2100 Pennsylvania Avenue NW
Washington, DC 20037
202-293-5960

Down's syndrome

Down's Syndrome Congress
1640 West Roosevelt Road
Chicago, IL 60608
312-226-0416

The Michael Fund: International
Foundation for Genetic Research
400 Penn Ct. Boulevard, #1022
Pittsburgh, PA 15235
412-325-3801

National Down Syndrome Society
70 West 40th Street
New York, NY 10018
800-221-4602

dwarfism

See growth disorders.

dysautonomia

Dysautonomia Foundation, Inc.
370 Lexington Avenue, #1504
New York, NY 10017
212-889-0300

See also genetic disorders.

dyslexia

Orton Dyslexia Society
724 York Road
Baltimore, MD 21204
301-296-0232

dystonia

Dystonia Foundation
425 Broad Hollow Road
Melville, NY 11747
516-249-7799

Dystonia Medical Research Foundation
9615 Brighton Way, #416
Beverly Hills, CA 90210
213-272-9880

See also genetic disorders.

dystrophic epidermolysis bullosa

DEBRA: Dystrophic Epidermolysis
Bullosa Research Association of America
2936 Avenue W
Brooklyn, NY 11229
718-774-8700

ear and hearing disorders

Alexander Graham Bell Association for
the Deaf, Inc.
International Parents' Organization
3417 Volta Place NW
Washington, DC 20007
202-337-5220

American Tinnitus Association
PO Box 5
Portland, OR 97207
503-248-9985

Hearing and Tinnitus Help Association
PO Box 231
Iselin, NJ 08830

International Association of Parents of the
Deaf
814 Thayer Avenue
Silver Spring, MD 20910
301-585-5400

John Tracy Clinic
806 West Adams Boulevard
Los Angeles, CA 90007
213-748-5481

National Association for Hearing and
Speech Action
10801 Rockville Pike
Rockville, MD 20852
800-638-8255

National Hearing Aid Society
20361 Middlebelt
Livonia, MI 48152
800-521-5247

National Information Center on Deafness
Gallaudet College
800 Floria Avenue
Washington, DC 20002
202-651-5109

Self Help for Hard of Hearing People,
Inc. (SHHH)
4848 Battery Lane, #100
Bethesda, MD 20814
301-657-2248

ectodermal dysplasias

National Foundation for Ectodermal
Dysplasias
108 North First Street, #311
Mascoutah, IL 62258
618-566-2020

education

Association for Children and Adults with
Learning Disabilities
4156 Library Road
Pittsburgh, PA 15234
412-341-1515

Council for Exceptional Children
1920 Association Drive
Reston, VA 22091
703-620-3660

National Committee/Arts for the
Handicapped (NCAH)
1825 Connecticut Avenue NW
Washington, DC 20006
202-332-6960

National Library Service for the Blind and
Physically Handicapped
Library of Congress
Washington, DC 20542
202-287-5100

Recording for the Blind
20 Roszel Road
Princeton, NJ 08540
609-452-0606

emotional disturbance

See mental illness/health.

epidermolysis bullosa

See dystrophic epidermolysis bullosa.

epilepsy

Epilepsy Foundation of America
4351 Garden City Drive
Landover, MD 20785
301-459-3700

extrophy

National Support Group for Extrophy
5075 Medhurst Street
Solon, OH 44139
216-248-6851

eye and vision disorders

American Council of the Blind Parents
1121 Connecticut Avenue NW, #506
Washington, DC 20036
800-424-8666

American Foundation for the Blind
15 West 16th Street
New York, NY 10011
212-620-2000

Association for Macular Diseases
PO Box 469
Merrick, NY 11566
516-883-3147

International Institute for Visually
Impaired, 0–7, Inc.
1975 Rutgers
East Lansing, MI 48823
517-332-2666

National Association for Parents of the
Visually Impaired, Inc.
PO Box 180806
Austin, TX 78718
512-459-6651

National Association for the Visually
Handicapped
305 East 24th Street
New York, NY 10010
212-889-3141

National Federation of the Blind
Newsletter for Parents
Box 552
Jefferson City, MO 65102
301-659-9341

National Retinitis Pigmentosa
Foundation
8331 Mindale Circle
Baltimore, MD 21207
301-655-1011

Optic Nerve Hypoplasia Parent Group
1730 Adler Drive
Great Falls, MT 59404
406-452-0696

facial deformities

See craniofacial deformities.

facial paralysis

Association for Congenital Facial
Paralysis, Inc.
928 Hanover Lane
Dyer, IN 46311
219-322-3389

Freeman-Sheldon syndrome

Freeman-Sheldon Parent Support Group
1459 East Maple Hills Drive
Bountiful, UT 84010
801-298-3149

Gaucher's disease

Gaucher's Disease Registry
4418 East Chapman, #139
Orange, CA 92669
714-532-2212

genetic disorders

Association of Birth Defect Children, Inc.
3201 E. Crystal Lake Avenue
Orlando, FL 32806
305-898-5342

March of Dimes Birth Defects Foundation
1275 Mamaroneck Avenue
White Plains, NY 10605
914-428-7100

National Foundation for Jewish Genetic
Diseases
250 Park Avenue, #1000
New York, NY 10177
212-682-5550

National Genetics Foundation
555 West 57th Street
New York, NY 10019
212-586-5800

See also rare disorders.

glycogen storage disease

Association for Glycogen Storage Disease
Box 896
Durant, IA 52747
319-785-6038

government agencies

Clearinghouse on the Handicapped
U.S. Department of Education
Switzer Building #3119
Washington, DC 20202
202-732-1241

National Health Information
Clearinghouse
PO Box 1133
Washington, DC 20013-1133
800-336-4797

National Information Center for
Handicapped Children and Youth
Box 1492
Washington, DC 20013

National Maternal and Child Health
Clearinghouse
3520 Prospect Street NW
Washington, DC 20057
202-625-8410

growth disorders

Little People of America
PO Box 633
San Bruno, CA 94066
415-589-0695

See also Turner's syndrome.

Guillain-Barré syndrome

Guillain-Barré Syndrome Support Group
Box 262
Wynnewood, PA 19096
215-649-7837

hair disorders

Alopecia Areata Foundation
PO Box 5027
Mill Valley, CA 94941
415-383-3444

Cartilage Hair Hypoplasia Foundation
3500 South 37th Street
Lincoln, NE 68506
402-488-7047

handicaps

See physical disabilities.

heart disorders

American Heart Association
7320 Greenville Avenue
Dallas, TX 75231
214-750-5300

See also Marfan syndrome.

hemochromatosis

Hemochromatosis Research Foundation
PO Box 8569
Albany, NY 12208
518-489-0972

hemodialysis and transplantation

National Association of Patients on
Hemodialysis and Transplantation
(NAPTH)
156 William Street
New York, NY 10038
212-619-2727

hemophilia

National Hemophilia Foundation
19 West 34th Street, #1204
New York, NY 10001
212-563-0211

hospice

See death and bereavement.

human growth

Human Growth Foundation
5701 Normandale Road
Edina, MN
612-962-5534

humanizing health care

The Association for the Care of Children's
Health
3615 Wisconsin Avenue NW
Washington, DC 20016
202-244-1801

Pediatric Projects
PO Box 1880
Santa Monica, CA 90406
213-459-7710

Huntington's disease

Huntington's Disease Foundation of
America
250 West 57th Street, #2016
New York, NY 10107
212-757-0443

National Huntington's Disease Association
1182 Broadway, #402
New York, NY 10001
212-684-2781

hydrocephalus

Guardians of Hydrocephalus Research
Foundation
2618 Avenue Z
Brooklyn, NY 11235
718-648-0025

Hydrocephalus Parent Support Group
225 Dickinson Street, #H-893
San Diego, CA 92103
619-294-6812

Know Problems of Hydrocephalus
Box 97
Minnok, IL 60447
815-467-6548

hyperactivity

See behavioral disorders.

hypopigmentation

See albinism.

ileitis

National Foundation for Ileitis and
Colitis, Inc.
444 Park Avenue South
New York, NY 10016
212-685-3440

immune deficiency

Immune Deficiency Foundation
PO Box 586
Columbia, MD 21045
301-997-7919

intraventricula hemorrhage

IVH Parents
PO Box 56-1111
Miami, FL 33156
305-232-0381

iron overload diseases

Iron Overload Diseases Association, Inc.
5409 Harriet Place
West Palm Beach, FL 33407
305-689-6968

See also hemochromatosis.

Jewish genetic disorders

See genetic disorders or the specific disorder.

Joseph diseases

International Joseph Diseases
Foundation, Inc.
PO Box 2550
Livermore, CA 94550
415-455-0706

kidney disorders

National Kidney Foundation, Inc.
2 Park Avenue
New York, NY 10016
212-889-2210

laryngectomy

International Association of
Laryngectomees
777 Third Avenue
New York, NY 10017
212-371-2900

learning disabilities

See education; dyslexia.

leukemia

Leukemia Society of America
733 Third Avenue, 14th floor
New York, NY 10017
212-573-8484

See also cancer.

leukodystrophy

United Leukodystrophy Foundation, Inc.
2304 Highland Drive
Sycamore, IL 60178
815-895-3211

See also adrenoleukodystrophy.

liver disorders

American Liver Foundation
998 Pompton Avenue
Cedar Grove, NJ 07009
201-857-2626

Children's Liver Foundation, Inc.
28 Highland Avenue
Maplewood, NJ 07040
201-761-1111

Lowe's syndrome

Lowe's Syndrome Association
607 Robinson Street
West Lafayette, IN 47906
317-743-3634

lung disorders

American Lung Association
1740 Broadway
New York, NY 10019
212-245-8000

lupus

American Lupus Society
23751 Madison Street
Torrance, CA 90505
213-373-1335

Lupus Foundation of America, Inc.
11673 Holly Springs Drive
St. Louis, MO 63146
314-872-9036

National Lupus Erythematosis Foundation
5430 Van Nuys Boulevard, #206
Van Nuys, CA 91401
213-885-8787

Systemic Lupus Erythematosis
Foundation
95 Madison Avenue, #1402
New York, NY
212-685-4118

lymphatic and venous disorders

National Lymphatic and Venous
Foundation, Inc.
PO Box 80
Cambridge, MA 02140
617-359-7632

maple syrup urine disease

Families with Maple Syrup Urine Disease
Route 2, Box 24-A
Flemingsburg, KE 41041
606-849-4679

Marfan syndrome

National Marfan Foundation
54 Irma Avenue
Port Washington, NY 11050
516-883-8712

mental illness/health

American Mental Health Fund
PO Box 17389
Washington, DC 20041
703-790-8570

Mental Health Law Project
2021 L Street NW, #800
Washington, DC 20036
202-467-5730

National Alliance for the Mentally Ill
1234 Massachusetts Avenue NW, #721
Washington, DC 20005
202-280-2878

National Clearinghouse for Mental Health
Information
Public Inquiries Section, #15C-17
5600 Fischers Lane
Rockville, MD 20957
301-443-4513

Recovery Inc: The Association of Nervous
and Former Mental Patients
802 North Dearborn
Chicago, IL 60603
312-337-5661

mental retardation/delayed development

Association for Retarded Citizens of the
United States
2501 Avenue J
Arlington, TX 76011
817-640-0204

Mental Retardation Association of
America, Inc.
211 East 300 South, #212
Salt Lake City, UT 84111
801-328-1575

People First International, Inc.
PO Box 12362
Salem, OR 97309
503-362-0336

See also specific disorder.

midget

See growth disorders.

mucopolysaccharidosis

March of Dimes National Registry of
MPS/ML Disorders
53 W. Jackson Boulevard, #1-50
Chicago, IL 60604
312-341-1370

muscoviscidosis

See cystic fibrosis.

muscular dystrophy

Muscular Dystrophy Association of
America
810 Seventh Avenue
New York, NY 10019
212-586-0808

myasthenia gravis

Myasthenia Gravis Foundation
15 East 26th Street, #1603
New York, NY
212-889-8157

narcolepsy

American Narcolepsy Association
PO Box 5846
Stanford, CA 94305
415-591-7979

Narcolepsy and Cataplexy Foundation of
America
1410 York Avenue, #32-D
New York, NY 10021
212-628-6315

neurofibromatosis

National Neurofibromatosis Foundation
70 West 40th Street
New York, NY 10018
212-869-9034

neurometabolic disorders

Association for Neurometabolic Disorders
5223 Brookfield Lane
Sylvania, OH 43506
419-885-1497

organic acidemias

Organic Acidemias Support Group
1532 South 87th Street
Kansas City, KS 66111
913-422-7080

osteogenesis imperfecta

American Brittle Bone Society
1256 Merrill Drive
West Chester, PA 19380
215-692-6248

Osteogenesis Imperfecta Foundation, Inc.
PO Box 838
Manchester, NH 03105
603-623-0934

osteoporosis

See osteogenesis imperfecta.

ostomy

United Ostomy Association, Inc.
2001 W. Beverly Boulevard
Los Angeles, CA 90057
213-413-5510

paralysis

See spinal cord injury.

parent support groups

Candlelighters Childhood Cancer
Foundation
2025 Eye Street NW, # 1011
Washington, D.C. 20006
202-659-5136

Families Together
Box 926
Lawrence, KS 66044
913-841-7241

Parentele
1301 East 38th Street
Indianapolis, IN 46205
317-926-4142

Parents Helping Parents, Inc.
47 Maro Drive
San Jose, CA 95127
408-272-4774

Pilot Parents
121 East Voltaire Avenue
Phoenix, AR 80522
692-863-4048

patient support groups

Center for Attitudinal Healing
19 Main Street
Tiburon, CA
415-435-5022

Make a Wish Foundation of America
4601 North 16th Street, #205
Phoenix, AZ 85016
602-234-0960

phenylketonuria

PKU Parents
518 Paco Drive
Los Altos, CA 94022
415-941-9799

physical disabilities

National Easter Seal Society
2023 West Ogden Avenue
Chicago, IL 60612
312-243-8400

See also severe handicaps.

Prader-Willi syndrome

Prader-Willi Syndrome Association
5515 Malibu Drive
Edina, MN 55436
612-933-0113

premature infants

Parents of Premature and High-Risk
Infants International, Inc.
33 West 42nd Street, #1227
New York, NY 10036
212-840-1259

progeria

Progeria International Registry
1050 Forest Hill Road
Staten Island, NY 10314
212-494-5231

radiation

National Association of Radiation Survivors
78 El Camino Real
Berkeley, CA 94705
415-652-4400

rare disorders

National Organization for Rare Disorders
1182 Broadway, #402
New York, NY 10001
212-686-1057

See also genetic disorders.

recreation

For a complete list of organizations see *Sports
and Recreational Programs for the Child and
Young Adult with Physical Disability,* listed
in "Suggested Reading" for Chapter 13.

rehabilitation engineering

National Institute for Rehabilitation
Engineering
97 Decker Road
Butler, NJ 07405
201-838-2500

rehabilitation information

National Rehabilitation Information
Center
Catholic University of America
4407 Eighth Street NE
Washington, DC 20017
202-635-5826

retardation

See mental retardation/delayed development.

retinal degeneration

See eye and vision disorders.

retinitis pigmentosa

See eye and vision disorders

Reye's syndrome

National Reye's Syndrome Foundation
PO Box RS
7045 Traverse Avenue
Benzonia, MI 49616
616-882-5521

scoliosis

National Scoliosis Foundation, Inc.
48 Stone Road
Belmont, MA 02178
617-489-0888

Scoliosis Association, Inc.
183 Main Street East, #1428
Rochester, NY 14604
716-546-1814

severe handicaps

The Association for the Severely
Handicapped (TASH)
7010 Roosevelt Way NE
Seattle, WA 98103
206-523-8446

sexuality

Coalition on Sexuality and Disability, Inc.
122 East 23rd Street
New York, NY 10010
212-677-7400

Planned Parenthood Federation of
America
810 Seventh Avenue
New York, NY 10019
212-541-7800

Sex Information and Education Council
80 Fifth Avenue, #801
New York, NY 10011
212-929-2300

short stature

See growth disorders.

sibling support groups

Sibling Information Network
Department of Educational Psychology
University of Connecticut
Storrs, CT 06268
203-466-4032

sickle cell disease

National Association for Sickle Cell
Disease, Inc. (NASCD)
3460 Wilshire Boulevard, #1012
Los Angeles, CA 90010
213-731-1166

National Sickle Cell Clinics Foundation
211 North Whitfield Street, #742
Pittsburgh, PA 15206
412-441-6116

skeletal dysplasia

See growth disorders.

spina bifida

Spina Bifida Association of America
343 South Dearborn, #317
Chicago, IL 60604
800-621-3141

spinal cord injury

American Paralysis Association
4100 Spring Valley Road, #104, LB 3
Dallas, TX 75234
800-527-0321

National Spinal Cord Injury Association
369 Elliot Street
Newton Upper Falls, MA 02164
617-964-0521

Spinal Cord Society
6203 Bellaire Avenue
North Hollywood, CA 91606
213-761-2931

spinal muscular atrophy

Families of Spinal Muscular Atrophy
PO Box 1465
Highland Park, IL 60035
312-432-5551

substance abuse

National Clearinghouse for Alcohol
Information
PO Box 2345
Rockville, MD 20852
301-468-2600

National Council on Alcoholism, Inc (NCA)
733 Third Avenue
New York, NY 10017
212-986-4433

National Federation of Parents for
Drug-Free Youth
1820 Franwall Avenue #16
Silver Spring, MD 20902
800-544-KIDS

Tay-Sachs syndrome

National Tay-Sachs and Allied Diseases
Association
92 Washington Avenue
Cederhurst, NY 11516
516-569-4300

See also genetic disorders.

teeth problems
See dental problems.

terminal illness
See death and bereavement.

thasselemia
See Cooley's anemia.

thromocytopina absent radius syndrome

Thromocytopina Absent Radius
Syndrome Association (TARSA)
312 Sherwood Drive
Linwood, NJ 08821
609-927-0418

Tourette syndrome

Tourette Syndrome Association, Inc.
41-02 Bell Boulevard
Bayside, NY 11361
718-224-2999

travel

Rehabilitation USA (Access to the Skies
Program)
Flying Ridge
Newtown, CT 06470

Society for the Advancement of Travel for
the Handicapped (SATH)
26 Court Street
Brooklyn, NY 11222
718-858-5483

Travel Information Center
Moss Rehabilitation Hospital
12th Street and Tabor Road
Philadelphia, PA 19141
215-329-5715

trisomy 18/13

Support Organization for Trisomy 18/13
478 Terrace Lane
Tooele, UT 84074
801-882-6635

trisomy 21
See Down's syndrome.

transplants
See hemodialysis and transplantation.

tuberous sclerosis

National Tuberous Sclerosis Association
Box 612
Winfield, IL 60190
312-668-0787

Tuberous Sclerosis Association of America
339 Union Street
PO Box 44
Rockland, MA 02370
617-878-5528

Turner's syndrome

Turner's Syndrome Society
York University
Behavioral Sciences Building #101
4700 Keele Street
Downsview, Ontario
Canada M3J 1P3
416-667-3773

See also growth disorders.

venous disorders

See lymphatic and venous disorders.

ventilator and technology dependent children

SKIP: Sick Kids Need Involved People
216 Newport Drive
Severna Park, MD 21146
301-647-0164

vision disorders

See eye and vision disorders.

Werdnig Hoffmann's syndrome

See muscular dystrophy; spinal muscular atrophy.

Williams syndrome

National Organization for Parents of
Williams
3254 Clairemont Drive
San Diego, CA 92117

Wilson's disease

Foundation for the Study of Wilson's
Disease, Inc.
5447 Palisade Avenue
Bronx, NY 10471
212-430-2091

Wilson's Disease Association
PO Box 489
Dumfries, VA 22026
703-221-5532

Medical Procedures Index

Index

Page numbers in italics indicate figures.